I0074508

Cell Biology and Genetics

THE AUTHORS

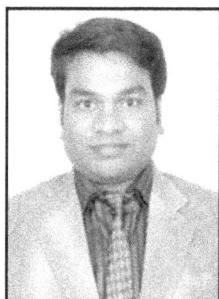

Dr. Ashok K. Rathoure has received his master degree from C.S.J.M. University Kanpur (M.Sc.) in 2005 followed by H.N.B. Garhwal University (M.Tech.) in 2007 and doctorate degree (Doctor of Philosophy) from H.N.B. Garhwal University Srinagar-Garhwal, (Central University) in Biotechnology. He has also done Diploma in Human Resource Management from Algappa University Karaikudi Tamilnadu. His area of research is environmental biotechnology and research publication includes 57 full length research papers in international and national journals of repute, 6 Course books, 5 Research books and 4 Book chapters in Springer verlag, I.K. Publishers, Mumbai and Daya Publishers New Delhi, respectively. He had reviewed more than 60 research manuscript for many international journals. He is member of APCBEES (Hong Kong), IACSIT (Singapore), EFB (Spain), Society for Conservation Biology (Washington) and founder member of Scientific Planet Society (Dehradun). He has supervised 24 research scholars (UG PG and Diploma). He has more than 4 years of teaching and more than 2 years of industry experience. He is also serving as Editor-in-Chief for Octa Journal of Environmental Research, Managing Editor for Octa Journal of Biosciences and Executive Editor for Scientific India Magazine.

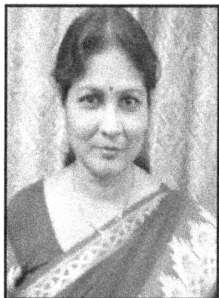

Dr. Meena Srivastava is associate professor in Department of Zoology Maharana Pratap Government Postgraduate College, Hardoi, Uttar Pradesh. She has an exhaustive teaching experience for 20 years at undergraduate and 15 years at postgraduate level. After securing top position in M.Sc. Zoology (Entomology) in 1979 she joined her PhD under Professor Y.N. Singh at Allahabad University wherein the same was awarded in 1986. She has also received UGC fellowship and work with Late Professor U.S. Srivastava. Dr. Srivastava is instrumental in carrying out various experiments and has a through experience of 5 years in different laboratory techniques and instruments handling at Forensic Science Laboratory, Lucknow. She has also received pertinent training on Electrophoretic Techniques in field of Forensic science. She has published many National and International research papers in the field of Neuroendocrinology, Developmental Entomology and Environmental Biology to her credit.

Cell Biology and Genetics

Authors

Dr. Ashok K. Rathoure

Dr. Meena Srivastava

2015

Daya Publishing House®

A Division of

Astral International Pvt. Ltd.

New Delhi - 110 002

© 2015 AUTHORS

Publisher's note:

Every possible effort has been made to ensure that the information contained in this book is accurate at the time of going to press, and the publisher and author cannot accept responsibility for any errors or omissions, however caused. No responsibility for loss or damage occasioned to any person acting, or refraining from action, as a result of the material in this publication can be accepted by the editor, the publisher or the author. The Publisher is not associated with any product or vendor mentioned in the book. The contents of this work are intended to further general scientific research, understanding and discussion only. Readers should consult with a specialist where appropriate.

Every effort has been made to trace the owners of copyright material used in this book, if any. The author and the publisher will be grateful for any omission brought to their notice for acknowledgement in the future editions of the book.

All Rights reserved under International Copyright Conventions. No part of this publication may be reproduced, stored in a retrieval system, or transmitted in any form or by any means, electronic, mechanical, photocopying, recording or otherwise without the prior written consent of the publisher and the copyright owner.

Cataloging in Publication Data--DK
  Courtesy: D.K. Agencies (P) Ltd. <docinfo@dkagencies.com>

  Rathoure, Ashok K.
Cell biology and genetics / authors, Ashok K. Rathoure, Meena Srivastava.
    p.   cm.
    Includes bibliographical references (p.   ).

    ISBN 9789351302957 (International edition)

    1. Cytology. 2. Genetics. 3. Cell organelles. 4. Biomolecules.   I. Srivastava, Meena, joint author. II. Title.

DDC 571.6   23

Published by   :   **Daya Publishing House®**
A Division of
Astral International Pvt. Ltd.
– ISO 9001:2008 Certified Company –
House No. 96, Gali No. 6,
Block-C, 30ft Road, Tomar Colony, Burari
New Delhi-110 084
E-mail: info@astralint.com
Website: www.astralint.com

Sales Office   :   4760-61, 23 Ansari Road, New Delhi-110002
                        Ph. 011-23245578, 23244987

Laser Typesetting: **SSMG Computer Graphics,** Delhi - 110 084

Printed at   :   **Thomson Press India Limited**

This book is dedicated to
My Lovely Daughter
"ELA"
(Anika A. Rathoure),
Parents
&
Teachers
(By Dr. Ashok K. Rathoure

Acknowledgements

"This book is first and foremost dedicated to the glory of God, who in His infinite grace and mercy has sought to bring us together as family of believers,inspired us with His world, and strengthened us though His Means of Grace."

It's our immense pleasure to thank Dr. Naved Bahaar Khan, Director Higher Education, Uttar Pradesh (India) for motivation to write this manuscript. We express our sincere gratitude to Prof. Akhilesh Kumar, Principal, M.P. Govt. (PG) College, Hardoi (UP) India, Prof. N. Singh Dept. of Biotechnology and Zoology, Prof. S.C. Tiwari and Prof. J.P. Mehta, Dept. of Microbiology and Botany HNBGU (A Central University), Srinagar-Garhwal (Uttarakhand), India for their critical suggestions and inspirations. Our special thanks to Prof. B.S. Bisht, Dept. of Zoology, HNBGU (A Central University), SRT Campus Badshahithaul Tehri (Uttarakhand) India, Dr. I.D. Singh, Ex Head, Dept. of Botany, M. P. Govt (PG) College Hardoi (UP) India, Dr. V.D. Joshi, Principal, Govt. PG College Purola, Uttarkashi (Uttarakhand) India, Dr. Harish Chandra and Dr. Manoj Bhatt, Dept. of Biotechnology, G.B. Pant Engineering College Pauri-Garhwal, Dr. Arun Kumar, Director Research, Dolphin Institute of Biomedical and Natural Sciences, Dr. A.K. Singh, Scientist E, Wadia Institute of Himalayan Geology, Dehradun, Dr. S.P. Goyal, Scientist F and Head, Forensic Science Laboratory, Wild Life Institute of India, Dehradun, Mr. P. Dwivedi Dept. of Biotechnology, Amity Institute Noida, India, Dr. Saswat Katiyar Dept. of Biochemistry, CSJMU Kanpur (UP) India, Dr. Sandip Kumar and Dr. Sandip Tripathi, NIMS University Jaipur India, Dr. Ashish Thapliyal, Scientist State Biotech Program Utterakhand, Dr. N. Rai Dept. of Biotech, GEU Dehradun, Dr. Aftab Ahmad, Director Beehive College Dehradun, Dr. G. Sunil Babu, Dept. of Env. Biotech. BRA University Lucknow (U.P.), Dr. M.S. Khan, Dept. of Microbiology AMU Aligarh, Dr. A. K. Chopra, Dr. P.C. Joshi, Dept. of Zoology, Gurukul Kangari University Haridwar, Dr. R. Kumar, Scientist, IARI Delhi, Dr. Sanjay Gupta Dept. of Biotech, SBS College Dehradun, Prof. Neelima Gupta, Dept of Animal Science, MJP Rohelkhand University, Bareilly (Uttar Pradesh); Prof. P. Soni. Retd. Scientist-G & Head Ecology & Environment, FRI, Dehradun; Prof. U.K. Atheya. Ex.

Head, Dept of Animal Science, G.B. Pant University of Sciences and Technology Pantnagar (Uttarakhand); Prof. R.P. Singh, School for Environmental Sciences Babasaheb Bhimrao Ambedkar University, Lucknow; Dr Vinod Kumar, Assistant Prof., Dept. of Lifescience, Beehive College of Ad. Studies, Dehradun (Uttarakhand); Dr. Arun Bhatt, Associate Professor (Genetics and Plant Breeding), Officer Incharge Department of Crop Improvement, College of Forestry and Hill Agriculture, Ranichauri ,Tehri Garhwal-249199; Dr. Ashish Chauhan, Jr. Scientist, National Institute of Pharmaceutical Education and Research (NIPER), Sector 67, Phase 10, S.A.S Nagar, Mohali, Punjab 160 062; Dr. G. Awasthi, Assistant Prof., Dept of Biochemistry, Dolphin Institute of Natural Sciences, Dehradun (Uttarakhand); Dr. M.K. Tripathi, Senior Scientist (Biochemistry), APPD, CIAE, Bhopal; Dr. Manoj Eledath, Ecology and Biodiversity Expert and Proprietor, Ananthsree Ecocare Meghna Complex, Bhatar Char Rasta Surat Gujrat; Dr. Manoj Kumar Upadhyay, Scientist C & Quality Manager, Biotech Park Lucknow; Dr. Pankaj Chauhan, Professor, Dept of Biotechnology, Soolani University (HP); Dr. R. Ramachandran, MBA Dept. Shivaji University, Kohlapur, (Maharashtra); Dr. Rajib Roychowdhury, Centre for Biotechnology, Visva-Bharati Santiniketan-731235, West Bengal; Dr. Rekha Rani, Assistant Professor, Depts. of Zoology, Navyug Kanya PG College, Rajendra Nager, Lucknow; Dr. Tejpal Dhewa, Asst. Professor, Dept of Microbiology, BCAS, Delhi University of Delhi, Sector-2, Phase-1, Dwarka, New Delhi-110075; Dr Vishal Rajput, Assistant Prof. Dept. of Biotechnology and Biochemistry, Post Graduate Institute of Biomedical Science & Research Balawala Dehradun, (Uttarakhand) for discussions and valuable comments which have helped to improve the matter.

We also thankful to Dr. I. O. Agbagwa, Department of Plant Sciences and Plant Biotechnology, University of Port Hartcourt, Nigeria; Dr. Idress Hamad Attitalla, Associate Professor, Botany Department, Faculty of Science, Omar Al-Mukhtar University, Al- Bayda, Libya; Prof. Badar Alam Iqbal, Former Fulbright Visiting Professor; Claflin University; South Carolina; USA; Prof. M Ekin Uddin, State University of Bangladesh, 77 Satmasjid Road, Dhanmondi, Dhaka–1205, Bangladesh; Prof. Nelson Duran, Environmental Biotechnology and Pharmacology, Chemical Institute, UNICAMP, Campinas, SP, Brazil; Prof. Paulo Jubilut, Sao Paulo State University, UNESP Rua Quirino de Andrade, 215 - Centro Sao Paulo, 01049010, Brazil; Prof. S. Choi, Dept. of Molecular Biology and Bioinformatics, Pusan National University, Pusan South Korea; Prof. Silas Granato Villas-Boas, Industrial Microbiology, University of Aukland, New Zealand; Prof. Tanvir Shams Qureshi, Dept of Civil Engineering, Department of Civil Engineering, Bangladesh University, Bondorbazar, Sylhet; Prof. Nathalie Gravel, Geography Division, Université Laval, Quebec City, 2325, rue de l' Universite, Québec (Quebec) G1V 0A6 Canada; Prof. G T. P. Wong, Research Centre for Environmental Changes, Academia Sinica, Academia Rd. Nankang, Taipei, Taiwan; Prof. Welington Luiz de Araujo, Biotechnology of Microorganisms, Microbiology Institute, Universidade Estadual de Sao Paulo Brazil for their critics and valuable suggestions.

We thank our colleagues Drs. Kiran Yadav, Archana Rajan, Anju Agarwal, Sangeeta Awasthi, Pankaj Chauhan, Pankaj Dhiman, Dinesh Kumar and Navneet Kumar and for their scientific discussions and valuable company to keep cheerful and focused. We sincerely appreciate the help and support rendered by Mrs. Kanchan Prabha Rathoure, Mr. Jitendra Kumar and Mr. Atul Kumar Singh. Our sincere thanks to all other friends and colleagues whose names we have not mentioned here. We also thanks the team of Astral International Pvt Ltd. for composing, typsetting, designing of cover page, figures etc.

Thank you all forever!!!

Authors

Preface

With the ever changing scenario and development of new course contents as laid down by regulatory bodies for Indian Universities in the course outline for undergraduate and postgraduate students of zoology, biotechnology and biosciences, a basic need to cater the complete syllabus into one umbrella has laid down the foundation stone and blueprint of the present book entitled *"Cell Biology and Genetics"* aims to cover a wide area of cell biology and Mendelian genetics in a form especially suitable for first year undergraduates for unified syllabus of all Indian universities. The overall theme for the book is the cell as the unit of life and its components. We begin by describing the history and components of the cell as seen under the microscope in chapter 1. Further, we turn to the theories and plasma membrane structure and its function. The next chapter describes structure and function of cell organelles. The aim of chapter 3 to describe the biomolecules with structure of chromosomes, Watson and Crick model of DNA, differences between DNA and RNA. We have discussed cell cycle and cell division in detail in chapter 4 whereas Mendelian genetics and sex linkage with various examples given in chapter 5. The chapter 6 discusses various aspects of sex determination, sex differentiation, prenatal detection of genetic diseases (amniocentesis), sex linked characters, genetic diseases and abnormalities, chromosomal aberrations, eugenics and molecular evolution describes the last section. To conclude the book, summary is given at the end of each section for reader to review. Boxed material throughout the book is divided into examples to illustrate the topics covered in the main text, explanations of the medical relevance of the material and in depth sections that extend the coverage beyond the content of the main text. This book will extensively assist students, teachers and academicians to further extend their knowledge beyond the course work and related subject matter but onto the practical application to gain insights of what happening new in the present era of applied science. We shall, in any cases, welcome any suggestions/ criticisms for further improvement, since there surely remains a limitless scope for the same.

Authors

Contents

Chapter 1

Introduction to Cell Biology

Introduction

The earth surrounded by the living and non living things. The living things are regarded as organisms. The living organisms are complicated and highly organized and are composed of many cells, typically of many types. These cells possess sub-cellular structures or organelles, which are complex assemblies of very large polymeric molecules or macromolecules. Crucial events in biomineral formation such as compartmentalization, supersaturation, precipitation, export of macromolecules and cessation require a referee who can control these events with precision and fidelity. This job falls to the cell and in particular, a specialized cell, such as an osteoblast, odontoblast, mantle epithelium or bacterium who has evolved or differentiated into a molecular factory that generates and controls the biomineralization process. All organisms are composed of structural and functional units of life called cells. The study of cell and its organelles is called cytology derived from Greek word kytos meaning container. This includes their physiological properties, their structure organelles they contain, interactions with their environment, their life cycle, division and death. This is done both on a microscopic and molecular level. Cell biology research extends to both the great diversity of single celled organisms like bacteria and the many specialized cells in multicellular organisms like humans. Knowing the composition of cells and how cells work is fundamental to all of the biological sciences. Appreciating the similarities and differences between cell types is particularly important to the fields of cell and molecular biology. These fundamental similarities and differences provide a unifying theme, allowing the principles learned from studying one cell type to be extrapolated and generalized to other cell types. Research in cell biology is closely related to genetics, biochemistry, molecular biology and developmental biology.

The body of some organisms like bacteria, protozoans and some algae is made up of a single cell while the body of fungi, plants and animals are composed of many cells. Human body is built of about one trillion cells. Cells vary in size and structure as they are specialized to perform different functions. But the basic components of the cell are common to all cells. Both living and non-living things are composed of molecules made from chemical elements such as Carbon, Hydrogen, Oxygen and Nitrogen. The organization of these molecules into cells is one feature that distinguishes living things from all other matter. A cell may be defined as a unit of protoplasm bounded by a plasma or cell membrane and possessing a nucleus. It is the basic unit of life. Microorganisms such as bacteria, yeast and amoebae exist as single cells. By contrast, the adult human is made up of about 30 trillion cells (1 trillion = 10^{12}) which are mostly organized into collectives called tissues. Cells are, with a few notable exceptions, small with lengths measured in micrometers (μm, where 1000 μm = 1 mm) and their discovery stemmed from the conviction of a small group of seventeenth-century microscope makers that a new and undiscovered world lay beyond the limits of the human eye. These pioneers set in motion a science and an industry that continues to the present day. Protoplasm is the life giving substance and includes the cytoplasm and the nucleus. The cytoplasm has ribosomes, Mitochondria, Golgi bodies, plastids, lysosomes and endoplasmic reticulum etc. Plant cells have in their cytoplasm large vacuoles containing non-living inclusions like crystals, pigments etc. The bacteria have neither organelles nor a well formed nucleus.

But every cell has three major components-

a) Plasma membrane

b) Cytoplasm

c) DNA (naked in bacteria and covered by a membrane in all other organisms).

Landmarks in cell study

Anton van Leewenhock invented the microscope, soon after discovery of microscope, Robert Hooke (1665) observed a piece of cork under the microscope and found it to be made of small compartments which he called *cella* (open spaces), later it was known as cells (Latin cell = small room). But the colossus of this era of discovery was a Dutchman, Anton van Leeuwenhoek (1632–1723), a man with no university education but with unrivaled talents as both a microscope maker and as an observer and recorder of the microscopic living world. Anton van Leeuwenhoek was a contemporary and friend of the Delft artist Johannes Vermeer (1632–1675) who pioneered the use of light and shade in art at the same time that Anton van Leeuwenhoek was exploring the use of light to discover the microscopic world. In 1672, Leewenhock observed bacteria, sperm and red blood corpuscles, all of which were cells. In 1831, Robert Brown, an Englishman observed that all cells had a centrally positioned body which he termed the nucleus.

After 156 years of discovery of cell, in 1838, the botanist Matthias Schleiden and the zoologist Theodor Schwann proposed that all living organisms are composed of cells. Their cell theory was a milestone in the development of modern biology.

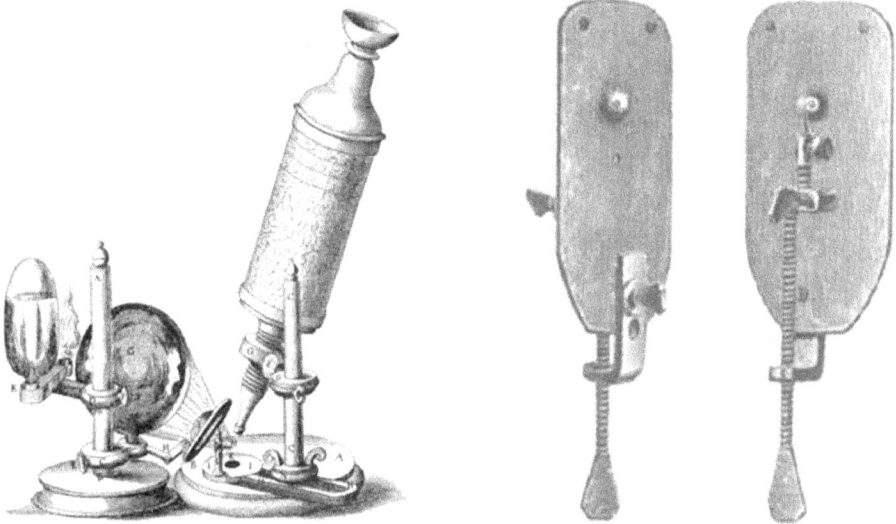

Figure 1.1 : Early Microscope

Nevertheless general acceptance took many years, in large part because the plasma membrane, the membrane surrounding the cell that divides the living inside from the nonliving extracellular medium is too thin to be seen using a light microscope.

a) Anaximander

A member of the Greeks in the sixth century B.C. who resided on the Ionian Islands, he is credited with coming up with the primary thoughts of evolution. His perspective was that creatures from the sea were forced to come ashore, thereby evolving into land creatures.

b) Plato

Plato did not directly aid in the progress of biological thinking. His view was not experimental, but more philosophical. Many of his students went on to influence the progression of biological studies in the field of classification.

c) Aristotle

Aristotle (384-322 BC) was known for his experimental approach and numerous dissections. He was drawn to animal classification in order to discover aspects of connection between the soul and the human body. Some of his animal classifications still stand today. One of his famous thoughts is a foreshadowing of Mendelian genetics concepts:

"It is evident that there must be something or other really existing, corresponding to what we call by the name of Nature. For a given germ does not give rise to any random living being, nor spring from any chance one, but each germ springs from a definite parent and gives rise to a predictable progeny. And thus it is the germ that is the ruling influence and fabricator of the offspring."

d) Leonardo Da Vinci, Rene Descartes and William Harvey

These three scientific figures, thought not all living during the same time period, can be accredited with much of the advancement of anatomical thought following the Dark Ages, such as discovering the circulation of blood.

e) Robert Hooke

This English naturalist (1635-1703) coined the term cell after viewing slices of cork through a microscope. The term came from the Latin word *cella* which means storeroom or small container. He documented his work in the Micrographia written in 1665.

f) Jean-Baptiste De Lamarck

The majority of this Frenchman's work (1744 - 1829) dealt with animal classification and evolution. He is credited with taking steps towards the creation of the cell theory with this saying:

"Every step which Nature takes when making her direct creations consists in organizing into cellular tissue the minute masses of viscous or mucous substances that she finds at her disposal under favourable circumstances."

g) Rudolf Virchow

German pathologist Rudolf Virchow (1821-1902) altered the thought of cellular biology with his statement that every cell comes from a cell. Not even twenty years after this statement, processes of cell reproduction were being described-Virchow had completed the thought behind the basic cell theory.

Table 1.1: Landmarks in Study of Cell Biology

S.No.	Year	Landmarks
1.	1595	Jansen credited with 1st compound microscope
2.	1626	Redi postulated that living things do not arise from spontaneous generation.
3.	1655	Hooke described 'cells' in cork.
4.	1674	Leeuwenhoek discovered protozoa. He saw bacteria some 9 years later.
5.	1833	Brown descibed the cell nucleus in cells of the orchid.
6.	1838	Schleiden and Schwann proposed cell theory.
7.	1840	Albrecht von Roelliker realized that sperm cells and egg cells are also cells.
8.	1856	N. Pringsheim observed how a sperm cell penetrated an egg cell.
9.	1858	Rudolf Virchow (physician, pathologist and anthropologist) illustrates his famous conclusion: *omnis cellula e cellula that* is *cells develop only from existing cells.*
10.	1857	Kolliker described mitochondria.
11.	1869	Miescher isolated DNA for the first time.
12.	1879	Flemming described chromosome behavior during mitosis.
13.	1883	Germ cells are haploid, chromosome theory of heredity.
14.	1898	Golgi described the golgi apparatus.

Contd....

Table 1.1 Contd.....

S.No.	Year	Landmarks
15.	1926	Svedberg developed the first analytical ultracentrifuge.
16.	1938	Behrens used differential centrifugation to separate nuclei from cytoplasm.
17.	1939	Siemens produced the first commercial transmission electron microscope.
18.	1941	Coons used fluorescent labeled antibodies to detect cellular antigens.
19.	1952	Gey and co-workers established a continuous human cell line.
20.	1953	Crick, Wilkins and Watson proposed Structure of DNA double-helix.
21.	1955	Eagle systematically defined the nutritional needs of animal cells in culture.
22.	1957	Meselson, Stahl and Vinograd developed density gradient centrifugation in cesium chloride solutions for separating nucleic acids.
23	1965	Ham introduced a defined serum-free medium. Cambridge Instruments produced the first commercial scanning electron microscope.
24.	1976	Sato and colleagues publish papers showing that different cell lines require different mixtures of hormones and growth factors in serum-free media.
25.	1981	Transgenic mice and fruit flies are produced. Mouse embryonic stem cell line established.
26.	1987	First knockout mouse created.
27.	1998	Mice are cloned from somatic cells.
28.	1999	Hamilton and Baulcombe discover siRNA as part of post-transcriptional gene silencing (PTGS) in plants
29.	2000	Human genome DNA sequence draft
30.	2003	Human Genome completely sequenced with other seven organisms

Cell Theory/Docterine

M.J. Schleiden and Theodore Schwann formulated the cell theory in 1838. The idea predates other great paradigms of biology including Darwin's theory of evolution (1859), Mendel's laws of inheritance (1865) and the establishment of comparative biochemistry (1940). Ultrastructural research and modern molecular biology have added many tenets to the cell theory, but it remains as the preeminent theory of biology. The Cell Theory is to Biology as Atomic Theory is to Physics. The cell theory maintains that all organisms are composed of cells. Cell is the structural and functional unit of life and cells arise from pre-existing cells. Cell theory consists of three principles:

a) The cell is the unit of structure, physiology and organization in living things.

b) The cell retains a dual existence as a distinct entity and a building block in the construction of organisms.

c) Cells form by free-cell formation, similar to the formation of crystals (spontaneous generation).

It is known today that the first two doctrines are correct, but the third is clearly wrong. The correct interpretation of cell formation by division was finally promoted by others and formally enunciated in Rudolph Virchow's powerful dictum (1858), *Omnis cellula e cellula i.e.* all cells only arise from pre-existing cells.

Moden Cell Theory

The modern tenets of the Cell Theory include:

i.   All known living things are made up of cells.

ii. The cell is structural and functional unit of all living things.

iii. All cells come from pre-existing cells by division.

iv. Cells contain hereditary information which is passed from cell to cell during cell division.

v.   All cells are basically the same in chemical composition.

vi. All energy flow (metabolism and biochemistry) of life occurs within cells.

This theory also contains two exceptions:

i.   Viruses are considered by some to be alive, yet they are not made up of cells.

ii. The first cell did not originate from a preexisting cell.

History of Cell Theory

The first scientist to recognize the commonality of structure in making up both plants and animals was Charles François Brisseau de Mirbel who in 1809 stated that Plants are made up of cells, all parts of which are in continuity and form one and the same membranous tissue. The naturalist Jean-Baptiste Lamarck also recognized that living things were made of cells, extending the idea beyond plants to all living organisms. Both Mirbel and Lamarck saw living things as being made of cells but did not see cells as a distinct primary part of living structures but rather thought of cells as the mebranes surrounding the spaces rather than the spaces themselves.. The idea of cells were separable into individual units was proposed by Ludolph Christian Treviranus and Johann Jacob Paul Moldenhawer. Credit for developing Cell Theory is usually given to two scientists, Theodor Schwann, a zoologist and Matthias Jakob Schleiden, a botanist. In 1839 these two scientists suggested that cells were the basic unit of life. Their theory accepted the first two tenets of modern cell theory. However the cell theory of Schleiden differered from modern cell theory in that it proposed a method of spontaneous crystallization that he called Free Cell Formation. In 1858, Rudolf Virchow concluded that all cells come from pre-existing cells thus completing the modern theory.

Cell Diversity

There are many types of cell sfound in the living system having a huge diversity. Even cells within the same organism show enormous diversity in size, shape and internal organization. Human body contains 10^{13} to 10^{14} cells around 300 different cell types. There is a wide variation in the number of cells in different organisms.

Cell Shape and Size

The shapes of cells are quite varied with some being longer than they are wide such as neurons and others such as parenchyma, a common type of plant cell and erythrocytes, red blood cells being equidimensional. The cells may be spherical, cylindrical, discoidal, oval, columnar, circular, elliptical, cuboidal, spindle-shaped, polyhedral, bean-shaped, flattened, biconcave, biconvex, branched, fibrous, etc. Muscle cells are elongated in shape. Some cells are encased in a rigid wall, which constrains their shape, while others have a flexible cell membrane and no rigid cell wall. Cells range in size from small bacteria to large, unfertilized eggs laid by birds and dinosaurs. The size of cells is also related to their functions. They may be microscopic like mycoplasma or PPLO measuring only about 0.3 μ (0.0003 mm) and longest bacterium cell is 3 μ to 10 μ of *Bacillus anthracis*. Eggs or ova are very large, often being the largest cells an organism produces. Egg of the ostrich is the largest cell (75 mm). Nerve cells of animals have long extensions. They can be several feet in length. The large size of many eggs is related to the process of development that occurs after the egg is fertilized, when the contents of the egg (zygote) are used in a rapid series of cellular divisions, each requiring tremendous amounts of energy that is available in the zygote cells. Human egg is about 100 μ in diameter and human sperm is about 50 μ long. RBC measures 6.5 μ to 8 μ and WBC measure about 6 μ to 20 μ in diameter. *Acetabularia* algae may reach upto 10 cm in length and some species of *Caulerpa* may attain a length upto 1 meter.

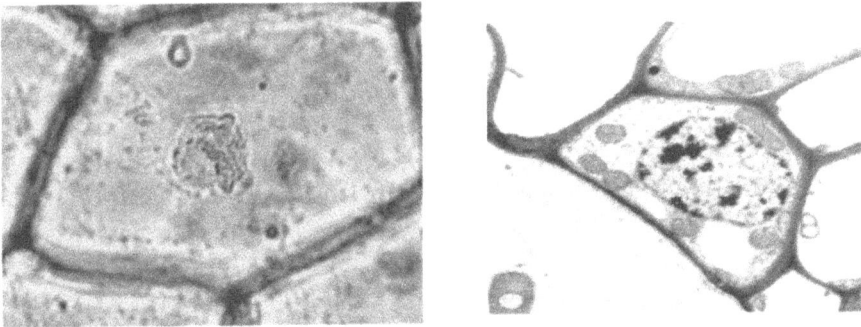

Figure 1.2: Microscopic View of Cell

In science, the metric system is used for measuring. There are some measurements and conversions listed below:

1 meter = 100 cm = 1,000 mm = 1,000,000 μm = 1,000,000,000 nm

1 centimenter (cm) = 1/100 meter = 10 mm

1 millimeter (mm) = 1/1000 meter = 1/10 cm

1 micrometer (μm) = 1/1,000,000 meter = 1/10,000 cm

1 nanometer (nm) = 1/1,000,000,000 meter = 1/10,000,000 cm

Internal Organization

Life exhibits varying degrees of organization. Atoms are organized into molecules, molecules into organelles and organelles into cells and so on. According to the Cell Theory, all living things are composed of one or more cells and the functions of a multicellular organism are a consequence of the types of cells it has. Cells fall into two broad groups: prokaryotes and eukaryotes. Prokaryotic cells are smaller and lack much of the internal compartmentalization and complexity of eukaryotic cells. No matter which type of cell we are considering, all cells have certain features in common, such as a cell membrane, DNA and RNA, cytoplasm and ribosomes. Eukaryotic cells have a great variety of organelles and structures. There is following

i. The cell of living systems contains a variety of internal structures called organelle *e.g.* mitochondria, plastid, golgybody, etc.

ii. An organelle is a cell component that performs a specific function.

iii. The cytoplasm is the cell contents with the exception of the nucleus including the membrane.

iv. There are many different cells; there are certain features common to all cells.

v. The entire cell is surrounded by a thin cell membrane. The plasma membrane encloses the cell, defines its boundaries and maintains the essential differences between the cytosol and the extracellular environment.

vi. Organelles have their own membranes these membranes have a similar structure. Endoplasmic reticulum, Golgi apparatus, mitochondria and other membrane-enclosed organelles maintain the characteristic differences between the contents of each organelle and the cytosol.

vii. The nucleus, mitochondria and chloroplasts all have double membranes, called envelopes.

viii. Ion gradients across membranes, established by the activities of specialized membrane proteins to drive the transmembrane movement of selected solutes or in nerve and muscle cells, to produce and transmit electrical signals. Proteins in the membrane can be used to transport substances across the membrane *e.g.* by facilitated diffusion or by active transport.

ix. The most abundant membrane lipids are the phospholipids. These have a polar head group and two hydrophobic hydrocarbon tails. Most types of lipid molecules in cell membranes are randomly mixed in the lipid monolayer in which they reside.

x. Biological membranes consist of a continuous double layer of lipid molecules in which membrane proteins are embedded. This lipid bilayer is fluid, with individual lipid molecules able to diffuse rapidly within their own monolayer. The membrane lipid molecules are amphipathic. The most numerous are the phospholipids. When placed in water they assemble spontaneously into bilayers, which form sealed compartments that reseal if torn.

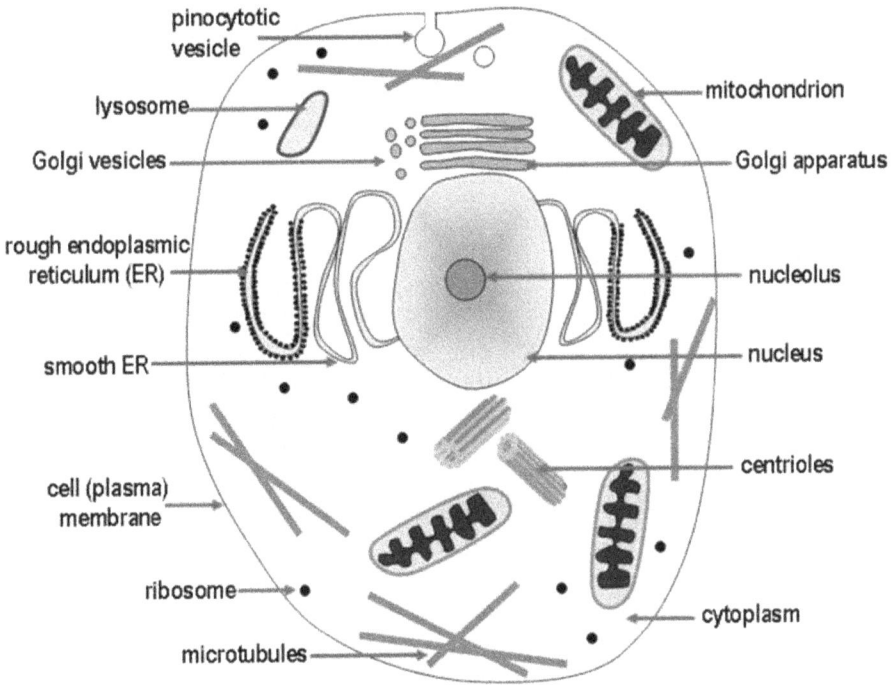

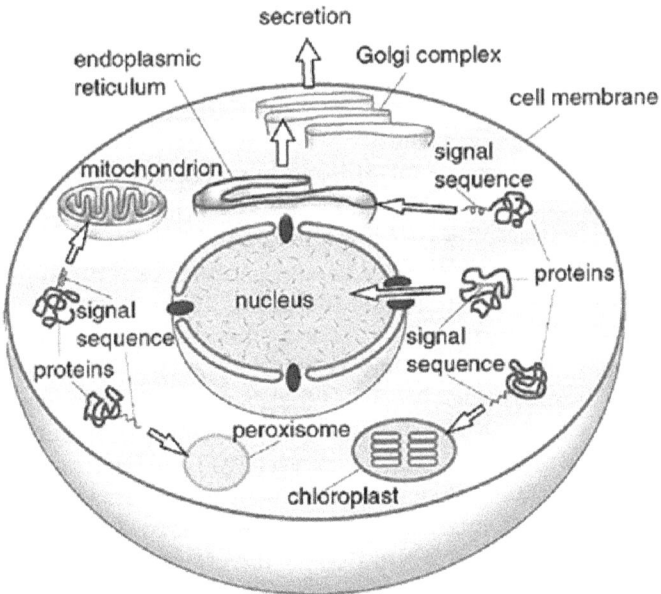

Figure 1.3: Cell and its Organelles

Table 1.2: Componnt of Cell (%dry weight)

S. No.	Elements	Dry Weight (%)
1.	C	50
2.	O	20
3.	N	14
4.	H	8
5.	P	3
6.	S	1
7.	K	1
8.	Na	1
9.	Ca	0.5
10.	Mg	0.5
11.	Cl	0.5
12.	Fe	0.2
13.	Others	0.3

Formula for Cell: $CH_{1.8}O_{0.5}N_{0.2}$

BOX 1.1

MYCOPLASMA

Mycoplasmas are the smallest and simplest self-replicating bacteria. The mycoplasma cell contains the minimum set of organelles essential for growth and replication: a plasma membrane, ribosomes and a genome consisting of a double stranded circular DNA molecule. Unlike all other prokaryotes, the mycoplasmas have no cell walls and they are consequently placed in a separate class Mollicutes (mollis menaing soft; cutis menaing skin). The trivial term mollicutes is frequently used as a general term to describe any member of the class, replacing in this respect the older term mycoplasmas. Mycoplasma is a genus of bacteria which lack a cell wall. Without a cell wall, they are unaffected by many common antibiotics such as penicillin or other beta-lactam antibiotics that target cell wall synthesis. They can be parasitic or saprotrophic. Several species are pathogenic in humans, including *M. pneumoniae*, which is an important cause of atypical pneumonia and other respiratory disorders and *M. genitalium* which is believed to be involved in pelvic inflammatory diseases. There are over 100 recognized species of the genus Mycoplasma, one of several genera within the bacterial class Mollicutes. As a group, Mollicutes have small genomes (0.58-1.38 megabase-pairs), lack a cell wall and have a low GC-content (18-40%). Mollicutes are parasites or commensals of humans, other animals including insects and plants; the genus Mycoplasma is by definition restricted to vertebrate hosts. Cholesterol is required for the growth of species of the genus Mycoplasma as well as certain other genera of mollicutes. Their optimum growth temperature is often the temperature of their host if warmbodied *e. g.* 37° C in humans or ambient temperature if the host is unable to regulate its own internal temperature. Analysis of 16S ribosomal RNA sequences as well as gene content strongly suggest that the mollicutes including the mycoplasmas are closely related to either the Lactobacillus or the Clostridium branch of the phylogenetic tree.

Cell Wall Structure: The bacteria of the genus Mycoplasma and their close relatives are largely characterized by lack of a cell wall. Despite this, the shapes of these cells often conform to one of several possibilities with varying degrees of intricacy *e.g.* members of the genus Spiroplasma assume an elongated helical shape without the aid of a rigid structural cell envelope. These cell shapes presumably contribute to the ability of mycoplasmas to thrive in their respective environments. *M. pneumoniae* cells possess an extension called tip-structure, protruding from the coccoid cell body. This structure is involved in adhesion to host cells, in movement along solid surfaces and in cell division. *M. pneumoniae* cells are of small size and pleomorphic, but with a rough shape in longitudinal cross-section resembling that of a round-bottomed flask.

Morphology: Mycoplasma is flask-shaped and most likely descended from Gram-positive bacteria. Due to their seriously degraded genome they cannot perform many metabolic functions, such as cell wall production or synthesis of purines. As such stripped down organisms they are considered the perfect model of the minimalist cell. Meaning they are believed to contain the absolute minimum machinery necessary for survival and are considered the model organisms for the essential functions of all living cells. The Mycoplasma cell is built of a minimum set of organelles including a plasma membrane, ribosomes and a highly coiled circular chromosome.

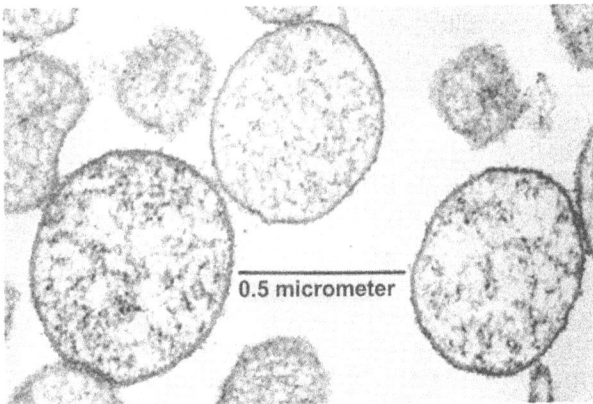

Mycoplasma cells: Cells are bounded by a single membrane showing in section the characteristic trilaminar shape.

The coccus is the basic form of all mycoplasmas in culture. The diameter of the smallest coccus capable of reproduction is about 300 nm. In most mycoplasma cultures, elongated or filamentous forms (up to 100 μm long and about 0.4 μm thick) also occur. The filaments tend to produce truly branched mycelioid structures, hence the name mycoplasma (myces, a fungus; plasma, a form). Mycoplasmas reproduce by binary fission, but cytoplasmic division frequently may lag behind genome replication, resulting in formation of multinuclear filaments

Classification: The medical and agricultural importance of members of the genus Mycoplasma and related genera has led to the extensive cataloging of many of these organisms by culture, serology and small subunit rRNA gene and whole genome sequencing. A recent focus in the sub-discipline of molecular phylogenetics has both clarified and confused certain aspects of the organization of the class Mollicutes and while a truce of sorts has been reached, the area is still somewhat of a moving target. The name mollicutes is derived from the Latin mollis (soft) and cutes (skin) and all of these bacteria do lack a cell wall and the genetic capability to synthesize peptidoglycan. While the trivial name mycoplasma has commonly denoted all members of this class, this usage is somewhat imprecise and will not be used as such here. Despite the lack of a cell wall, Mycoplasma and relatives have been classified in the phylum Firmicutes consisting of low G+C Gram-positive bacteria based on 16S rRNA gene analysis. The cultured members of Mollicutes are currently arranged into four orders: Acholeplasmatales, Anaeroplasmatales, Entomoplasmatales and Mycoplasmatales. The order Mycoplasmatales contains a single family, Mycoplasmataceae, which contains two genera: Mycoplasma and Ureaplasma. A limiting criterion for inclusion within the genus Mycoplasma is that the organism has a vertebrate host. In fact, the type species, *M. mycoides*, along with other significant mycoplasma species like *M. capricolum*, is evolutionarily more closely related to the genus Spiroplasma in the order Entomoplasmatales than to the other members of the Mycoplasma genus. This and other discrepancies will likely remain unresolved because of the extreme confusion that change could engender among the medical and agricultural communities. The remaining species in the genus Mycoplasma are divided into three non-taxonomic groups, hominis, pneumoniae and fermentans, based on 16S rRNA gene sequences. The hominis group contains the phylogenetic clusters of *M. bovis*, *M. pulmonis* and *M. hominis*, among others. The pneumoniae group contains the clusters of *M. muris* and *M. fastidiosum*, the currently unculturable haemotrophic mollicutes, informally referred to as haemoplasmas and the *M. pneumoniae* cluster. This cluster contains the species *M. alvi* (bovine), *M. amphoriforme* (human), *M. gallisepticum* (avian), *M. genitalium* (human), *M. imitans* (avian), *M. pirum* (uncertain/human), *M. testudinis* (tortoises) and *M. pneumoniae* (human).

Reproduction: Cells may either divide by binary fission or first elongate to multinucleate filaments, which subsequently breakup to coccoid bodies. Some mycoplasmas possess unique attachment organelles, which are shaped as a tapered tip in *M. pneumoniae* and *M genitalium*. Mycoplasma pneumoniae is a pathogen of the respiratory tract, adhering to the respiratory epithelium, primarily through the attachment organelle. Interestingly, these two human mycoplasmas exhibit gliding motility on liquid-covered surfaces. The tip structure always leads, again indicating its importance in attachment. One of the most useful distinguishing features of mycoplasma is their peculiar fried-egg colony shape, consisting of a central zone of growth embedded in the agar and a peripheral one on the agar surface.

Sectioned Colony

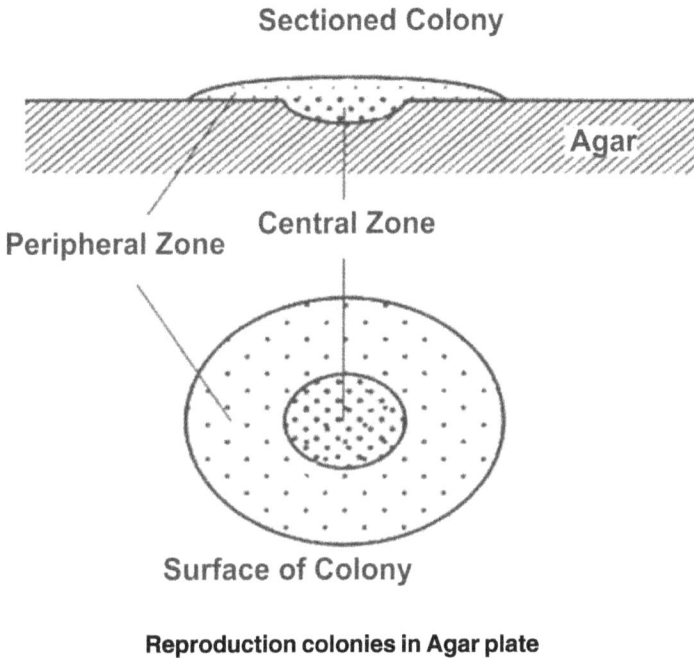

Peripheral Zone   Central Zone

Surface of Colony

Reproduction colonies in Agar plate

Svedberg Unit

When the cell is fractionated or broken down into its components rotating in an ultracentrifuge at different speed the ribosomes of eukaryotic and prokaryotic sediment (settle down) at different speed. The coefficient of sedimentation is represented in Svedberg unit and depicted as S.

BOX 1.2

MICROSCOPY

Microscopes make small objects appear bigger. A light microscope can magnify an image up to 1500 times its original size. Electron microscopes can achieve magnifications up to 1 million times. However, bigger is only better when more details are revealed. The fineness of detail of any object revealed by the resolving power of microscope. Resolving power is defined as the smallest distance that two objects can approach one another yet still is recognized as being separate. The resolution is mainly a function of the wavelength of the illu-mination source it employs. The smaller the wavelength, the smaller the object that cause diffraction and the better the resolving power. The light microscope, because it uses visible light of wavelength around 500 nanometers (nm, where 1000 nm = 1 μm), can distinguish objects as small as about half this: 250 nm. Therefore, it can be used to visualize the smallest cells and the major intracellular structures or organelles. The microscopic study of cell structure organization is known as cytology. An electron microscope is required to reveal the ultrastructure (the fine detail) of the organelles and other cytoplasmic structures. The wavelength of an electron beam is about 100,000 times less than that of white light. In theory, this should lead to a corresponding increase in resolution. In practice, the electron microscope can distinguish structures about 1000 times smaller than is possible in the light microscope, that is, down to about 0.2 nm in size.

Light Microscope

A light microscope consists of a light source, which may be the sun or an artificial light, plus three glass lenses: a condenser lens to focus light on the specimen, an objective lens to form the magnified image and a projector lens, usually called the eyepiece, to convey the magnified image to the eye. Depending on the focal length of the various lenses and their arrangement, a given magnification is achieved. In bright-field microscopy, the image that reaches the eye consists of the colors of white light less that absorbed by the cell. Most living cells have little color (plant cells are an exception) and are therefore largely transparent to transmitted light. This problem can be overcome by cytochemistry, the use of colored stains to selectively highlight particular structures and organelles. However, many of these compounds are highly toxic and to be effective they often require that the cell or tissue is first subjected to a series of harsh chemical treatments. The fine structure of living cells can be studied by phase-contrast microscopy. This relies on the fact that light travels at different speeds through regions of the cell that differ in composition. The phase-contrast microscope converts these differences in refractive index into differences in contrast and considerably more detail is revealed. Light microscopes come in a number of physical orientations upright, inverted, etc. but whatever the orientation of the microscope the optical principles are the same.

Electron Microscope

The most commonly used type of electron microscope in biology is called the transmission electron microscope because electrons are transmitted through the specimen to the observer. The transmission electron microscope has essentially the same design as a light microscope is electromagnets that bend beams of electrons. An electron gun generates a beam of electrons by heating a thin, V-shaped piece of tungsten wire to 3000°C. A large voltage accelerates the beam down the microscope column, which is under vacuum because the electrons would be slowed and scattered if they collided with air molecules. The magnified image can be viewed on a fluorescent screen that emits light when struck by electrons. While the electron microscope offers great improvements in resolution, electron beams are potentially highly destructive and biological material must be subjected to a complex processing schedule before it can be examined. A small piece of tissue (~1 mm^3) is immersed in glutaraldehyde and osmium tetroxide. These chemicals bind all the component parts of the cells together; the tissue is said to be fixed. It is washed thoroughly. The transmission electron microscope produces a detailed image but one that is static, two dimensional and highly processed. Electron microscopes are large and require a skilled operator. Nevertheless they are the main source of information on the structure of the cell at the nanometer scale called the ultrastructure. Whereas the image in a transmission electron microscope is formed by electrons transmitted through the specimen, in the scanning electron microscope it is formed from electrons that are reflected back from the surface of a specimen as the electron beam scans rapidly back and forth over it. These reflected electrons are processed to generate a picture on a display monitor. The scanning electron microscope operates over a wide magnification range, from 10X to 100,000X. Its greatest advantage is a large depth of focus that gives a three dimensional image. The scanning electron microscope is particularly useful for providing topographical information on the surfaces of cells or tissues. Modern instruments have a resolution of about 1 nm.

Noble Prize in Microscopy

Frits Zernike was awarded the Nobel prize for physics in 1953 for the development of phase-contrast microscopy and Ernst Ruska the same award in 1986 for the invention of the transmission electron microscope. Ruska's prize marks one of the longest gaps between a discovery in 1930s in the labs of Siemens Corporation in Berlin and award of a Nobel prize. Anton van Leeuwenhoek died almost two centuries before the Nobel prizes were introduced in 1901 and the prize is not awarded posthumously.

Type of Cells

There are two basic types of cells are found in typical living systesa. Organisms which do not possess a well formed nucleus are prokaryotes and cells of those organisms are called as prokaryotic (meaning before nucleus) such as the bacteria, because they have very little visible internal organization so that the genetic material is free within the cell. They are also small and the vast majority being 1–2 μm in length. All others possess a well defined nucleus, covered by a nuclear membrane. They are eukaryotes and cells of organisms are called eukaryotic (menaing with a nucleus) cells. These are generally larger (5–100 μm), although some eukaryotic cells are large enough to be seen with the naked eye and structurally more complex. Eukaryotic cells contain a variety of specialized structures known collectively as organelles, surrounded by a viscous substance called cytosol. The largest organelle, the nucleus, contains the genetic information stored in the molecule deoxyribonucleic acid (DNA).

Prokaryotic cell (Pro = early/primitive; karyon= nucleus)

The prokaryotic cells such as bacteria are simpler in their organization. They possess few internal membrane bound organelles and do not have a cytoskeletal network. Therefore, in those prokayotes with no internal organelles, all intracellular processes are combined together within cell cytoplasm and are not partitioned. Prokaryotes are bounded by a cell wall and in some cases, a cell membrane which is surrounded by the cell wall. Procaryotic structural components consist of macromolecules such as DNA, RNA, proteins, polysaccharides, phospholipids or some combination thereof. The macromolecules are made up of primary subunits such as nucleotides, amino acids and sugars. It is the sequence in which the subunits are put together in the macromolecule called the primary structure that determines many of the properties. Thus, the genetic code is determined by specific nuleotide base sequences in chromosomal DNA; the amino acid sequence in a protein determines the properties and function of the protein and sequence of sugars in bacterial lipopolysaccharides determines unique cell wall properties for pathogens. The primary structure of a macromolecule will drive its function and differences within the primary structure of biological macromolecules accounts for the immense diversity of life.

BOX 1.3

NEURONS

Neurons or nerve cells are electrically excitable cells in the nervous system that process and transmit information. In vertebrate animals, neurons are the core components of the brain, spinal cord and peripheral nerves. Neurons are typically composed of a soma or cell body, a dendritic tree and an axon. The majority of vertebrate neurons receives input on the cell body and dendritic tree and transmits output via the axon. However, there is great heterogeneity throughout the nervous system and the animal kingdom, in the size, shape and function of neurons. Neurons communicate via chemical and electrical synapses, in a process known as synaptic transmission. The fundamental process that triggers synaptic transmission is the action potential, a propagating electrical signal that is generated by exploiting the electrically excitable membrane of the neuron. This is also known as a wave of depolarization. The neuron's place as the primary functional unit of the nervous system was first recognised in the early 20th century through the work of the Spanish anatomist Santiago Ramón y Cajal. Cajal proposed that neurons were discrete cells that communicated with each other via specialized junctions or spaces, between cells. This became known as the neuron doctrine, one of the central principles of modern neuroscience. To observe the structure of individual neurons, Cajal used a silver staining method developed by his rival, Camillo Golgi. The Golgi stain is an extremely useful method for neuroanatomical investigations because, for reasons unknown, it stains a very small percentage of cells in a tissue, so one is able to see the complete microstructure of individual neurons without much overlap from other cells in the densely packed brain. Neurons are highly specialized for the processing and transmission of cellular signals. Given the diversity of functions performed by neurons in different parts of the nervous system, a wide variety in the shape, size and electrochemical properties of neurons *e.g.* the soma of a neuron can vary from 4 to 100 micrometers in diameter.

In the early days, it was thought that bacteria and other procaryotes were essentially bags of enzymes with no inherent cellular architecture. This was changed with the development of electron microscope in 1950s which revealed the distinct anatomical features of bacteria and confirmed the suspicion that they lacked a nuclear membrane. Procaryotes are cells of relatively simple construction, especially if compared to eucaryotes. Whereas eucaryotic cells have a preponderance of organelles with separate cellular functions, procaryotes carry out all cellular functions as individual units. A prokaryotic cell has five essential structural components such as nucleoid (DNA), ribosomes, cell membrane, cell wall and some sort of surface layer, which may or may not be an inherent part of the wall. Structurally, there are three architectural regions such as appendages in the form of flagella and pili or fimbriae; a cell envelope consisting of a capsule, cell wall and plasma membrane and a cytoplasmic region that contains the cell chromosome (DNA) and ribosomes and various sorts of inclusions.

Table 1.3: Macromolecule of Cell

S.No.	Macromolecule	Primary Subunits	Location
1	Proteins	Amino acids	Flagella, pili, cell walls, cytoplasmic membranes, ribosomes, cytoplasm
2	Polysaccharides	Sugars (carbohydrates)	Capsules, inclusions (storage), cell walls
3	Phospholipids	fatty acids	Membranes
4	Nucleic Acids	Nucleotides	DNA: nucleoid (chromosome), (DNA/RNA) plasmids rRNA: ribosomes; mRNA, tRNA: cytoplasm

Eukaryotic cell (eu = true, karyon = nucleus)

The eukaryotic cell can be characterized by a high degree of internal organization, as evidenced by the presence of intracellular organelles *i.e.* compartmentalized structures which perform specialized functions for cellular function. The cell boundary itself is delineated by a cell membrane; consisting of a protein-containing lipid bilayer the area within the cell is called the cytoplasm or cytosol. The endoplasmic reticulum, Golgi apparatus, vesicles and mitochondria are also bound by a membrane bilayer. However, the nucleus is actually bound by a double membrane bilayer. Membrane bilayers compartmentalize each organelle such that important functions are isolated and regulated. Within the nucleus are the chromosomes *i.e.* protein-bound deoxyribonucleic acid (DNA) complexes which contain genetic information (genes). The chromosomal DNA gives rise to heterogeneous nuclear ribonucleic acid RNA (hnRNA) via a process called transcription. The hnRNA is processed into messenger RNA (mRNA), which is exported out to the cytoplasm for translation of the genetic code into proteins *i.e.*, protein synthesis. The nucleolus is a large diffuse structure within the nucleus; it is the site of ribosome-specific RNA synthesis (rRNA) and the assembly of ribosomes. Within the cytoplasm, the cell generates energy via metabolic conversion of molecules. Part of the metabolic cycle concerned with oxygen reduction to water (aerobic metabolism) takes place within membrane bound organelles called mitochondria. Mitochondria also possess their own DNA and RNA.

Table 1.4: Comparison of Structures between Animal and Plant cells

Typical Animal cell	Typical Plant cell
Nucleus	Nucleus
Nucleolus(within nucleus)	Nucleolus (within nucleus)
Rough endoplasmic reticulum	Rough endoplasmic reticulum(ER)
endoplasmic reticulum (ER)	Smooth endoplasmic reticulum (ER)
Smooth endoplasmic reticulum(ER)	Ribosomes
Ribosomes	Cytoskeleton
Cytoskeleton	Golgi apparatus (dictiosomes)
Golgi apparatus	Cytoplasm
Cytoplasm	Mitochondria
Mitochondria	Plastids and its derivatives
Vesicles	Vacuole(s)
Lysosomes	Cell wall
Centrosome	
Centrioles	

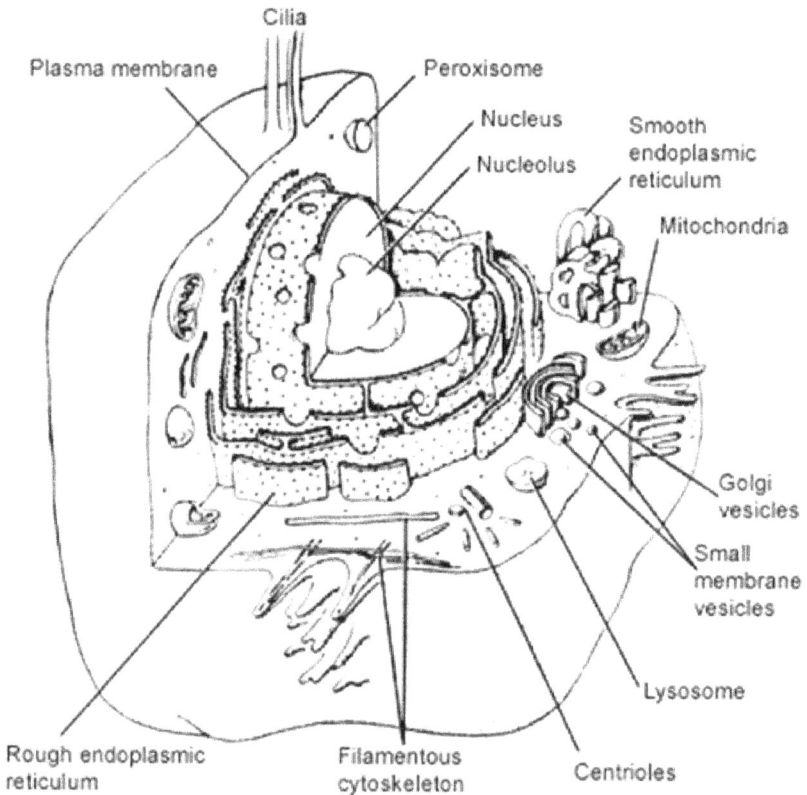

Figure 1.4: Structure of Animal cell [Darnell and Lodish (1986)]

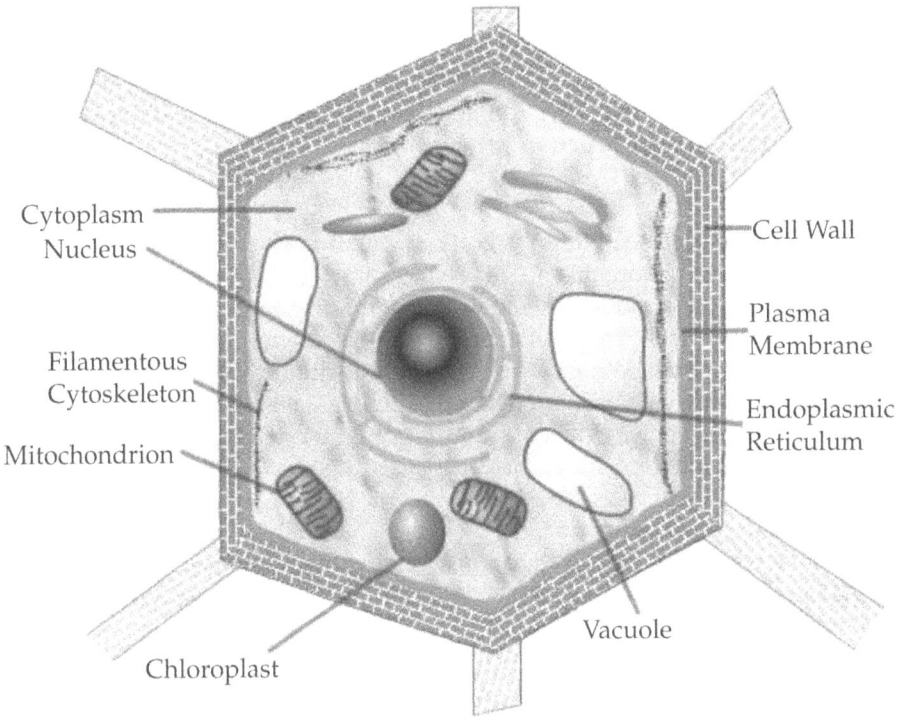

Figure 1.5: Structure of Typical Plant Cell

Other organelles such as the endoplasmic reticulum and Golgi apparatus are sites for protein synthesis for export, oligosaccharide and lipid synthesis, membrane growth and post-translational modification of proteins. The cytoplasm membrane itself is highly dynamic and experiences budding off to form membrane vesicles, sometimes termed matrix vesicles, as well as fusion of intracellular membrane vesicles and subsequent release of vesicle contents to the extracellular space (exocytosis) or engulfment of extracellular materials and their transport into the cytoplasm (endocytosis). Specialized vesicles, such as peroxisomes and lysosomes, are membrane-bound compartments that form from either the Golgi apparatus or from the cell membrane and these contain hydrolytic and oxidative enzymes. The cell is motile, *i.e.* it can move through media or on surfaces. To do this, the cell relies on a cytoskeletal network of contractile and support proteins that connect the cell membrane internally. Examples of cytoskeletal proteins include actin (actin filaments), tubulin (microtubules) and intermediate filament proteins. The cytoskeletal proteins attach to the cell membrane and are concentrated near the nuclear membrane. These contractile proteins provide shape to the cell and allow the membrane edges of the cell to extend/retract at various points, providing the cell with locomotion. Moreover, the cytoskeletal network also facilitates cytoplasmic streaming, *i.e.* movement or flow of the cytoplasm throughout the cell interior. The exterior of the cell membrane itself contains receptor proteins which allow the cell to adhere to surfaces and/or detect extracellular molecules. One type of mineral-producing eukaryotic cell that features different cell architecture is plant cells. The plant cell possesses a rigid polysaccharide containing coating called the cell wall which surrounds the cell membrane bilayer. Additionally, plant cells possess intracellular membrane-bound organelles known as chloroplasts. These organelles contain the chlorophyll-based photosynthetic apparatus utilized in O_2 production.

Plant Cell

Plant cells are enclosed within a rigid cell wall that gives shape to the cell and structural rigidity to the organism. This is in contrast to the flexible boundaries of animal cells. Plant cells frequently contain one or more vacuoles that can occupy up to 75% of the cell volume. Vacuoles accumulate a high concentration of sugars and other soluble compounds. Water enters the vacuole to dilute these sugars, generating hydrostatic pressure that is counterbalanced by the rigid wall. In this way the cells of the plant become stiff or turgid, in the same way that when an inner tube is inflated inside a bicycle tire the combination becomes stiff. Vacuoles are often pigmented and the spectacular colors of petals and fruit reflect the presence of compounds such as the purple anthocyanins in the vacuole. Cells of photosynthetic plant tissues contain a special organelle, the chloroplast that houses the light-harvesting and carbohydrate-generating systems of photosynthesis. Plant cells lack centrosomes although these are found in many algae.

Origin of Eukaryotic Cells

Prokaryotic cells are simpler and more primitive in their organization than eukaryotic cells. According to the fossil record, prokaryotic organisms antedate, by at least 2 billion years, the first eukaryotes that appeared some 1.5 billion years ago. It seems highly likely that eukaryotes evolved from prokaryotes and the most likely explanation of this process is the endosymbiotic theory. The basis of this hypothesis is that some eukaryotic organelles originated as free living prokaryotes that were engulfed by larger cells in which they established a mutually beneficial relationship *e.g.* mitochondria would have originated as free living aerobic bacteria and chloroplasts as cyanobacteria, photosynthetic prokaryotes formerly known as blue green algae. The endosymbiotic theory provides an attractive explanation for the fact that both mito-chondria and chloroplasts contain DNA and ribosomes of the prokaryotic type. The case for the origin of other eukaryotic organelles is less persuasive. While it is clearly not perfect, most biologists are now prepared to accept that the endosymbiotic theory pro-vides at least a partial explanation for the evolution of the eukaryotic cell from a prokaryotic ancestor. Unfortunately, living forms having a cellular organization intermediate between prokaryotes and eukaryotes are rare. Some primitive protists possess a nucleus but lack mitochondria and other typical eukaryotic organelles. They also have the prokaryotic type of ribosomes. These organisms are all intracellular parasites and they include Microspora, an organism that infects AIDS patients.

BOX 1.4

VIRUSES

Viruses occupy a unique space between the living and nonliving worlds. On one hand they are made of the same molecules as living cells. On the other hand they are incapable of independent existence, being completely dependent on a host cell to reproduce. Almost all living organisms have viruses that infect them. Human viruses include polio, influenza, herpes, rabies, ebola, smallpox, chickenpox and the AIDS (acquired immunodeficiency syndrome) virus HIV (human immunodeficiency virus). Viruses are submicroscopic parti-cles consisting of a core of genetic material enclosed within a protein coat called the capsid. Some viruses have an extra membrane layer called the envelope. Viruses are metabolically inert until they enter a host cell, whereupon the viral genetic material directs the host cell machinery to produce viral protein and viral genetic material. Viruses often insert their genome into that of the host, an ability that is widely made use of in molecular genetics. Bacterial viruses, called bacteriophages, are used by scientists to transfer genes between bacterial strains. Human viruses are used as vehicles for gene therapy. By exploiting the natural infection cycle of a virus such as adenovirus, it is possible to introduce a functional copy of a human gene into a patient suffering from a genetic disease such as cystic fibrosis.

Cell Specialization

All the body cells that comprise a single organism share the same set of genetic instructions in their nuclei. However, the cells are not all identical. Rather, plants and animals are composed of different tissues, groups of cells that are specialized to carry out a common function. This specialization occurs because different cell types read out different parts of the DNA blueprint and therefore make different proteins. In animals there are four major tissue types: epithelium, connective tissue, nervous tissue and muscle.

Table 1.5: Structure and Function Cell Components

S.No.		Structure Function(s)	Chemical composition
1.	Flagella	Swimming movement	Protein
		Pili	
2.	Sex pilus	Stabilizes mating bacteria during DNA transfer by conjugation	Protein
3.	Common pili or fimbriae	Attachment to surfaces; protection against phagotrophic engulfment	Protein
4.	Capsules (includes slime layers and glycocalyx)	Attachment to surfaces; protection against phagocytic engulfment, occasionally killing or digestion; reserve of nutrients or protection against desiccation	Usually polysaccharide; occasionally polypeptide

Contd...

Table 1.5 : Contd...

S.No.		Structure Function(s)	Chemical composition
		Cell wall	
5.	Gram-positive bacteria	Prevents osmotic lysis of cell protoplast and confers rigidity and shape on cells	Peptidoglycan (murein) complexed with teichoic acids
6.	Gram-negative bacteria	Peptidoglycan prevents osmotic lysis and confers rigidity and shape; outer membrane is permeability barrier; associated LPS and proteins have various functions	Peptidoglycan (murein) surrounded by phospholipid protein-lipopolysaccharide outer membrane
7.	Plasma membrane	Permeability barrier; transport of solutes; energy generation; location of numerous enzyme systems	Phospholipid and protein
8.	Ribosomes	Sites of translation (protein synthesis)	RNA and protein
9.	Inclusions	Often reserves of nutrients; additional specialized functions	Highly variable; carbohydrate, lipid, protein or inorganic
10.	Chromosome	Genetic material of cell	DNA
11.	Plasmid	Extrachromosomal genetic material	DNA

Table 5: Comparision between Prokaryotic and Eukaryotic Cell

S. No.	Features	Prokaryotes	Eukaryotes
1	Typical organisms	bacteria, archaea	protists, fungi, plants, animals
2	Typical size	~ 1–10 μm	~ 10–100 μm (sperm cells, apart from the tail, are smaller)
3	Type of nucleus	nucleoid region; no real nucleus	real nucleus with double membrane
4	DNA	circular (usually)	linear molecules (chromosomes) with histone proteins
5	RNA-/protein-synthesis	coupled in cytoplasm	RNA-synthesis inside the nucleus-protein synthesis in cytoplasm
6	Ribosomes	50S+30S	60S+40S
7	Cytoplasmatic structure	very few structures	highly structured by endomembranes and a cytoskeleton
8	Cell movement	flagella made of flagellin	flagella and cilia containing microtubules; lamellipodia and filopodia containing actin
9	Mitochondria	none	one to several thousand (though some lack mitochondria)
10	Chloroplasts	none	in algae and plants
11	Organization	usually single cells	single cells, colonies, higher multicellular organisms with specialized cells
12	Cell division	Binary fission (simple division)	Mitosis (fission or budding)Meiosis
13	First appeared	3.5×10^9 years ago	1.5×10^9 years ago

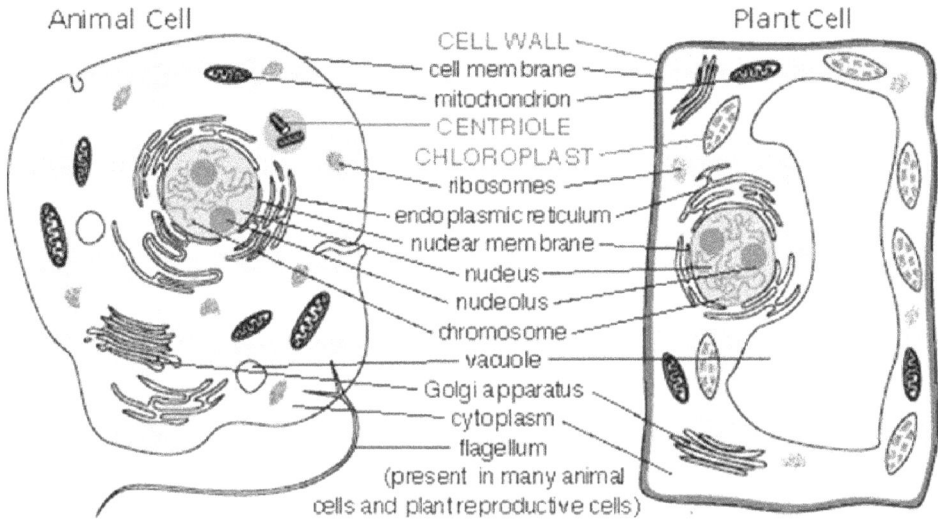

Figure 1.6 Comparism between Animal and Plant Cell

Ultra structure of Plasma membrane

The plasma membrane or cell membrane or cytoplasmic membrane is a biological membrane that separates the interior of all cells from the outside environment. The cell membrane is selectively permeable to ions and organic molecules and controls the movement of substances in and out of cells. It basically protects the cell from outside forces. It consists of the lipid bilayer with embedded proteins. Cell membranes are involved in a variety of cellular processes such as cell adhesion, ion conductivity and cell signaling and serve as the attachment surface for several extracellular structures, including the cell wall, glycocalyx and intracellular cytoskeleton. The plasma membrane is the most dynamic structure of a prokaryotic cell. Its presence was presumably visualized by Naegeli and Cramer in 1855, but is was confirmed in 1899 by E. Overton on the basis of his experimental studies on plant root hair cells and mammalian red blood cells. It is only 70-100 angstrom (7-10 mm) thick and invisible under light microscope. Its main function is as a selective permeability barrier that regulates the passage of substances into and out of the cell. The plasma membrane is the definitive structure of a cell since it sequesters the molecules of life in a unit, separating it from the environment. The bacterial membrane allows passage of water and uncharged molecules up to mw of about 100 Daltons, but does not allow passage of larger molecules or any charged substances except by means special membrane transport processes and transport systems. Bacterial membranes are composed of 40 percent phospholipid and 60 per cent protein. The phospholipids are amphoteric molecules with a polar hydrophilic glycerol head attached via an ester bond to two nonpolar hydrophobic fatty acid tails, which naturally form a bilayer in aqueous environments. Dispersed within the bilayer are various structural and enzymatic proteins which carry out most membrane functions. At one time, it was thought that the proteins were neatly organized along the inner and outer faces of the membrane and that this accounted for the double track appearance of the membrane in electron micrographs. However, it is now known that while some membrane proteins are located and functions on one side or another of the membrane, most proteins are partly inserted into the membrane or possibly even traverse the membrane as channels from the outside to the inside. It is possible that proteins can move laterally along a surface of the membrane, but it is thermodynamically unlikely that proteins can be rotated within a membrane, which discounts early theories of how transport systems might work. The membranes of Bacteria are structurally similar to the cell membranes of eucaryotes, except that bacterial membranes consist of saturated or monounsaturated fatty acids and do not normally contain sterols. The membranes of Archaea form bilayers functionally equivalent to bacterial membranes, but archaeal lipids are saturated, branched, repeating isoprenoid subunits that attach to glycerol via an ether linkage as opposed to the ester linkage found in glycerides of eukaryotic and bacterial membrane lipids. The structure of archaeal membranes is thought to be an adaptation to their existence and survival in extreme environments.

History of Plasma Membrane

Before the advent of electron microscopy, all efforts to illucidate the structure and composition of plasma membrane were indirect approaches based on physic-chemical properties of the membrane. Some efforts are made by the scientist to describe the structure of plasma membrane is given hereunder:

a) **Concept of Water insoluble Barrier (E. Overton):** Experiments conducted by E. Overton on permeability properties of cell boundries of plant root hair cells and mammalian red blodd cells during 1890s gave birth to the idea that plasma membrane is a relatively soild and water insoluble barrier through which lipid soluble molecules enter into cells mre readily than water soluble molecules. This suggested that lipids make up considerable part of plasma membrane.

b) **Concept of Biomolecular Lipid Layer (Gorter and Grendel):** Two important discoveries of early 19th century immensely helped in elucidation of the basic structure of plasma membrane. Firstly, it was discovered that lipids were the most common non polar, water repelling components of cells. Secondly, I. Langmuir discovered that when an amphipathic lipid molecuale having a polar head group was placed in water, it oriented with its polar head projecting into water and non polar tail part projecting away from the water at right angles to water surface.

By combining Langmuir's technique with microscopy, E Gorter and F. Grendel found that the surface area of red blood cells is about half of the surface area of a lipid monolayer that formed when lipid molecules obtained from the plasma membrane of RBC was placed in water. These workers postulated a bimolecular lipid layer model of the structure of plasma membrane in 1925, which explain that the plasma membrane has two layers of lipid.

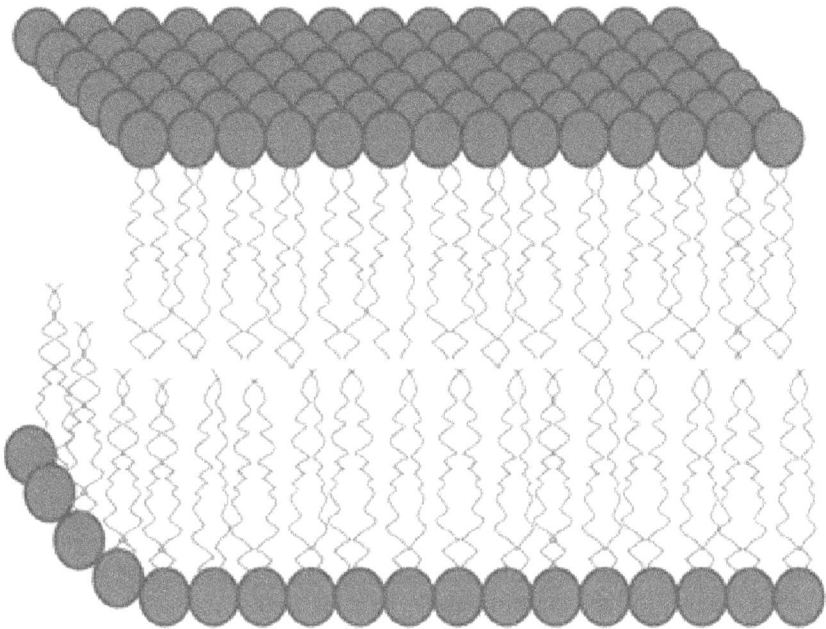

Figure 1.7: Lipid Bilayer Model

c) **Sandwich Model of Davson and Danielli:** On the basis of the comparative data of surface tensions of lipid layers and cell surfaces, collected during early 1930s, H Davson and J Danielli (1935) concluded that the plasma membrane contains a good amount of proteins in addition to the lipid bilayer. They hypothesized that:

(i) The polar heads of inner lipid layer are embedded in the surface of the aqueous extracellular medium.

(ii) The non polar fatty acid tails of the lipid molecules of both layers are directed away from the respective aqueous phases. Hence these faces eah other and form the middle core region of the plasma membrane

(iii) The polar heads of both lipid layers are coated by hydropprotiens which form almost continuous layers.

Therefore, Davson and Danielli proposed a Sandwich Model of plasma membrane with bimolecular lipid layer being sandwiched between two protein layers. Later (1954), Danielli further proposed that the lipid layer is performed by pores which are lined by protein moleculaes and which serve as diffusion channels for polar molecules and ions.

d) **Unit Membrane Concept of Robertson:** The plsam membrane was actually observed for the first time with the help of electron microscope during early 1950s. It was found to be a three layered structure showing two dark staining lines separated by a middle light staining line in a dark light dark railway track pattern. Each dark line represents a continuous sheet of mostly small and globular hydrophilic proteins together with the underlying polar heads of lipid molecules, whereas the middle light line represents a bilayer of non polar fatty acid tails of lipid molecules of both layers. It was also found that the proteins of external and internal layers are dissimilar so that the trilaminar structure is assymetrical. Since certain cell organelles are surrounded by two concentric membranes, each having this trilaminar structure, J.D. Robertson (1957) proposed that the trilaminar represents a unit membrane. This concept confirms that the plsam membrane is a water insoluble barrier so that only lipid soluble substances can pass directly through it.

e) **Fluid Mosaic Model of Singer and Nicolson:** Advances in electron microscopy and biophysical chemistry during 1960s led to a revision of the unit membrane concept on the basis of three types of new evidences:

(i) Besides the hydrophilic surface proteins, certain other proteins are found embedded in the hydrophobic interiror of the plasma membrane, interrupting the continuity of the lipid bilayer. These integral proteins are amphipathic, having both hydrophobic and hydrophilic regions.

(ii) The lipids of the membrane always remain in fluid state and can move about in the plane of the membrane.

(iii) The integral proteins are asymmetrically distributed in the pattern of a mosaic and can freely move about in the fluid lipid layer in the plane of the membrane. These evidences led J.S. Singer and G. Nicolson to propose a fluid mosaic model (1972) of plasma membrane structure. This model was confirmed by Bretscher (1985) and is currently accepted by biologists. The Fluid Mosaic Model predicts that plasma membrane is flexible, quasifluid and dynamic boundry in which component molecules can move about and can interact with each other as well as with the molecules of extracellular medium and cytosol as required for the various functions of the membrane.

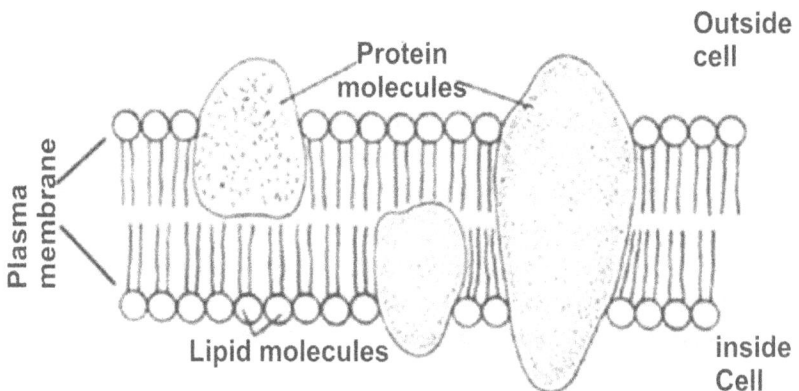

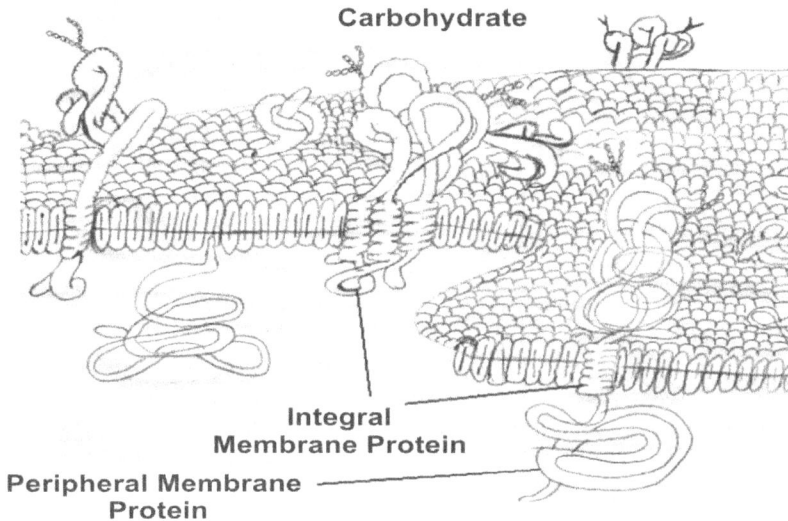

Figure 1.8: Fluid Mosaic Model

Chemical Composition of Plasma Membrane

By weight, the plasma membrane of animal cell is about 55% proteins, 40% lipids and 5% carbohydrates. Cell membranes contain a variety of biological molecules, notably lipids and proteins. Material is incorporated into the membrane or deleted from it, by a variety of mechanisms:

- Fusion of intracellular vesicles with the membrane (exocytosis) not only excretes the contents of the vesicle but also incorporates the vesicle membrane's components into the cell membrane. The membrane may form blebs around extracellular material that pinch off to become vesicles (endocytosis).

- If a membrane is continuous with a tubular structure made of membrane material, then material from the tube can be drawn into the membrane continuously.

- Although the concentration of membrane components in the aqueous phase is low (stable membrane components have low solubility in water), there is an exchange of molecules between the lipid and aqueous phases.

Lipids:The cell membrane consists of three classes of amphipathic lipids: phospholipids, glycolipids and cholesterols. The amount of each depends upon the type of cell, but in the majority of cases phospholipids are the most abundant. In RBC studies, 30% of the plasma membrane is lipid. The fatty chains in phospholipids and glycolipids usually contain an even number of carbon atoms, typically between 16 and 20. The 16- and 18-carbon fatty acids are the most common. Fatty acids may be saturated or unsaturated, with the configuration of the double bonds nearly always *cis*. The length and the degree of unsaturation of fatty acid chains have a profound effect on membrane fluidity as unsaturated lipids create a kink, preventing the fatty acids from packing together as tightly, thus decreasing the melting temperature of the membrane. The ability of some organisms to regulate the fluidity of their cell membranes by altering lipid composition is called homeoviscous adaptation.

The entire membrane is held together via non-covalent interaction of hydrophobic tails; however the structure is quite fluid and not fixed rigidly in place. Under physiological conditions phospholipid molecules in the cell membrane are in the liquid crystalline state. It means the lipid molecules are free to diffuse and exhibit rapid lateral diffusion along the layer in which they are present. However, the exchange of phospholipid molecules between intracellular and extracellular leaflets of the bilayer is a very slow process. Lipid rafts and caveolae are examples of cholesterol-enriched microdomains in the cell membrane. In animal cells cholesterol is normally found dispersed in varying degrees throughout cell membranes, in the irregular spaces between the hydrophobic tails of the membrane lipids, where it gives stiffening and strengthening effect on the membrane.

Phospholipids forming Lipid Vesicles :Lipid vesicles or liposomes are circular pockets that are enclosed by a lipid bilayer. These structures are used in laboratories to study the effects of chemicals in cells by delivering these chemicals directly to the cell, as well as getting more insight into cell membrane permeability. Lipid vesicles and liposomes are formed by first suspending a lipid in an aqueous solution then agitating the mixture through sonication, resulting in a uniformly circular vesicle. By measuring the rate of efflux from that of the inside of the vesicle to the ambient solution, allows us to better understand membrane permeability. Vesicles can be formed with molecules and ions inside the vesicle by forming the vesicle with the desired molecule or ion present in the solution. Proteins can also be embedded into the membrane through solubilizing the desired proteins in the presence of detergents and attaching them to the phospholipids in which the liposome is formed.

Carbohydrates : Plasma membranes also contain carbohydrates, predominantly glycoproteins, but with some glycolipids (cerebrosides and gangliosides). For the most part, no glycosylation occurs on membranes within the cell; rather generally glycosylation occurs on the extracellular surface of the plasma membrane.The glycocalyx is an important feature in all cells, especially epithelia with microvilli. Recent data suggest the glycocalyx participates in cell adhesion, lymphocyte homing and much other. The penultimate sugar is galactose and the terminal sugar is sialic acid, as the sugar backbone is modified in the golgi apparatus. Sialic acid carries a negative charge, providing an external barrier to charged particles.

Proteins: Proteins within the membrane are key to the functioning of the overall membrane. These proteins mainly transport chemicals and information across the membrane. Every membrane has a varying degree of protein content. Proteins can be in the form of peripheral or integral.

Table 6: Protein of Plasmamebrane

S. No.	Type	Description	Examples
1	Integral proteinsor transmembrane proteins	Span the membrane and have a hydrophilic cytosolic domain, which interacts with internal molecules, a hydrophobic membrane-spanning domain that anchors it within the cell membrane and a hydrophilic extracellular domain that interacts with external molecules. The hydrophobic domain consists of one, multiple or a combination of á-helices and â sheet protein motifs.	Ion channels, proton pumps, G protein-coupled receptor
2	Lipid anchored proteins	Covalently bound to single or multiple lipid molecules; hydrophobically insert into the cell membrane and anchor the protein. The protein itself is not in contact with the membrane.	G proteins
3	Peripheral proteins	Attached to integral membrane proteins or associated with peripheral regions of the lipid bilayer. These proteins tend to have only temporary interactions with biological membranes and once reacted the molecule dissociate to carry on its work in the cytoplasm.	Some enzymes, some hormones

The cell membrane plays host to a large amount of protein that is responsible for its various activities. The amount of protein differs between species and according to function, however the typical amount in a cell membrane is 50%. These proteins are undoubtedly important to a cell: Approximately a third of the genes in yeast code specifically for them and this number is even higher in multicellular organisms. The cell membrane, being exposed to the outside environment, is an important site of cell-cell communication. As such, a large variety of protein receptors and identification proteins, such as antigens, are present on the surface of the membrane. Functions of membrane proteins can also include cell-cell contact, surface recognition, cytoskeleton contact, signaling, enzymatic activity or transporting substances across the membrane.Most membrane proteins must be inserted in some way into the membrane. For this to occur, an N-terminus signal sequence of amino acids directs proteins to the endoplasmic reticulum, which inserts the proteins into a lipid bilayer. Once inserted, the proteins are then transported to their final destination in vesicles, where the vesicle fuses with the target membrane.

Variation in Plasma Membrane

The cell membrane has different lipid and protein compositions in distinct types of cells and may have therefore specific names for certain cell types:

- Sarcolemma in myocytes,

- Oolemma in oocytes,

- Historically, the plasma membrane was also referred to as the plasmalemma.

Permeability

The permeability of a membrane is the ease with which molecules pass through it. These molecules are known as permeant molecules. Permeability depends mainly on the electric charge of the molecule and to a lesser extent the molar mass of the molecule. Due to the cell membrane's hydrophobic nature, electrically neutral and small molecules pass through the membrane easier than charged, large ones. The inability of charged molecules to pass through the cell membrane results in pH parturition of substances throughout the fluid compartments of the body.

Function of Plasma Membrane

The cell membrane surrounds the cytoplasm of a cell and, in animal cells, physically separates the intracellular components from the extracellular environment. Fungi, bacteria and plants also have the cell wall which provides a mechanical support for the cell and precludes the passage of larger molecules. The cell membrane also plays a role in anchoring the cytoskeleton to provide shape to the cell and in attaching to the extracellular matrix and other cells to help group cells together to form tissues. The membrane is differentially permeable and able to regulate what enters and exits the cell, thus facilitating the transport of materials needed for survival. The movement of substances across the membrane can be passive, occurring without the input of cellular energy or active, requiring the cell to expend energy in transporting it. The membrane also maintains the cell potential. The cell membrane thus works as a selective filter that allows only certain things to come inside or go outside the cell. To do so, the membrane employs a number of transport mechanisms:

a. **Diffusion:** Some substances (small molecules, ions) such as carbon dioxide (CO_2), oxygen (O_2) and water can move across the plasma membrane by diffusion, which is a passive transport process.

b. **Osmosis:** Because the membrane acts as a barrier for certain molecules and ions, they can occur in different concentrations on the two sides of the membrane. Such a concentration difference across a semipermeable membrane can set up the osmotic flow for the solvent, in this case water. Water can thus be transported across the membrane by osmosis.

c. **Mediated Transport:** Nutrients such as sugars and materials of growth such as amino acid must enter the cell and the waste of metabolism must leave. Such molecules are moved across the membrane by special proteins called transport proteins or permeases. Permeases form a small passageway through the membrane, enabling the solute molecule to cross the phospholipid bilayer. Permeases are usually quite specific, recognizing and transporting only a limited group of chemical substances, often even only a single substance.

d. **Endocytosis:** Endocytosis is the process in which cells absorb molecules by engulfing them. The plasma membrane creates a small deformation inward, called an invagination, in which the substance to be transported is captured. The deformation then pinches off from the membrane on the inside of the cell, creating a vesicle containing the captured substance. Endocytosis is a pathway for internalizing solid particles (cell eating or phagocytosis), small molecules and ions (cell drinking or pinocytosis) and macromolecules. Endocytosis requires energy and is thus a form of active transport.

e. **Exocytosis:** Just as material can be brought into the cell by invagination and formation of a vesicle, the membrane of a vesicle can be fused with the plasma membrane, extruding its contents to the surrounding medium. This is the process of exocytosis. Exocytosis occurs in various cells to remove undigested residues of substances brought in by endocytosis, to secrete substances such as hormones and enzymes and to transport a substance completely across a cellular barrier. In the process of exocytosis, the undigested waste-containing food vacuole or the secretory vesicle budded from Golgi apparatus, is first moved by cytoskeleton from the interior of the cell to the surface. The vesicle membrane comes in contact with the plasma membrane. The lipid molecules of the two bilayers rearrange themselves and the two membranes are, thus, fused. A passage is formed in the fused membrane and the vesicles discharge its contents outside the cell.

Since procaryotes lack any intracellular organelles for processes such as respiration or photosynthesis or secretion, the plasma membrane includes these processes for the cell and consequently has a variety of functions in energy generation and biosynthesis *e.g.* electron transport system that couples aerobic respiration and ATP synthesis is found in the procaryotic membrane. The photosynthetic chromophores that harvest light energy for conversion into chemical energy are located in the membrane. Hence, the plasma membrane is the site of oxidative phosphorylation and photophosphorylation in procaryotes, analogous to the functions of mitochondria and chloroplasts in eukaryotic cells. Besides transport proteins that selectively mediate the passage of substances into and out of the cell, procaryotic membranes may contain sensing proteins that measure concentrations of molecules in the environment or binding proteins that translocate signals to genetic and metabolic machinery in the cytoplasm. Membranes also contain enzymes involved in many metabolic processes such as cell wall synthesis, septum formation, membrane synthesis, DNA replication, CO_2 fixation and ammonia oxidation.

Summary

1. All organism from the smallest to the largest are composed of tiny structures called Cell. G. Loewy and P. Siekevitz (1963) defined the cell as "A unit of biological activity delimited by a semipermiable membrane and capable of self-reproduction in a medium free of other living systems".

2. Robert Hooke first examined cork and used the term Cell to describe its basic unit.

3. Antony Van Leeuwenhoek first observed nuclei and unicellular organisms, including bacteria: in 1676, bacteria were described for the first time as animalcules.

4. J.B. Lamarck showed the importance of cell in living organisms.

5. J.E. Purkinje introduced the term protoplasm.

6. Robert Brown described described the nucleus as a characteristic spherical body in plant cells.

7. In 1838, a German botanist, M. Jakob Schleiden and in 1839, a German zoologist, Theodore Schwann recognized the cells with nuclei as the fundamental unit of all living beings- Animal and Plants. The concept that the cell is basic unit of life is known as cell theory.

8. Rudolf Virchow, a German physician, in 1858 extended the cell theory and suggested that all living cells arise from pre-existing living cells.

9. Cells of all organisms have close similarities in structure, molecular organmism and biological activities.

10. Cells need a constant flow of ordered energy for maintaining their organized structure and functions. The source of this energy is the sun.

11. Cells regulate their life processes with the help of continual flow of information. The flow of information takes two routes. The first is the flow of genetic information and the second is the flow of extrinsic information.

12. There two basic types of cells depending on the degree of internal organization. Prokaryotic cell, characteristic of bacteria and cyanobacteria, is simple in morphology.

13. The cytoplasm lacks membrane bound organelles and the respiratory or photosynthetic enzymes are located in the plasma membrane. The cytoplasm contains many membranous compartments and membrane bound organelles *e.g.* mitochondria, lysosomes, chloroplasts, etc.

14. The genetic material, DNA, is not organized into distinct chromosomes.

15. The cell membrane shows comparatively more selective permeability. DNA is located in chromosomes and the nucleus has a distinct nuclear envelope.

16. Eukaryotic cell, characteristic of all organisms other than bacteria and cyanobacteria, is complicated in morphology.

17. Animal cells generally do not posses a cell wall.

18. There is great variety in size, from, structure and function of cells.

19. Prokaryotes have only a limited repertoire of organelles in their cytoplasm and these are generally nonmembranous like ribosomes. They lack cilia, centrioles, microfilaments and microtubules.

20. Eukaryotes are rich in the numbers and kinds of organelles and they include both membranous and non-membranous types.

21. In plant cells, fungi and bacteria, the plasma membrane is enclosed within an extraneous coat of non-living material that usually confers some rigidity to the cell it surrounds.

22. There are general layers of the cell wall: middle layer, primary wall and secondary wall. The middle lamella is present between two primary walls of adjacent cells. Micelles from the framework of the cell wall within the cell wal matrix.

23. In many protistian and animals cell membranes are not enclosed by cellulosic walls.

24. The glycocalyx contains receptors that bind with a variety of external substances controlling internal cell activity.

25. In many cells, special structures are formed that anchor the cells firmly together.

26. The cell membrane is the outer layer of the living cell. The main role of the cell membrane is to separate protoplast from the environment.

27. The unit membrane hypothesis describes the membrane as inner and outer dense protein layer surrounding a thicker but less dense phospholipids layer.

28. S.J. Singer and Nicholson (1972) introduced the Fluid Mosaic Model.

29. The jelly like fluid protoplasmic matrix which surrounds the nucleus and constitutes the true internal milieu of the cell is called cytoplasm.

30. Nucleus discovered by Robert Brown in 1833. The nucleus is universal and prominent feature of all cells except the members of the kingdom Monera.

31. Plastids are cytoplasmic organelles present in eukaryotic plant cell. The term was first used in 1885 by A. F. W. Schimper to include the cell organelles which are primarily involved in the synthesis and storage of carbohydrates. Plastids are of three type *viz.* green chloroplsts, colourless leucoplast are disc shaped structures measuring 4-10 µm in length and 1-3 µm in breadth.

32. Each chloroplast is enclosed by a double membrane of lipo-protein which 40-60 Å thick.

33. The cytoplasm of the cell is interlaced by an elaborate membrane bound vesicular system is known as Endoplasmic reticulum. Rough ER is concerned with transport of proteins whereas smooth ER plays an especially important role in the synthesis and assembly of gycolipids.

34. Golgi complex discovered by Camillo Gogi in 1898. It consists of a system of stacks of flat circular cisternae, each bound by a smooth unit membrane.

35. Lysosome is found in most eukaryotic cells but is particularly abundant in animal cells exhibiting phagocytic activity. They commonly knew as Suicidle bags. They are sac like structure, about 0.2-0.5 µm in diameter, bounded by a single membrane.

36. Microbodies are small bodies, 0.5-1.5 µm in diameter which occur in the cytoplasm of a variety of tissue. Peroxisomes are microbodies in liver cells and leaf parenchyma cells.

37. Microvilli are finger like extension of the cell surface membrane that increases of the cell surface membrane that increases the surface area by as much as 25 times.

38. Cilia are short, motile structures, generally present in large numbers covering the cell, whereas flagella are larger than cilia.

39. Centrioles are non membranous small hollow cylinders that occur in pairs in most animal and lower plant cell.

40. Vacuoles are discrete, clear regions within the cell that contain water and dissolved salts.

Chapter 2

Cell Organelles: Structure and Function

Introduction

The vast majority of the reactions that cells carry out take place in water. Eukaryotic cells are carrying out an enormous range of such chemical manipulations: these reactions are collectively called as metabolism. In much the same way that our homes are divided into rooms that are adapted for particular activities, the eukaryotic cells contain distinct compartments or organelles to house specific functions. The term organelle is used rather loosely, at one extreme, some scientists use it to mean any distinct cellular structure that has a more or less well-defined job to do; at the other are scientists who would reserve the name organelle for those cellular compartments that contain their own DNA and have some limited genetic autonomy. Three cell organelles *i.e.* the nucleus, mitochondrion and the chloro-plast (in plant cells), share two distinctive features. They are all enclosed within an envelope consisting of two parallel membranes (double mebrane) and they all contain the genetic material DNA. Other cell organelles *e.g.* ribosomes, ER, Golgi apparatus, lysosomes, peroxisomes etc have single membrane and do not have own DNA. The structure and function of cell organelles is given hereunder:

Cell Membrane (for more detail see chapter 1)

The cell membrane functions as a semi-permeable barrier, allowing a very few molecules across it while fencing the majority of organically produced chemicals inside the cell. Electron microscopic examinations of cell membranes have led to the development of the lipid bilayer model also referred to as the fluid-mosaic model. The most common molecule in the model is the phospholipid, which has a polar (hydrophilic) head and two nonpolar (hydrophobic) tails. These phospholipids are aligned tail to tail so the nonpolar areas form a hydrophobic region between the hydrophilic heads on the inner and outer surfaces of the membrane. This layering is termed a bilayer since an electron microscopic technique known as freeze fracturing is able to split the bilayer.

Cholesterol is another important component of cell membranes embedded in the hydrophobic areas of the inner (tail-tail) region. Most bacterial cell membranes do not contain cholesterol. Cholesterol aids in the flexibility of a cell membrane. Proteins are suspended in the inner layer, although the more hydrophilic areas of these proteins stick out into the cells interior as well as outside the cell. These proteins function as gateways that allow certain molecules to cross into and out of the cell by moving through open areas of the protein channel. These integral proteins are sometimes known as gateway proteins. The outer surface of the membrane tends to be rich in glycolipids, which have their hydrophobic tails embedded in the hydrophobic region of the membrane and their heads exposed outside the cell. These are thought to function in the self recognition *i.e.* a sort of cellular identification system.

Cell Wall

Most notably animals and many of the more animal-like protistans do not have cell wall. Bacteria have cell walls containing the chemical peptidoglycan. Plant cells have a variety of chemicals incorporated in their cell walls. Cellulose, a nondigestible polysaccharide, is the most common chemical in the plant primary cell wall. Some plant cells also have lignin and other chemicals embedded in their secondary walls. The cell wall is located outside the plasma membrane. Plasmodesmata are connections through which cells communicate chemically with each other through their thick walls. Fungi and many protists have cell walls although they do not contain cellulose, rather a variety of chemicals (chitin for fungi). Animal cells lack a cell wall and must instead rely on their cell membrane to maintain the integrity of the cell. Many protistans also lack cell walls; using variously modified cell membranes act as a boundary to the inside of the cell.

Nucleus

The nucleus derived from Latin nucleus or nuculeus meaning kernel, is the most prominent cell organelle. The nucleus is a membrane enclosed organelle found in eukaryotic cells. It occurs only in eukaryotic cells. It contains most of the cell's genetic material organized as multiple long linear DNA molecules in complex with a large variety of proteins, such as histones, to form chromosomes. The genes within these chromosomes are the cell's nuclear genome. Danish biologist Joachim Hammerling carried out an important experiment in 1943. His work showed the role of the nucleus in controlling the shape and features of the cell. The function of the nucleus is to maintain the integrity of these genes and to control the activities of the cell by regulating gene expression the nucleus is, therefore, the control center of the cell. The main structures making up the nucleus are the nuclear envelope, a triple cell membrane and membrane that enclose the entire organelle and unify its contents from the cellular cytoplasm and the nucleoskeleton which includes nuclear lamina, a meshwork withithe nucleus that adds mechanical support, much like the cytoskeleton, which supports the cell as a whole. Because the nuclear membrane is impermeable to most molecules, nuclear pores are required to allow movement of molecules across the envelope. These pores cross both of the membranes, providing a channel that allows free movement of small molecules and ions. The movement of larger molecules such as proteins is carefully controlled and requires active transport regulated by carrier proteins. Nuclear transport is crucial to cell function, as movement through the pores is required for both gene expression and chromosomal maintenance. The interior of the nucleus does not contain any membrane-bound subcompartments, its contents are not uniform and a number of subnuclear bodies exist, made up of unique proteins, RNA molecules and particular parts of the mitochondria. The best known of these is the nucleolus, which is mainly involved in the assembly of ribosomes. After being produced in the nucleolus, ribosomes are exported to the cytoplasm where they translate mRNA.

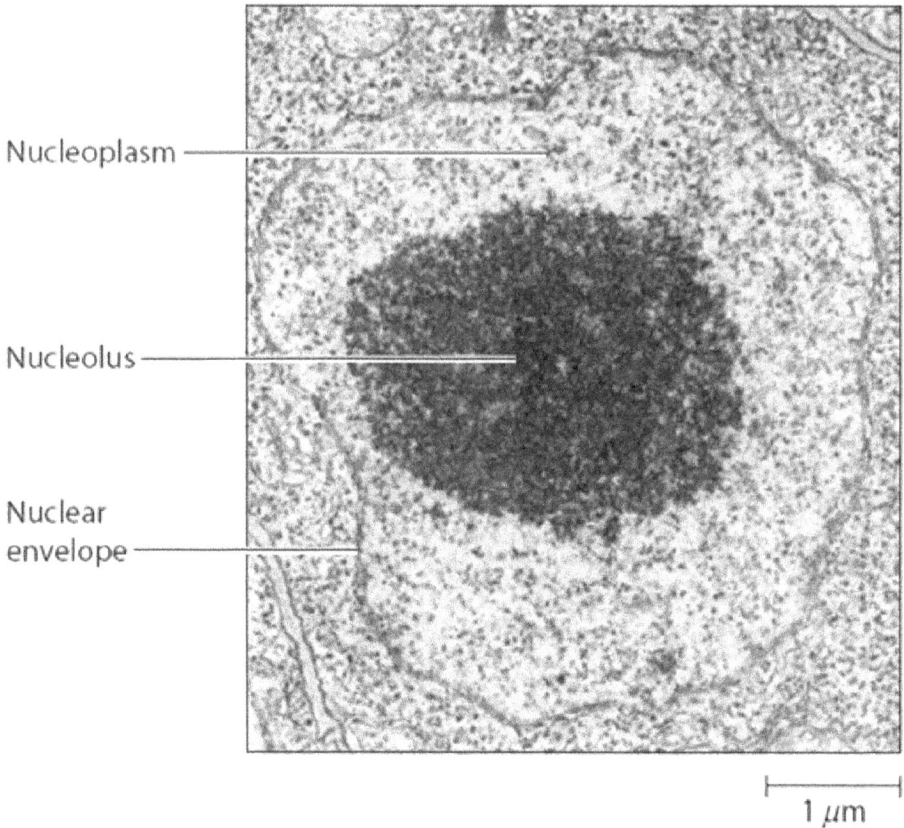

Figure 2.1: Structure of Nucleus

Outer membrane
Inner membrane
Nucleoplasm
Nucleolus
Chromatin
Nuclear envelope
Pore in nuclear envelope

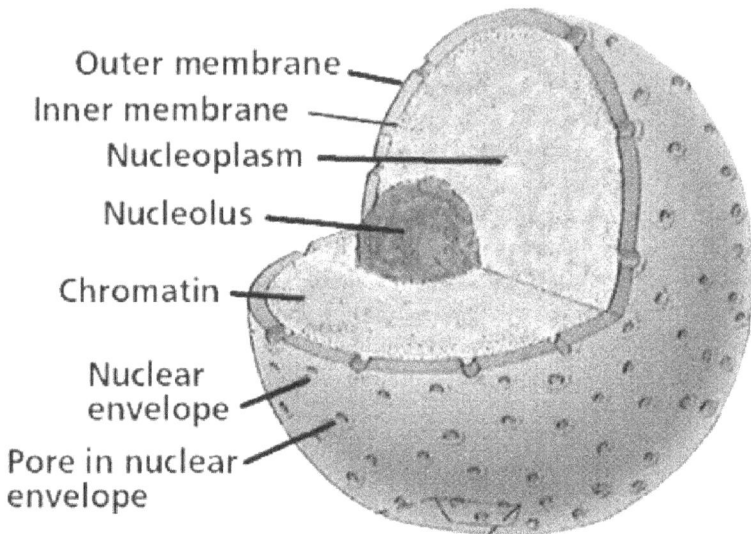

Figure 2.2: Nucleus

History of Nucleaus

The nucleus was the first organelle to be discovered. Possibly the oldest preserved sketch is of drawn by Antonie van Leeuwenhoek (1632–1723). He observed a Lumen in the red blood cells of salmon. Unlike mammalian red blood cells, those of other vertebrates still possess nuclei. The nucleus was also described by Franz Bauer in 1804 by Scottish botanist Robert Brown in 1831 in orchid cells. In 1838, Matthias Schleiden proposed that the nucleus plays a role in generating cells, thus he introduced the name Cytoblast (cell builder). He believed that he had observed new cells assembling around cytoblasts. Franz Meyen was a strong opponent of this view, having already described cells multiplying by division and believing that many cells would have no nuclei. The idea that cells can be generated de novo, by the cytoblast or otherwise, contradicted work by Robert Remak (1852) and Rudolf Virchow (1855) who decisively propagated the new paradigm that cells are generated solely by cells (*Omnis cellula e cellula*).

Oscar Hedwig published several studies on the fertilization of sea urchin eggs during 1877 and 1878 showing that the nucleus of the sperm enters the oocyte and fuses with its nucleus. This was the first time it was suggested that an individual develops from a single nucleated cell. This was in contradiction to Ernst Haeckel's theory that the complete phylogeny of a species would be repeated during embryonic development, including generation of the first nucleated cell from a Monerula, a structureless mass of primordial mucus *i.e.* Urschleim. Therefore, the necessity of the sperm nucleus for fertilization was discussed for quite some time. However, Hertwig

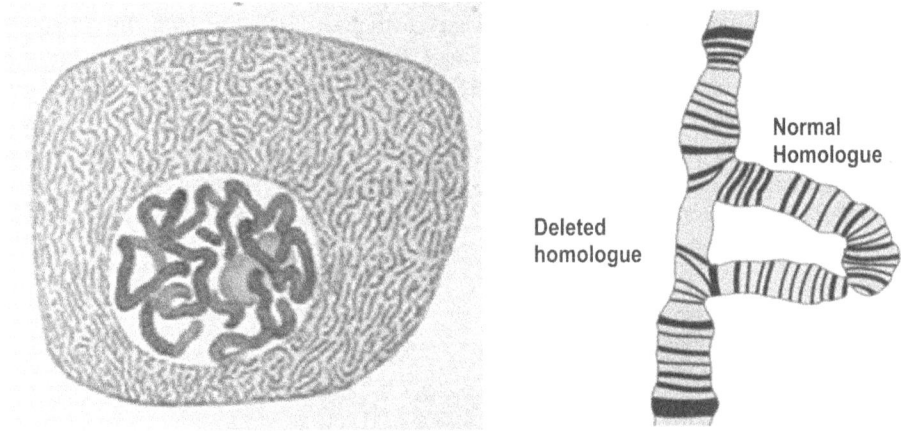

Figure 2.3a: Drawing of Chironomus salivary gland cell: Published by Walther Flemming in 1882. The nucleus contains polytene chromosomes.

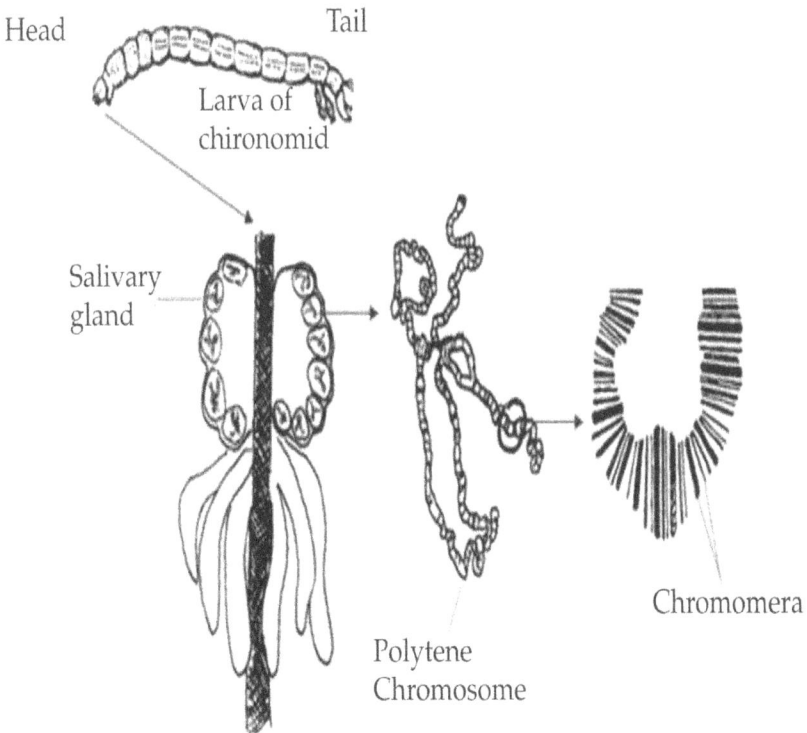

Figure 2.3b: Structure of polytene (giant) chromosome

confirmed his observation in other animal groups, e.g. amphibians and molluscs. Strasburger (1882) proved that nucleus arises from pre existing nucleus by division. Hertwig and van Beneden showed the role of nucleus in fertilization. Hammerling (1953) by his grafting experiments on Acetabularia (largest unicellular green, marine alga) proved the role of nucleus in heredity, growth and morphology. 1/10th of volume of cell is occupied by nucleus. In a cell, there is a definite nucleo cytoplasmic ratio. The function of the nucleus as carrier of genetic information became clear only later, after mitosis was discovered and the Mendelian rules were rediscovered at the beginning of the 20th century; the chromosome theory of heredity was developed.

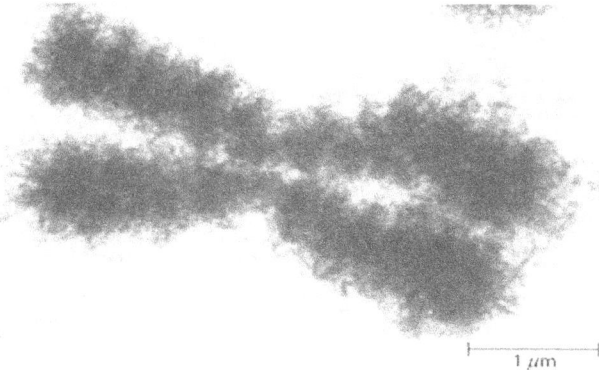

Figure 2.4. Eukaryotic chromosome

Structure of Nucleus

The cell nucleus acts like the brain of the cell. It helps control eating, movement and reproduction. The nucleus is the largest cellular organelle found in animals. In mammalian cells, the average diameter of the nucleus is approximately 6 micrometers (6 ìm), which occupies about 10% of the total cell volume. The viscous liquid within it is called nucleoplasm and is similar in composition to the cytosol found outside the nucleus. It appears as a dense, roughly spherical organelle.

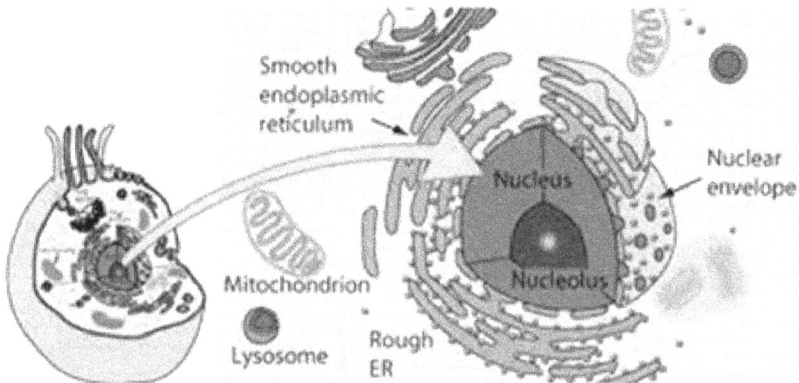

Figure 2.5: Componeuts of Nucleus

Nuclear Envelope and Pores :The outer envelope otherwise known as nuclear membrane consists of two cellular membranes, an inner and an outer membrane, arranged parallel to one another and separated by 10 to 50 nanometers (nm). The nuclear envelope completely encloses the nucleus and separates the cell's genetic material from the surrounding cytoplasm, serving as a barrier to prevent macromolecules from diffusing freely between the nucleoplasm and the cytoplasm. The outer nuclear membrane is continuous with the membrane of the rough endoplasmic reticulum (RER) and is similarly studded with ribosomes. The space between the membranes is called the perinuclear space and is continuous with the RER lumen.

Nuclear pores, which provide aqueous channels through the envelope, are composed of multiple proteins, collectively referred to as nucleoporins. The pores are about 125 million daltons in molecular weight and consist of around 50 in yeast to 100 proteins in vertebrates. The pores are 100 nm in total diameter; however, the gap through which molecules freely diffuse is only about 9 nm wide, due to the presence of regulatory systems within the center of the pore. This size allows the not-free passage of small water-soluble molecules while preventing larger molecules, such as nucleic acids and larger proteins, from inappropriately entering or exiting the nucleus. These large molecules must be actively transported into the nucleus instead. The nucleus of a typical mammalian cell will have about 3000 to 4000 pores throughout its envelope, each of which contains a donut-shaped, eightfold-symmetric ring-shaped structure at a position where the inner and outer membranes fuse. The structure attached to the ring is called the nuclear basket that extends into the nucleoplasm and a series of filamentous extensions that reach into the cytoplasm both structures serve to mediate binding to nuclear transport proteins.

Most proteins, ribosomal subunits and some DNAs are transported through the pore complexes in a process mediated by a family of transport factors known as karyopherins. Those karyopherins that mediate movement into the nucleus are also called importins, whereas those that mediate movement out of the nucleus are called exportins. Most karyopherins interact directly with their cargo, although some use adaptor proteins. Steroid hormones such as cortisol and aldosterone, as well as other small lipid soluble molecules involved in intercellular signaling, can diffuse through the cell membrane and into the cytoplasm, where they bind nuclear receptor proteins that are trafficked into the nucleus. There they serve as transcription factors when bound to their ligand; in the absence of ligand, many such receptors function as histone deacetylases that repress gene expression.

Nuclear Lamina : In animal cells, two networks of intermediate filaments provide the nucleus with mechanical support. The nuclear lamina forms an organized meshwork on the internal face of the envelope, while less organized support is provided on the cytosolic face of the envelope. Both systems provide structural support for the nuclear envelope and anchoring sites for chromosomes and nuclear pores. The nuclear lamina is composed mostly of lamin proteins. Like all proteins, lamins are synthesized in the cytoplasm and later transported into the nucleus interior, where they are assembled before being incorporated into the existing network of nuclear lamina. Lamins found on the cytosolic face of the membrane, such as emerin and nesprin, bind to the cytoskeleton to provide structural support. Lamins are also found inside the nucleoplasm where they form another regular structure, known as the nucleoplasmic veil, which is visible using fluorescence microscopy. The actual function of the veil is not clear, although it is excluded from the nucleolus and is present during interphase. Lamin structures that make up the veil, such as LEM3, bind chromatin and disrupting their structure inhibits transcription of protein coding genes.

Like the components of other intermediate filaments, the lamin monomer contains an alpha-helical domain used by two monomers to coil around each other, forming a dimer structure called a coiled coil. Two of these dimer structures then join side by side, in an antiparallel arrangement, to form a tetramer called a protofilament. Eight of these protofilaments form a lateral arrangement that is twisted to form a ropelike filament. These filaments can be assembled or disassembled in a dynamic manner, meaning that changes in the length of the filament depend on the competing rates of filament addition and removal.

Mutations in lamin genes leading to defects in filament assembly are known as laminopathies. The most notable laminopathy is the family of diseases known as progeria, which causes the appearance of premature aging in its sufferers. The exact mechanism by which the associated biochemical changes give rise to the aged phenotype is not well understood. The cell nucleus contains the majority of the cell's genetic material in the form of multiple linear DNA molecules organized into structures called chromosomes. Each human cell contains 2m of DNA. During most of the cell cycle these are organized in a DNA-protein complex known as chromatin and during cell division the chromatin can be seen to form the well-defined chromosomes familiar from a karyotype. A small fraction of the cell's genes are located instead in the mitochondria.

There are two types of chromatin. Euchromatin is the less compact DNA form and contains genes that are frequently expressed by the cell. The other type, heterochromatin, is the more compact form and contains DNA that are infrequently transcribed. This structure is further categorized into facultative heterochromatin, consisting of genes that are organized as heterochromatin only in certain cell types or at certain stages of development and constitutive heterochromatin that consists of chromosome structural components such as telomeres and centromeres. During interphase the chromatin organizes itself into discrete individual patches, called chromosome territories. Active genes, which are generally found in the euchromatic region of the chromosome, tend to be located towards the chromosome's territory boundary. Antibodies to certain types of chromatin organization, in particular, nucleosomes, have been associated with a number of autoimmune diseases, such as systemic lupus erythematosus, these are known as anti-nuclear antibodies (ANA) and have also been observed in concert with multiple sclerosis as part of general immune system dysfunction. As in the case of progeria, the role played by the antibodies in inducing the symptoms of autoimmune diseases is not obvious.

Nucleolus : The nucleolus is a discrete densely stained structure found in the nucleus. It is not surrounded by a membrane and is sometimes called a suborganelle. It forms around tandem repeats of rDNA, DNA coding for ribosomal RNA (rRNA).

These regions are called nucleolar organizer regions (NOR). The main roles of the nucleolus are to synthesize rRNA and assemble ribosomes. The structural cohesion of the nucleolus depends on its activity, as ribosomal assembly in the nucleolus results in the transient association of nucleolar components, facilitating further ribosomal assembly and hence further association. This model is supported by observations that inactivation of rDNA results in intermingling of nucleolar structures. The first step in ribosomal assembly is transcription of the rDNA, by a protein called RNA polymerase I, forming a large pre-rRNA precursor. This is cleaved into the subunits 5.8S, 18S and 28S rRNA. The transcription, post-transcriptional processing and assembly of rRNA occurs in the nucleolus, aided by small nucleolar RNA (snoRNA) molecules, some of which are derived from spliced introns from messenger RNAs encoding genes related to ribosomal function. The assembled ribosomal subunits are the largest structures passed through the nuclear pores.

When observed under the electron microscope, the nucleolus can be seen to consist of three distinguishable regions: the innermost fibrillar centers (FCs), surrounded by the dense fibrillar component (DFC), which in turn is bordered by the granular component (GC). Transcription of the rDNA occurs either in the FC or at the FC-DFC boundary and, therefore, when rDNA transcription in the cell is increased, more FCs is detected. Most of the cleavage and modification of rRNAs occurs in the DFC, while the latter steps involving protein assembly onto the ribosomal subunits occur in the GC.

Table 2.1: Size of Subnuclear Bodies

S.No.	Subnuclear bodies	Diameter
1.	Cajal bodies	0.2–2.0 µm
2.	PIKA	5 µm
3.	PML bodies	0.2–1.0 µm
4.	Paraspeckles	0.2–1.0 µm
5.	Speckles	20–25 nm

Besides the nucleolus, the nucleus contains a number of other non-membrane-delineated bodies. These include Cajal bodies, Gemini of coiled bodies, polymorphic interphase karyosomal association (PIKA), promyelocytic leukaemia (PML) bodies, paraspeckles and splicing speckles. Although little is known about a number of these domains, they are significant in that they show that the nucleoplasm is not uniform mixture, but rather contains organized functional subdomains. Other subnuclear structures appear as part of abnormal disease processes *e.g.* presence of small intranuclear rods has been reported in some cases of nemaline myopathy. This condition typically results from mutations in actin and the rods themselves consist of mutant actin as well as other cytoskeletal proteins.

Cajal bodies and Gems: A nucleus typically contains between 1 and 10 compact structures called Cajal bodies or coiled bodies (CB), whose diameter measures between 0.2 µm and 2.0 µm depending on the cell type and species. When can see under an electron microscope, they resemble balls of tangled thread and are dense foci of distribution for the protein coilin. CBs are involved in a number of different roles relating to RNA processing, specifically small nucleolar RNA (snoRNA) and small nuclear RNA (snRNA) maturation and histone mRNA modification. Similar to Cajal bodies are Gemini of coiled bodies or gems, whose name is derived from the Gemini constellation in reference to their close twin relationship with CBs. Gems are similar in size and shape to CBs and in fact are virtually indistinguishable under the microscope. Unlike CBs, gems do not contain small nuclear ribonucleoproteins (snRNPs), but do contain a protein called survivor of motor neurons (SMN) whose function relates to snRNP biogenesis. Gems are believed to assist CBs in snRNP biogenesis, though it has also been suggested from microscopy evidence that CBs and gems are different manifestations of the same structure.

RAFA and PTF domains: RAFA domains or polymorphic interphase karyosomal associations were first described in microscopy studies in 1991. Their function was and remains unclear, though they were not thought to be associated with active DNA replication, transcription or RNA processing. They have been found to often associate with discrete domains defined by dense localization of the transcription factor PTF, which promotes transcription of snRNA.

PML bodies: Promyelocytic leukaemia bodies (PML bodies) are spherical bodies found scattered throughout the nucleoplasm, measuring around 0.2–1.0 μm. They are known by a number of other names, including nuclear domain 10 (ND10), Kremer bodies and PML oncogenic domains. They are seen in the nucleus in association with Cajal bodies and cleavage bodies. It has been suggested that they play a role in regulating transcription.

Paraspeckles: Paraspeckles are irregularly shaped compartments in the nucleus interchromatin space discovered by Fox in 2002. First documented in HeLa cells, where there are generally 10–30 per nucleus, paraspeckles are now known to also exist in all human primary cells, transformed cell lines and tissue sections. Their name is derived from their distribution in the nucleus; the para is short for parallel and the speckles refer to the splicing speckles to which they are always in close proximity. Paraspeckles are dynamic structures that are altered in response to changes in cellular metabolic activity. They are transcription dependent and in the absence of RNA Pol II transcription, the paraspeckle disappears and all of its associated protein components (PSP1, p54nrb, PSP2, CFI (m) 68 and PSF) form a crescent shaped perinucleolar cap in the nucleolus. This phenomenon is demonstrated during the cell cycle. In the cell cycle, paraspeckles are present during interphase and during all of mitosis except for telophase. During telophase, when the two daughter nuclei are formed, there is no RNA Pol II transcription so the protein components instead form a perinucleolar cap.

Splicing Speckles: Speckles are subnuclear structures that are enriched in pre-messenger RNA splicing factors and are located in the interchromatin regions of the nucleoplasm of mammalian cells. At the fluorescence-microscope level they appear as irregular, punctate structures, which vary in size and shape and when examined by electron microscopy they are seen a s clusters of interchromatin granules. Speckles are dynamic structures and both their protein and RNA-protein components can cycle continuously between speckles and other nuclear locations, including active transcription sites. Studies on the composition, structure and behaviour of speckles have provided a model for understanding the functional compartmentalization of the nucleus and the organization of the gene-expression machinery. Sometimes referred to as interchromatin granule clusters or as splicing-factor compartments, speckles are rich in splicing snRNPs and other splicing proteins necessary for pre-mRNA processing. Because of a cell's changing requirements, the composition and location of these bodies changes according to mRNA transcription and regulation via phosphorylation of specific proteins.

Function of Nucleus

The main function of the cell nucleus is to control gene expression and mediate the replication of DNA during the cell cycle. The nucleus provides a site for genetic transcription that is segregated from the location of translation in the cytoplasm, allowing levels of gene regulation that are not available to prokaryotes.

Cell Compartmentalization: The nuclear envelope allows the nucleus to control its contents and separate them from the rest of the cytoplasm where necessary. This is important for controlling processes on either side of the nuclear membrane. In some cases where a cytoplasmic process needs to be restricted, a key participant is removed to the nucleus, where it interacts with transcription factors to downregulate the production of certain enzymes in the pathway. This regulatory mechanism occurs in the case of glycolysis, a cellular pathway for breaking down glucose to produce energy. Hexokinase is an enzyme responsible for the first the step of glycolysis, forming glucose-6-phosphate from glucose. At high concentrations of fructose-6-phosphate, a molecule made later from glucose-6-phosphate, a regulator protein removes hexokinase to the nucleus, where it forms a transcriptional repressor complex with nuclear proteins to reduce the expression of genes involved in glycolysis. In order to control which genes are being transcribed, the cell separates some transcription factor proteins responsible for regulating gene expression from physical access to the DNA until they are activated by other signaling pathways. This prevents even low levels of inappropriate gene expression. In case of NF-êB-controlled genes, which are involved in most inflammatory responses, transcription is induced in response to a signal pathway such as that initiated by the signaling molecule TNF-á, binds to a cell membrane receptor, resulting in the recruitment of signalling proteins and eventually activating the transcription factor NF-êB. A nuclear localisation signal on the NF-êB protein allows it to be transported through the nuclear pore and into the nucleus, where it stimulates the transcription of the target genes. The compartmentalization allows the cell to prevent translation of unspliced mRNA. Eukaryotic mRNA contains introns that must be removed before being translated to produce functional proteins. The splicing is done inside the nucleus before the mRNA can be accessed by ribosomes for translation. Without the nucleus, ribosomes would translate newly transcribed (unprocessed) mRNA, resulting in misformed and nonfunctional proteins.

Gene Expression: Gene expression first involves transcription, in which DNA is used as a template to produce RNA. In the case of genes encoding proteins that RNA produced from this process is messenger RNA (mRNA), which then needs to be translated by ribosomes to form a protein. As ribosomes are located outside the nucleus, mRNA produced needs to be exported. Since the nucleus is the site of transcription, it also contains a variety of proteins that either directly mediates transcription or is involved in regulating the process. These proteins include helicases, which unwind the double-stranded DNA molecule to facilitate access to it, RNA polymerases, which synthesize the growing RNA molecule, topoisomerases, which change the amount of supercoiling in DNA, helping it wind and unwind, as well as a large variety of transcription factors that regulate expression.

Processing of pre-mRNA: Newly synthesized mRNA molecules are known as primary transcripts or pre-mRNA. They must undergo post-transcriptional modification in the nucleus before being exported to the cytoplasm; mRNA that appears in the cytoplasm without these modifications is degraded rather than used for protein translation. The three main modifications are 5' capping, 3' polyadenylation and RNA splicing. While in the nucleus, pre-mRNA is associated with a variety of proteins in complexes known as heterogeneous ribonucleoprotein particles (hnRNPs). Addition of the 5' cap occurs co-transcriptionally and is the first step in post-transcriptional modification. The 3' poly-adenine tail is only added after transcription is complete. RNA splicing, carried out by a complex called the spliceosome, is the process by which introns or regions of DNA that do not code for protein, are removed from the pre-mRNA and the remaining exons connected to re-form a single continuous molecule. This process normally occurs after 5' capping and 3' polyadenylation but can begin before synthesis is complete in transcripts with many exons. Many pre-mRNAs, including those encoding antibodies, can be spliced in multiple ways to produce different mature mRNAs that encode different protein sequences. This process is known as alternative splicing and allows production of a large variety of proteins from a limited amount of DNA.

Nuclear Transport: The entry and exit of large molecules from the nucleus is tightly controlled by the nuclear pore complexes. Although small molecules can enter the nucleus without regulation, macromolecules such as RNA and proteins require association karyopherins called importins to enter the nucleus and exportins to exit. Cargo proteins that must be translocated from the cytoplasm to the nucleus contain short amino acid sequences known as nuclear localization signals, which are bound by importins, while those transported from the nucleus to the cytoplasm carry nuclear export signals bound by exportins. The ability of importins and exportins to transport their cargo is regulated by GTPases, enzymes that hydrolyze the molecule guanosine triphosphate to release energy. The key GTPase in nuclear transport is Ran, which can bind either GTP or GDP (guanosine diphosphate), depending on whether it is located in the nucleus or the cytoplasm. Whereas importins depend on RanGTP to dissociate from their cargo, exportins require RanGTP in order to bind to their cargo. Nuclear import depends on the importin binding its cargo in the cytoplasm and carrying it through the nuclear pore into the nucleus. Inside the nucleus, RanGTP acts to separate the cargo from the importin, allowing the importin to exit the nucleus and be reused. Nuclear export is similar, as the exportin binds the cargo inside the nucleus in a process facilitated by RanGTP, exits through the nuclear pore and separates from its cargo in the cytoplasm. Specialized export proteins exist for translocation of mature mRNA and tRNA to the cytoplasm after post-transcriptional modification is complete. This quality-control mechanism is important due to the these molecules' central role in protein translation; mis-expression of a protein due to incomplete excision of exons or mis-incorporation of amino acids could have negative consequences for the cell, incompletely modified RNA that reaches the cytoplasm is degraded rather than used in translation.

Assembly and Disassembly: During its lifetime, a nucleus may be broken down, either in the process of cell division or as a consequence of apoptosis, a regulated form of cell death. During these events, the structural components of the nucleus the envelope and lamina can be systematically degraded. In most cells, the disassembly of the nuclear envelope marks the end of the prophase of mitosis. However, this disassembly of the nucleus is not a universal feature of mitosis and does not occur in all cells. Some unicellular eukaryotes *e.g.* yeasts undergo so-called closed mitosis, in which the nuclear envelope remains intact. In closed mitosis, the daughter chromosomes migrate to opposite poles of the nucleus, which then divides in two. The cells of higher eukaryotes, however, usually undergo open mitosis, which is characterized by breakdown of the nuclear envelope. The daughter chromosomes then migrate to opposite poles of the mitotic spindle and new nuclei reassemble around them.

At a certain point during the cell cycle in open mitosis, the cell divides to form two cells. In order for this process to be possible, each of the new daughter cells must have a full set of genes, a process requiring replication of the chromosomes as well as segregation of the separate sets. This occurs by the replicated chromosomes, the sister chromatids, attaching to microtubules, which in turn are attached to different centrosomes. The sister chromatids can then be pulled to separate locations in the cell. In many cells, the centrosome is located in the cytoplasm, outside the nucleus; the microtubules would be unable to attach to the chromatids in the presence of the nuclear envelope. Therefore the early stages in the cell cycle, beginning in prophase and until around prometaphase, the nuclear membrane is dismantled. Likewise, during the same period, the nuclear lamina is also disassembled, a process regulated by phosphorylation of the lamins by protein kinases such as the CDC_2 protein kinase. Towards the end of the cell cycle, the nuclear membrane is reformed and the nuclear lamina is reassembled by dephosphorylating the lamins around the same time. However, in dinoflagellates, the nuclear envelope remains intact, the centrosomes are located in the cytoplasm and the microtubules come in contact with chromosomes, whose centromeric regions are incorporated into the nuclear envelope the so called closed mitosis with extranuclear spindle. In many other protists *e.g.* ciliates, sporozoans and fungi, the centrosomes are intranuclear and their nuclear envelope also does not disassemle during cell division.

Apoptosis is a controlled process in which the cell's structural components are destroyed, resulting in death of the cell. Changes associated with apoptosis directly affect the nucleus and its contents in the condensation of chromatin and the disintegration of the nuclear envelope and lamina. The destruction of the lamin networks is controlled by specialized apoptotic proteases called caspases, which cleave the lamin proteins and thus, degrade the nucleus' structural integrity. Lamin cleavage is sometimes used as a laboratory indicator of caspase activity in assays for early apoptotic activity. Cells that express mutant caspase-resistant lamins are deficient in nuclear changes related to apoptosis, suggesting that lamins play a role in initiating the events that lead to apoptotic degradation of the nucleus. Inhibition of lamin assembly itself is an inducer of apoptosis. The nuclear envelope acts as a barrier that prevents both DNA and RNA viruses from entering the nucleus. Some viruses require access to proteins inside the nucleus in order to replicate and/or assemble. DNA viruses, such as herpesvirus replicate and assemble in the cell nucleus and exit by budding through the inner nuclear membrane. This process is accompanied by disassembly of the lamina on the nuclear face of the inner membrane.

Anucleated and Polynucleated Cells

Although most cells have a single nucleus, some eukaryotic cell types have no nucleus and others have many nuclei. This can be a normal process, as in the maturation of mammalian red blood cells or a result of faulty cell division. Anucleated cells contain no nucleus and are, therefore, incapable of dividing to produce daughter cells. The best-known anucleated cell is the mammalian red blood cell or erythrocyte, which also lacks other organelles such as mitochondria and serves primarily as a transport vessel to ferry oxygen from the lungs to the body's tissues. Erythrocytes mature through erythropoiesis in the bone marrow, where they lose their nuclei organelles and ribosomes. The nucleus is expelled during the process of differentiation from an erythroblast to a reticulocyte, which is the immediate precursor of the mature erythrocyte. The presence of mutagens may induce the release of some immature micronucleated erythrocytes into the bloodstream. Anucleated cells can also arise from flawed cell division in which one daughter lacks a nucleus and the other has two nuclei. Polynucleated cells contain multiple nuclei. Most Acantharean species of protozoa and some fungi in mycorrhizae have naturally polynucleated cells. Other examples include the intestinal parasites in the genus *Giardia*, which have two nuclei per cell. In humans, skeletal muscle cells, called myocytes, become polynucleated during development; the resulting arrangement of nuclei near the periphery of the cells allows maximal intracellular space for myofibrils. Multinucleated and Binucleated cells can also be abnormal in human; cells arising from the fusion of monocytes and macrophages, known as giant multinucleated cells, sometimes accompany inflammation and are also implicated in tumor formation.

Evolution of Nucleus

As the major defining characteristic of the eukaryotic cell, the nucleus' evolutionary origin has been the subject of much speculation. Four major theories have been proposed to explain the existence of the nucleus, although none have yet earned widespread support. The theory known as the syntrophic model proposes that a symbiotic relationship between the archaea and bacteria created the nucleus-containing eukaryotic cell. Organisms of the Archaea domain have no cell nucleus. It is hypothesized that the symbiosis originated when ancient archaea, similar to modern methanogenic archaea, invaded and lived within bacteria similar to modern myxobacteria, eventually forming the early nucleus. This theory is analogous to the accepted theory for the origin of eukaryotic mitochondria and chloroplasts, which are thought to have developed from a similar endosymbiotic relationship between proto-eukaryotes and aerobic bacteria. The archaeal origin of the nucleus is supported by observations that archaea and eukarya have similar genes for certain proteins, including histones. Observations that myxobacteria are motile, can form multicellular complexes and possess kinases and G proteins similar to eukarya, support a bacterial origin for the eukaryotic cell. A second model proposes that proto-eukaryotic cells evolved from bacteria without an endosymbiotic stage. This model is based on the existence of modern planctomycetes bacteria that possess a nuclear structure with primitive pores and other compartmentalized membrane structures. A similar proposal states that a eukaryote-like cell, the chronocyte, evolved first and phagocytosed archaea and bacteria to generate the nucleus and the eukaryotic cell. The most controversial model, known as viral eukaryogenesis, posits that the membrane-bound nucleus, along with other eukaryotic features originated from the infection of a prokaryote by a virus. The suggestion is based on similarities between eukaryotes and viruses such as linear DNA strands, mRNA capping and tight binding to proteins analogizing histones to viral envelopes. One version of the proposal suggests that the nucleus evolved in concert with phagocytosis to form an early cellular predator. Another variant proposes that eukaryotes originated from early archaea infected by poxviruses, on the basis of observed similarity between the DNA polymerases in modern poxviruses and eukaryotes. It has been suggested that the unresolved question of the evolution of sex could be related to the viral eukaryogenesis hypothesis. A very recent proposal suggests that traditional variants of the endosymbiont theory are insufficiently powerful to explain the origin of the eukaryotic nucleus. This model, termed the exomembrane hypothesis, suggests that the nucleus instead originated from a single ancestral cell that evolved a second exterior cell membrane; the interior membrane enclosing the original cell then became the nuclear membrane and evolved increasingly elaborate pore structures for passage of internally synthesized cellular components such as ribosomal subunits.

Cytoplasm

The cytoplasm was defined earlier as the material between the plasma membrane or cell membrane and the nuclear envelope. Fibrous proteins that occur in the cytoplasm, referred to as the cytoskeleton maintain the shape of the cell as well as anchoring organelles, moving the cell and controlling internal movement of structures. Microtubules function in cell division and serve as temporary scaffolding for other organelles. Actin filaments are thin threads that function in cell division and cell motility. Intermediate filaments are between the size of the microtubules and the actin filaments.

Vacuoles and Vesicles

Vacuoles are single membrane organelles that are essentially part of the outside that is located within the cell. The single membrane is known in plant cells as a tonoplast. Many organisms will use vacuoles as storage areas. Vesicles are much smaller than vacuoles and function in transporting materials both within and to the outside of the cell.

Ribosome

A ribosome is a component of cells that assembles the twenty specific amino acid molecules to form the particular protein molecule determined by the nucleotide sequence of an RNA molecule. One of the central tenets of biology, often referred to as

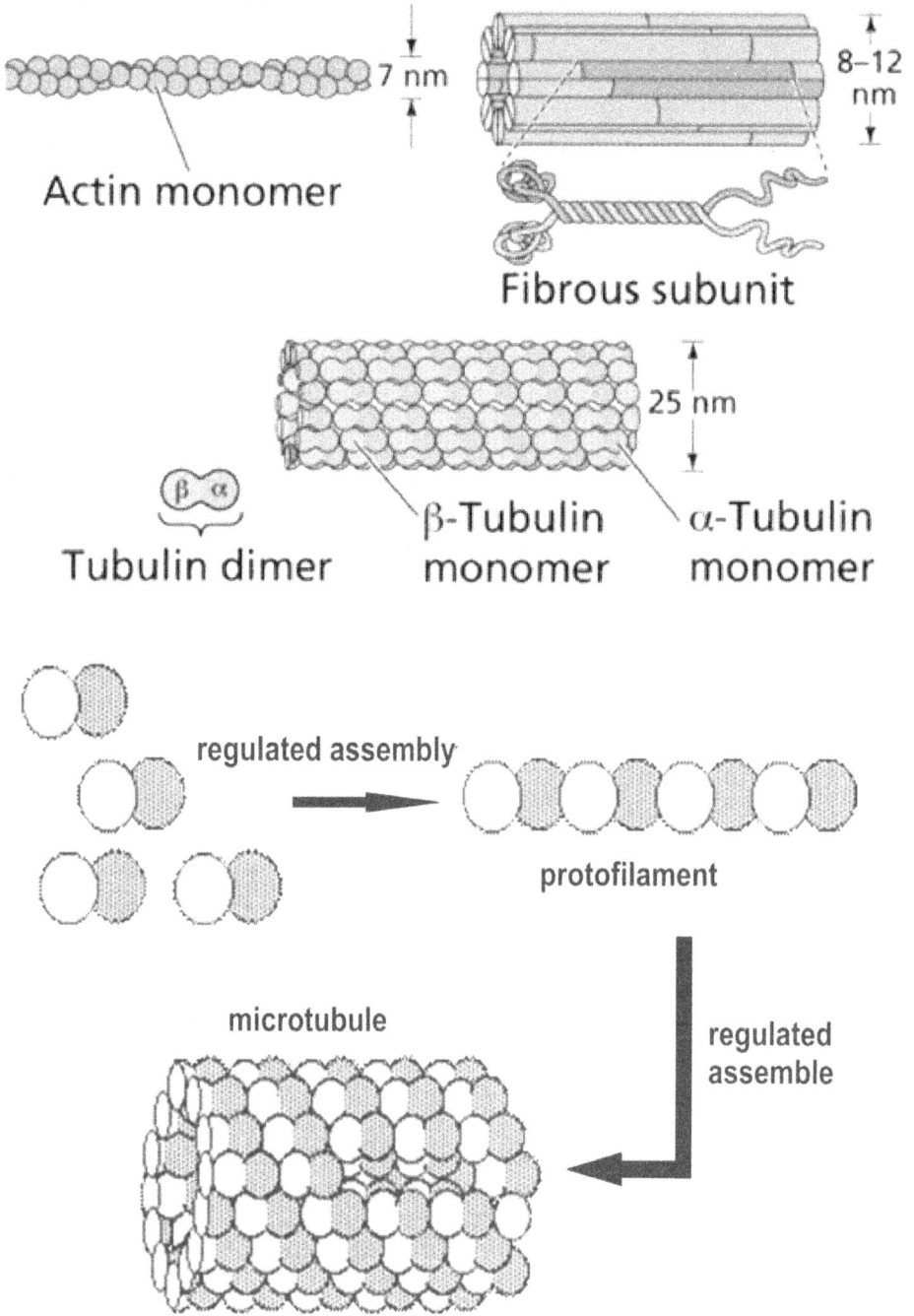

Actin monomer

7 nm

8–12 nm

Fibrous subunit

25 nm

Tubulin dimer

β-Tubulin monomer

α-Tubulin monomer

regulated assembly

protofilament

microtubule

regulated assemble

Figure 2.6: Microtubules

the central dogma of molecular biology, is that DNA is used to make RNA, which is used to make proteins. The DNA sequence in genes is copied into a messenger RNA (mRNA). Ribosomes then read the information in this mRNA and use it to create proteins. This process is known as translation; the ribosome translates the genetic information from the RNA into proteins. Ribosomes do this by binding to an mRNA and using it as a template for determining the correct sequence of amino acids in a particular protein. The amino acids are attached to transfer RNA (tRNA) molecules, which enter one part of the ribosome and bind to the messenger RNA sequence. The attached amino acids are then joined together by another part of the ribosome. The ribosome moves along the mRNA, reading its sequence and producing a corresponding chain of amino acids. Ribosomes are made from complexes of RNAs and proteins called ribonucleoproteins. Ribosomes are divided into two subunits. The smaller subunit binds to the mRNA, while the larger subunit binds to the tRNA and the amino acids. When a ribosome finishes reading an mRNA, these two subunits split apart. Ribosomes have been classified as ribozymes, because the ribosomal RNA seems to be most important for the peptidyl transferase activity that links amino acids together. Ribosomes from bacteria, archaea and eukaryotes have significantly different structures and RNA sequences. These differences in structure allow some antibiotics to kill bacteria by inhibiting their ribosomes, while leaving human ribosomes unaffected. The ribosomes in the mitochondria of eukaryotic cells functionally resemble in many features those in bacteria, reflecting the likely evolutionary origin of mitochondria. The word ribosome comes from ribonucleic acid and the Greek *soma* meaning body.

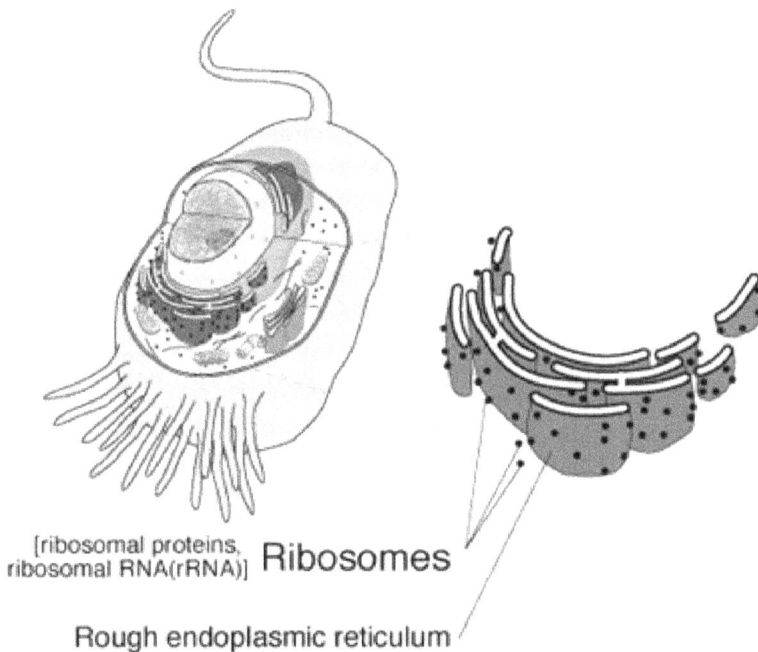

[ribosomal proteins, ribosomal RNA(rRNA)] Ribosomes

Rough endoplasmic reticulum

Figure 2.7: Endoplasmic Reticulum and Ribosomes

Archaeal, eubacterial and eukaryotic ribosomes differ in their size, composition and the ratio of protein to RNA. Because they are formed from two subunits of non-equal size, they are slightly longer in the axis than in diameter. Prokaryotic ribosomes are around 20 nm (200 ú) in diameter and are composed of 65% ribosomal RNA and 35% ribosomal proteins. Eukaryotic ribosomes are between 25 and 30 nm (250-300 angstroms) in diameter and the ratio of rRNA to protein is close to 1. Ribosomes translate messenger RNA (mRNA) and build polypeptide chains *e.g.* proteins using amino acids delivered by transfer RNA (tRNA). Their active sites are made of RNA, so ribosomes are now classified as ribozymes. Ribosomes build proteins from the genetic instructions held within messenger RNA. Free ribosomes are suspended in the cytosol; others are bound to the rough endoplasmic reticulum, giving it the appearance of roughness and thus its name or to the nuclear envelope. As ribozymes are partly constituted from RNA, it is thought that they might be remnants of the RNA world. Although catalysis of the peptide bond involves the C2 hydroxyl of RNA's P-site adenosine in a protein shuttle mechanism, other steps in protein synthesis such as translocation are caused by changes in protein conformations. Ribosomes are sometimes referred to as organelles, but the use of the term organelle is restricted to describing sub-cellular components that include a phospholipid membrane, which ribosomes do not. For this reason, ribosomes may sometimes be described as non-membranous organelles.

Ribosomes were first observed in the mid-1950s by Romanian cell biologist George Palade using an electron microscope as dense particles or granules for which he would win the Nobel Prize. The term ribosome was proposed by scientist Richard B. Roberts in 1958. During the course of the symposium a semantic difficulty became apparent. To some of the participants, microsomes mean the ribonucleoprotein particles of the microsome fraction contaminated by other protein and lipid material; to others, the microsomes consist of protein and lipid contaminated by particles. The phrase microsomal particles do not seem adequate and ribonucleoprotein particles of the microsome fraction are much too awkward. During the meeting, the word ribosome was suggested, which has a very satisfactory name and a pleasant sound. The present confusion would be eliminated if ribosome were adopted to designate ribonucleoprotein particles in sizes ranging from 35 to 100S.

Ribosomes consist of two subunits that fit together and work as one to translate the mRNA into a polypeptide chain during protein synthesis. Bacterial subunits consist of one or two and eukaryotic of one or three very large RNA molecules known as ribosomal RNA or rRNA and multiple smaller protein molecules. Crystallographic work has shown that there are no ribosomal proteins close to the reaction site for polypeptide synthesis. This suggests that the protein components of ribosomes act as a scaffold that may enhance the ability of rRNA to synthesize protein rather than directly participating in catalysis.

Biogenesis of Ribosomes

In bacterial cells, ribosomes are synthesized in the cytoplasm through the transcription of multiple ribosome gene operons. In eukaryotes, the process takes place both in the cell cytoplasm and in the nucleolus, which is a region within the cell

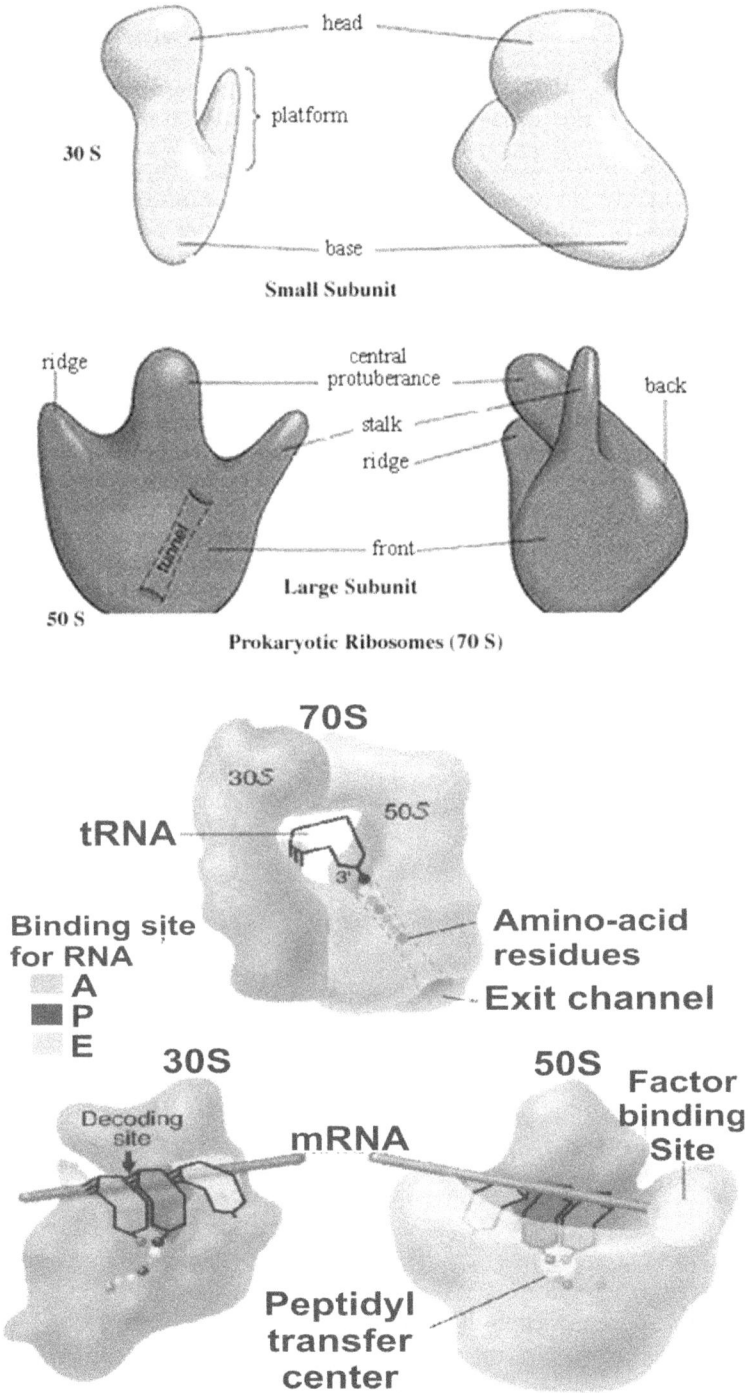

Figure 2.8: Structure of Ribosome subunits

nucleus. The assembly process involves the coordinated function of over 200 proteins in the synthesis and processing of the four rRNAs, as well as assembly of those rRNAs with the ribosomal proteins.

Distribution of Ribosomes

Ribosomes are found in almost all organisms except viruses. An *E.coli* cell may contain 15000 to 20000 ribosomes at any given time, but an active eukaryotic cell may have 10-20 times the number of prokaryotic cells. Oocytes of certain amphibians' posses' three million ribosomes per cell and the same is stored for the future use. While in prokaryotes, ribosomes are distributed through out the cell, eukaryotic cells contain different classes of ribosomes and they are located in different sites like cytoplasm, mitochondria and plastids. Cytoplasmic 80s ribosomes are either bound to endoplasmic membrane or freely.The majority of the so called free ribosomes are found located in the intersection of microtrabacular and actin filament network. On the contrary cellular organelles like chloroplast and mitochondria contain another class of ribosomes called *70s*, which are more or less similar to that of bacterial ribosomes. In the Oocytes of chicks and lizards, ribosomes are aggregated on membranes into crystalline structures. They remain inactive till they are required at some stage of development.

Ribosome Locations

Ribosomes are classified as being either free or membrane-bound. Free and membrane-bound ribosomes differ only in their spatial distribution; they are identical in structure. Whether the ribosome exists in a free or membrane-bound state depends on the presence of an ER-targeting signal sequence on the protein being synthesized, so an individual ribosome might be membrane-bound when it is making one protein, but free in the cytosol when it makes another protein.

Free Ribosomes

Free ribosomes can move about anywhere in the cytosol, but are excluded from the cell nucleus and other organelles. Proteins that are formed from free ribosomes are released into the cytosol and used within the cell. Since the cytosol contains high concentrations of glutathione and is a reducing environment. Proteins containing disulfide bonds cannot be produced in this compartment. They formed from oxidized cysteine residues.

Membrane bound Ribosomes

When a ribosome begins to synthesize proteins that are needed in some organelles, the ribosome making this protein can become membrane-bound. In eukaryotic cells this happens in a region of the endoplasmic reticulum (ER) called the rough ER. The newly produced polypeptide chains are inserted directly into the ER by the ribosome and are then transported to their destinations, through the secretory pathway. Bound ribosomes usually produce proteins that are used within the plasma membrane or are expelled from the cell via exocytosis.

Structure of Ribosome

The ribosomal subunits of prokaryotes and eukaryotes are quite similar. The unit of measurement is the Svedberg unit, a measure of the rate of sedimentation in centrifugation rather than size and accounts for why fragment names do not add up (70S is made of 50S and 30S). Prokaryotes have 70S ribosomes each consisting of a small (30S) and a large (50S) subunit. Their large subunit is composed of a 5S RNA subunit consisting of 120 nucleotides, a 23S RNA subunit (2900 nucleotides) and 34 proteins. The 30S subunit has a 1540 nucleotide RNA subunit (16S) bound to 21 proteins. Proteins involved in the initiation of translation, S1 and S21 are associated with the 3'-end of 16S ribosomal RNA. Eukaryotes have 80S ribosomes, each consisting of a small (40S) and large (60S) subunit. Their large subunit is composed of a 5S RNA (120 nucleotides), a 28S RNA (4700 nucleotides), a 5.8S subunit (160 nucleotides) and ~49 proteins. The 40S subunit has a 1900 nucleotide (18S) RNA and approximately 33 proteins. The ribosomes found in chloroplasts and mitochondria of eukaryotes also consist of large and small subunits bound together with proteins into one 70S particle. These organelles are believed to be descendants of bacteria and as such their ribosomes are similar to those of bacteria.

The various ribosomes share a core structure, which is quite similar despite the large differences in size. Much of the RNA is highly organized into various tertiary structural motifs, pseudoknots that exhibit coaxial stacking. The extra RNA in the larger ribosomes is in several long continuous insertions, such that they form loops out of the core structure without disrupting or changing it. All of the catalytic activity of the ribosome is carried out by the RNA; the proteins reside on the surface and seem to stabilize the structure. The differences between the bacterial and eukaryotic ribosomes are exploited by pharmaceutical chemists to create antibiotics that can destroy a bacterial infection without harming the cells of the infected person. Due to the differences in their structures, the bacterial 70S ribosomes are vulnerable to these antibiotics while the eukaryotic 80S ribosomes are not. Even though mitochondria possess ribosomes similar to the bacterial ones, mitochondria are not affected by these antibiotics because they are surrounded by a double membrane that does not easily admit these antibiotics into the organelle.

Class of Ribosomes

Ribosomes can be isolated by magnesium precipitation. If some ribosomes, obtained from a eukaryotic organism, are subjected to density gradient ultracentrifugation, ribosomes settle into two distinct bands. Based on the sedimentation values, determined by Svedberg, they can be distinguished into 70s and 80s ribosomes. The 80s ribosomes are found in cytoplasm, whereas 70s types are found in mitochondria and chloroplasts. The *70s* type are smaller and 80s are little larger. However, prokaryotes contain only one kind of ribosomes *i.e.* 70 type. The 80s and 70s ribosomes can be further distinguished by their sensitivity to chloramphenicol (CAP) and cycloheximide (CHI). The 70s ribosomal mediated protein synthesis is inhibited by chloramphenicol, while 80s ribosomal protein synthesis is inhibited by CHI.

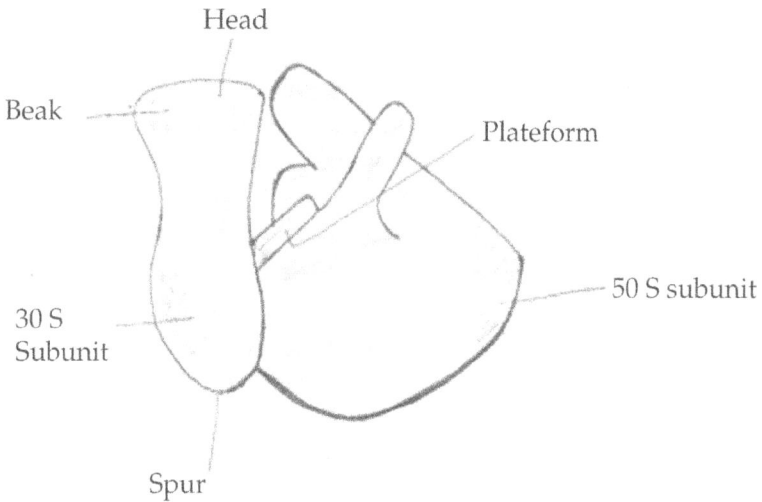

Figure 2.9: 70S Ribosomal subunits

The general molecular structure of the ribosome has been known since the early 1970s. In the early 2000s the structure has been achieved at high resolutions, on the order of a few Å. The first papers giving the structure of the ribosome at atomic resolution were published in rapid succession in late 2000. First, the 50S (large prokaryotic) subunit from the archaeon *Haloarcula marismortui* was published. Soon after, the structure of the 30S subunit from Thermus thermophilus was published. Shortly thereafter, a more detailed structure was published. These structural studies were awarded the Nobel Prize in Chemistry in 2009. Together with Albert Claude and Christian de Duve, George Emil Palade was awarded the Nobel Prize in Physiology or Medicine in 1974 for the discovery of the ribosomes. The Nobel Prize in Chemistry 2009 was awarded to Venkatraman Ramakrishnan, Thomas A. Steitz and Ada E. Yonath for studies of the structure and function of the ribosome.

Functions of Ribosomes

Ribosomes are the workhorses of protein biosynthesis. Protein biosynthesis is the process of translating mRNA into protein. The mRNA comprises a series of codons that dictate to the ribosome the sequence of the amino acids needed to make the protein. Using the mRNA as a template, the ribosome traverses each codon (3 nucleotides) of the mRNA, pairing it with the appropriate amino acid provided by a tRNA. Molecules of transfer RNA (tRNA) contain a complementary anticodon on one end and the appropriate amino acid on the other. The small ribosomal subunit, typically bound to a tRNA containing the amino acid methionine, binds to an AUG codon on the mRNA and recruits the large ribosomal subunit. The ribosome then contains three RNA binding sites, designated A, P and E. The A site binds an aminoacyl-tRNA and tRNA bound to an amino acid. The P site binds a peptidyl-

Table 2.2: Components of Ribosomes

S. No	Ribosome Types	RNA size	No. of proteins	Methylations	Functions
1	70 S			Coded by seven genes		
	30s subunits	16s RNA, 1540-1542 ntds	21 (s1 to s21)	10 at 2'OH, 2, methyl adenines, 2, dimethyl guanines	30 or more methylations
	50S subunits	23s RNA, 2900 ntds; 5s RNA, 120 ntds	31, L1 to L31	20 at 2'OH of sugars	Help in processing and folding
2	80S			Coded by hundreds of genes located on chromosomes 12, 13, 14, 21 and 22		>100 sites for methylations and 100 sites for pseudouridenylations
	40S subunits	18s RNA; (1843 or 1900 ntds)	33; S1 to s34	43 to 44 methylations at 2'OH	Yeast has 43 pseudo uridines
	60s subunits	28sRNA- (4718-4800 ntds)	49; L1 to L45-50	74 methylations at 2'OH of sugars,	
		5.8s RNA- (160 ntds)		Methylation at adenine,	
		5sRNA-(120 ntds)		Methylation at guanine, plus conversion of Uridine into pseudo-uridines	
3	mRibosome	Like 70s (general)	28s	-1560 ntds, 48 proteins	--	--
		Fungus-73s		-29 proteins		
		Maize-78s	12s			
4	cRibosome	70s	16s RNA	23sRNA, 5s RNA, 4.5s RNA	--	--

tRNA and tRNA bound to the peptide being synthesized. The E site binds a free tRNA before it exits the ribosome. Protein synthesis begins at a start codon AUG near the 5' end of the mRNA. The mRNA binds to the P site of the ribosome first. The ribosome is able to identify the start codon by use of the Shine Dalgarno sequence of the mRNA in prokaryotes and Kozak box in eukaryotes.

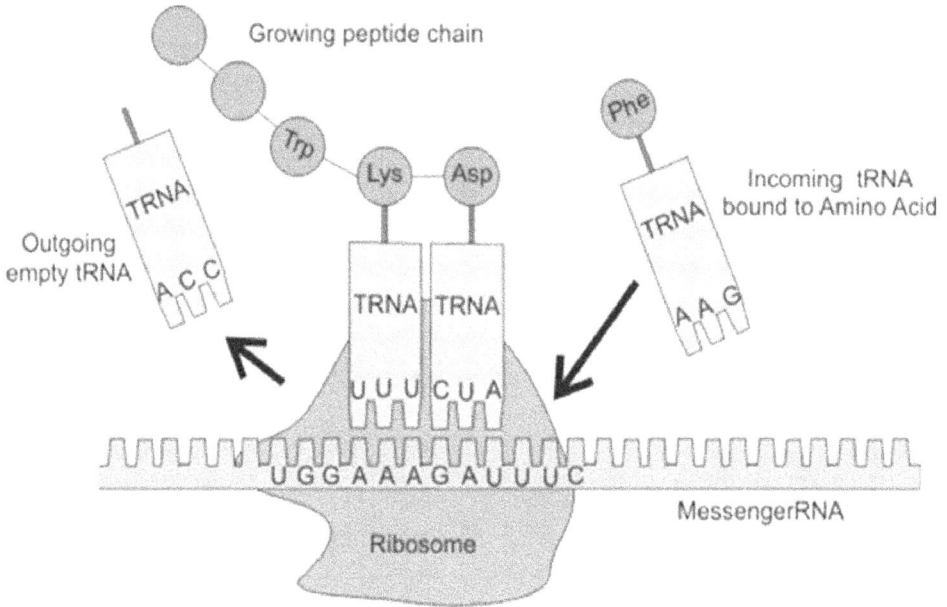

Figure 2.10: Translation of mRNA

In Figure 14, both ribosomal subunits (small and large) assemble at the start codon towards the 5' end of the mRNA. The ribosome uses tRNA that matches the current codon (triplet) on the mRNA to append an amino acid to the polypeptide chain. This is done for each triplet on the mRNA, while the ribosome moves towards the 3' end of the mRNA. Usually in bacterial cells, several ribosomes are working parallel on a single mRNA, forming what is called a polyribosome or polysome.

Endoplasmic Reticulum

Endoplasmic reticulum is a mesh of interconnected membranes that serve a function involving protein synthesis and transport. The endoplasmic reticulum (ER) is a eukaryotic organelle that forms an interconnected network of tubules, vesicles and cisternae within cells. Rough endoplasmic reticula synthesize proteins, while smooth endoplasmic reticula synthesize lipids and steroids, metabolize carbohydrates and steroids and regulate calcium concentration, drug metabolism and attachment of receptors on cell membrane proteins. Sarcoplasmic reticula solely regulate calcium levels. The lacey membranes of the endoplasmic reticulum were first seen by Keith R. Porter, Albert Claude and Ernest F. Fullam in 1945.

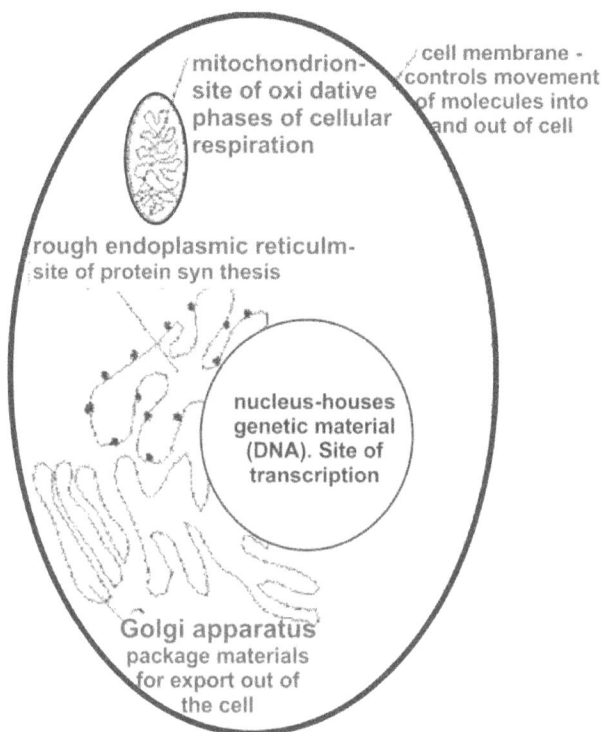

Figure 2.11: Position of ER in Cell

The endoplasmic reticulum (ER) is responsible for the production of the protein and lipid components of most of the cell's organelles. The ER contains a great amount of folds but the membrane forms a single sheet enclosing a single closed sac. This internal space is called the ER lumen. The ER is additionally responsible for moving proteins and other carbohydrates to the Golgi apparatus, to the plasma membrane, to the lysosomes or wherever else needed.

Structure of ER

The general structure of the endoplasmic reticulum is an extensive membrane network of cisternae (sac like structure) held together by the cytoskeleton. The phospholipid membrane encloses a space, the cisternal space or lumen, which is continuous with the perinuclear space but separate from the cytosol. The functions of the endoplasmic reticulum vary greatly depending on the exact type of endoplasmic reticulum and the type of cell in which it resides. The three varieties are called rough endoplasmic reticulum, smooth endoplasmic reticulum and sarcoplasmic reticulum. The quantity of RER and SER in a cell can quickly interchange from one type to the other, depending on changing metabolic needs. One type will undergo numerous changes including new proteins embedded in the membranes in order to transform.

Also, massive changes in the protein content can occur without any noticeable structural changes, depending on the enzymatic needs of the cell.

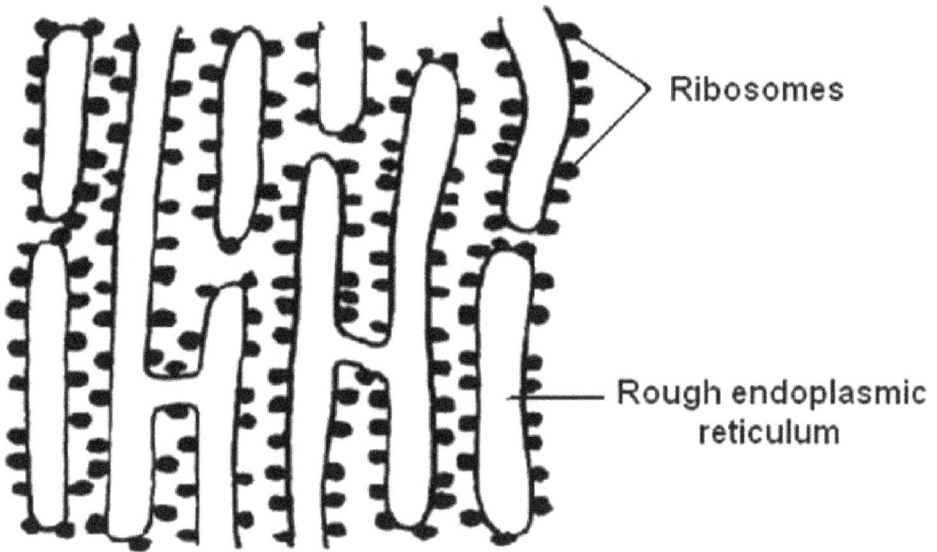

Figure 2.12: Endoplasmic Reticulum

Rough Endoplasmic Reticulum

The surface of the rough endoplasmic reticulum (RER) is studded with protein-manufacturing ribosomes giving it a rough appearance. However, the ribosomes bound to the RER at any one time are not a stable part of this organelle's structure as ribosomes are constantly being bound and released from the membrane. A ribosome binds to the ER only when it begins to synthesize a protein destined for the secretory pathway. Here, a ribosome in the cytosol begins synthesizing a protein until a signal recognition particle recognizes the pre-piece of 5-15 hydrophobic amino acids preceded by a positively charged amino acid. This signal sequence allows the recognition particle to bind to the ribosome, causing the ribosome to bind to the RER and pass the new protein through the ER membrane. The pre-piece is then cleaved off within the lumen of the ER and the ribosome released back into the cytosol. The membrane of the RER is continuous with the outer layer of the nuclear envelope. Although there is no continuous membrane between the RER and the Golgi apparatus, membrane-bound vesicles shuttle proteins between these two compartments. Vesicles are surrounded by coating proteins called COPI and COPII. COPII targets vesicles to the Golgi and COPI marks them to be brought back to the RER. The RER works in concert with the Golgi complex to target new proteins to their proper destinations. A second method of transport out of the ER is areas called membrane contact sites, where the membranes of the ER and other organelles are held closely together, allowing the transfer of lipids and other small molecules. The RER is key in multiple functions:

- Lysosomal enzymes with a mannose-6-phosphate marker added in the cis-Golgi network.

- Secreted proteins, either secreted constitutively with no tag or secreted in a regulatory manner involving clathrin and paired basic amino acids in the signal peptide.

- Integral membrane proteins that stay imbedded in the membrane as vesicles exit and bind to new membranes. Rab proteins are complementory in targeting the membrane while SNAP and SNARE proteins are used as key in the fusion event.

- Initial glycosylation as assembly continues. This is N-linked (O-linking occurs in the Golgi). If the protein is properly folded, glycosyltransferase recognizes the AA sequence NXS or NXT (with S/T residue phosphorylated) and adds a 14-sugar backbone (2-N-acetylglucosamine, 9-branching mannose and 3-glucose at the end) to the side-chain nitrogen of Asn is called N-linked glycosylation.

Endoplasmic Reticulum Stress: Disturbances in redox regulation, calcium regulation, glucose deprivation and viral infection can lead to ER stress. It is a state in which the folding of proteins slows leading to an increase in unfolded proteins. This ER stress is emerging as a potential cause of damage in hypoxia/ischemia, insulin resistance and other disorders.

Smooth Endoplasmic Reticulum

The smooth endoplasmic reticulum (SER) has functions in several metabolic processes, including synthesis of lipids and steroids, metabolism of carbohydrates, regulation of calcium concentration, drug detoxification, attachment of receptors on cell membrane proteins and steroid metabolism. It is connected to the nuclear envelope. Smooth endoplasmic reticulum is found in a variety of cell types both animal and plant and it serves different functions in each. The Smooth ER also contains the enzyme glucose-6-phosphatase, which converts glucose-6-phosphate to glucose, a step in gluconeogenesis. The SER consists of tubules and vesicles that branch forming a network. In some cells, there are dilated areas like the sacs of RER. The network of SER allows increased surface area for the action or storage of key enzymes and the products of these enzymes.

Sarcoplasmic Reticulum

The sarcoplasmic reticulum (SR) from the Greek sarx (flesh) is a special type of smooth ER found in smooth and striated muscle. The only structural difference between this organelle and the SER is the medley of proteins they have, both bound to their membranes and drifting within the confines of their lumens. This fundamental difference is indicative of their functions: The SER synthesizes molecules, while the SR stores and pumps calcium ions. The SR contains large stores of calcium, which it sequesters and then releases when the muscle cell is stimulated. The SR's release of calcium upon electrical stimulation of the cell plays a major role in excitation-contraction coupling.

Functions of ER

The endoplasmic reticulum serves many general functions, including the facilitation of protein folding and the transport of synthesized proteins in sacs called cisternae. Correct folding of newly-made proteins is made possible by several endoplasmic reticulum chaperone proteins, including protein disulfide isomerase (PDI), ERp29, the Hsp70 family member Grp78, calnexin, calreticulin and the peptidylpropyl isomerase family. Only properly-folded proteins are transported from the rough ER to the Golgi complex.

Transport of Proteins: Secretary proteins are moved across the endoplasmic reticulum membrane. Proteins that are transported by the endoplasmic reticulum and from there throughout the cell are marked with an address tag called a signal sequence. The N-terminus of a polypeptide chain *i.e.* a protein contains a few amino acids that work as an address tag, which are removed when the polypeptide reaches its destination. Proteins that are destined for places outside the endoplasmic reticulum are packed into transport vesicles and moved along the cytoskeleton toward their destination. The endoplasmic reticulum is also part of a protein sorting pathway. It is, in essence, the transportation system of the eukaryotic cell. The majority of endoplasmic reticulum resident proteins are retained in the endoplasmic reticulum through a retention motif. This motif is composed of four amino acids at the end of the protein sequence. The most common retention sequence is KDEL (lys-asp-glu-leu). However, variation on KDEL does occur and other sequences can also give rise to endoplasmic reticulum retention. It is not known whether such variation can lead to sub-endoplasmic reticulum localizations. There are three KDEL receptors in mammalian cells and they have a very high degree of sequence identity. The functional differences between these receptors remain to be established.

Other Functions

- **Insertion of proteins into the endoplasmic reticulum membrane:** Integral membrane proteins are inserted into the endoplasmic reticulum membrane as they are being synthesized (co-translational translocation). Insertion into the endoplasmic reticulum membrane requires the correct topogenic signal sequences in the protein.

- **Glycosylation**: Glycosylation involves the attachment of oligosaccharides.

- **Disulfide bond formation and rearrangement**: Disulfide bonds stabilize the tertiary and quaternary structure of many proteins.

- **Drug metabolism**: The smooth ER is the site at which some drugs are modified by microsomal enzymes, which include the cytochrome P450 enzymes.

Golgi apparatus

The Golgi apparatus also Golgi body or the Golgi complex is an organelle found in most eukaryotic cells. It was identified in 1897 by the Italian physician Camillo Golgi (Nobel Prize, 1906) after whom the Golgi apparatus is named. It processes and packages proteins after their synthesis and before they make their way to their destination; it is particularly important in the processing of proteins for secretion.

The Golgi apparatus forms a part of the cellular endomembrane system. Due to its fairly large size, the Golgi apparatus was one of the first organelles to be discovered and observed in detail. The apparatus was discovered in 1897 by Italian physician Camillo Golgi during an investigation of the nervous system. After first observing it under his microscope, he termed the structure the internal reticular apparatus. The structure was then renamed after Golgi not long after the announcement of his discovery in 1898. However, some doubted the discovery at first, arguing that the appearance of the structure was merely an optical illusion created by the observation technique used by Golgi. With the development of modern microscopes in the 20th century, the discovery was confirmed.

Structure of Golgi apparatus

The Golgi is composed of stacks of membrane-bound structures known as cisternae found within the cytoplasm of both plant and animal cells. An individual stack is sometimes called a dictyosome (diction means net and soma means body), especially in plant cells. A mammalian cell typically contains 40 to 100 stacks. Between four and eight cisternae are usually present in a stack in some protists as many as sixty have been observed. Each cisterna comprises a flat, membrane enclosed disc that includes special Golgi enzymes which modify or help to modify cargo proteins that travel through it. The cisternae stack has four functional regions; cis-Golgi network, medial-Golgi, endo-Golgi and trans-Golgi network. Vesicles from the endoplasmic reticulum via the vesicular tubular clusters fuse with the network and subsequently progress through the stack to the trans Golgi network, where they are packaged and sent to the required destination. Each region contains different enzymes which selectively modify the contents depending on where they reside. The cisternae carry structural proteins important for their maintenance as flattened membranes which stack upon each other.

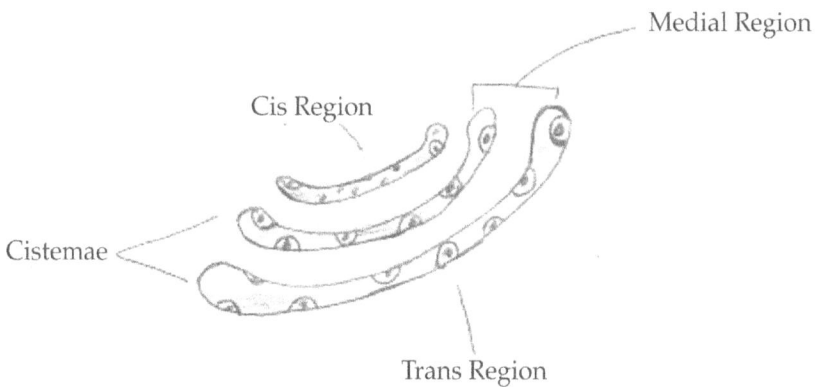

Figure 2.13: Golgi apparatus

Function of Golgi apparatus : Cells synthesise a large number of different macromolecules. The Golgi apparatus is integral in modifying, sorting and packaging these macromolecules for cell secretion (exocytosis) or use within the cell. It primarily modifies proteins delivered from the rough endoplasmic reticulum but is also involved in the transport of lipids around the cell and the creation of lysosomes. In this respect it can be thought of as similar to a post office; it packages and labels items which it then sends to different parts of the cell. Enzymes within the cisternae are able to modify the proteins by addition of carbohydrates (glycosylation) and phosphates (phosphorylation). In order to do so, the Golgi imports substances such as nucleotide sugars from the cytosol. These modifications may also form a signal sequence which determines the final destination of the protein *e.g.* Golgi apparatus adds a mannose-6-phosphate label to proteins destined for lysosomes. The Golgi plays an important role in the synthesis of proteoglycans, which are molecules present in the extracellular matrix of animals. It is also a major site of carbohydrate synthesis. This includes the production of glycosaminoglycans (GAGs), long unbranched polysaccharides which the Golgi then attaches to a protein synthesised in the endoplasmic reticulum to form proteoglycans. Enzymes in the Golgi polymerize several of these GAGs via a xylose link onto the core protein. Another task of the Golgi involves the sulfation of certain molecules passing through its lumen via sulphotranferases that gain their sulphur molecule from a donor called PAPs. This process occurs on the GAGs of proteoglycans as well as on the core protein. The level of sulfation is very important to the proteoglycans' signalling abilities as well as giving the proteoglycan its overall negative charge.

The phosphorylation of molecules requires that ATP is imported into the lumen of the Golgi and then utilised by resident kinases such as casein kinase 1 and casein kinase 2. One molecule that is phosphorylated in the Golgi is Apolipoprotein, which forms a molecule known as VLDL that is a constituent of blood serum. It is thought that the phosphorylation of these molecules is important to help aid in their sorting for secretion into the blood serum. The Golgi has a putative role in apoptosis, with several Bcl-2 family members localised there, as well as to the mitochondria.

Vesicular Transport

The vesicles that leave the rough endoplasmic reticulum are transported to the *cis* face of the Golgi apparatus, where they fuse with the Golgi membrane and empty their contents into the lumen. Once inside the lumen, the molecules are modified, sorted and shipped towards their final destination. The Golgi apparatus tends to be larger and more numerous in cells that synthesise and secrete large amounts of substances *e.g.* plasma B cells and the antibody-secreting cells of the immune system have prominent Golgi complexes. Those proteins destined for areas of the cell other than either the endoplasmic reticulum or Golgi apparatus are moved towards the trans face, to a complex network of membranes and associated vesicles known as the trans-Golgi network (TGN). This area of the Golgi is the point at which proteins are sorted and shipped to their intended destinations by their placement into one of at least three different types of vesicles, depending upon the molecular marker they carry.

Table 2.3: Funtion of Golgi body

Type	Description	Example
Exocytotic vesicles (continuous)	Vesicle contains proteins destined for extracellular release. After packaging the vesicles bud off and immediately move towards the plasma membrane, where they fuse and release the contents into the extracellular space in a process known as constitutive secretion.	Antibody release by activated plasma B cells
Secretory vesicles (regulated)	Vesicle contains proteins destined for extracellular release. After packaging, the vesicles bud off and are stored in the cell until a signal is given for their release. When the appropriate signal is received they move towards the This process membrane and fuse to release their contents. is known as regulated secretion.	Neurotransmitter release from neurons
Lysosomal vesicles	Vesicle contains proteins destined for the lysosome, an organelle of degradation containing many acid hydrolases or to lysosome-like storage organelles. These proteins include both digestive enzymes and membrane proteins. The vesicle first fuses with the late endosome and the contents are then transferred to the lysosome via unknown mechanisms.	Digestive proteases destined for the lysosome

Transport Mechanism

The transport mechanism which proteins use to progress through the Golgi apparatus is not yet clear; however a number of hypotheses currently exist. Until recently, the vesicular transport mechanism was favoured but now more evidence is coming to light to support cisternal maturation. The two proposed models may actually work in conjunction with each other, rather than being mutually exclusive. This is sometimes referred to as the combined model.

- **Cisternal maturation model**: The cisternae of the Golgi apparatus move by being built at the *cis* face and destroyed at the trans face. Vesicles from the endoplasmic reticulum fuse with each other to form a cisterna at the cis face, consequently this cisterna would appear to move through the Golgi stack when a new cisterna is formed at the *cis* face. This model is supported by the fact that structures larger than the transport vesicles, such as collagen rods, were observed microscopically to progress through the Golgi apparatus. This was initially a popular hypothesis, but lost favour in the 1980s. Recently it has made a comeback, as laboratories at the University of Chicago and the University of Tokyo have been able to use new technology to directly observe Golgi compartments maturing. Additional evidence comes from the fact that COPI vesicles move in the retrograde direction, transporting endoplasmic reticulum proteins back to where they belong by recognizing a signal peptide.

- **Vesicular transport model**: Vesicular transport views the Golgi as a very stable organelle, divided into compartments in the cis to trans direction.

Membrane bound carriers transport material between the endoplasmic reticulum and the different compartments of the Golgi. Experimental evidence includes the abundance of small vesicles known technically as shuttle vesicles in proximity to the Golgi apparatus. To direct the vesicles, actin filaments connect packaging proteins to the membrane to ensure that they fuse with the correct compartment.

Role of Golgi apparatus in Mitosis

In animal cells, the Golgi apparatus break up and disappear following the onset of mitosis or cellular division. During the telophase of mitosis, the Golgi apparatus reappears; however, it is still uncertain how this occurs. Intriguingly, the same is not true of plant or yeast Golgi stacks, which has been observed to remain intact throughout the cell cycle. The reason for this difference is not yet known, but it may, in part, be a consequence of golgin proteins.

Lysosome

Lysosomes are relatively large vesicles formed by the Golgi. Lysosomes are sometimes called cell stomachs because they contain enzymes that digest cellular components. Lysosomes are cellular organelles that contain acid hydrolase enzymes to break down waste materials and cellular debris. They are found in animal cells, while in yeast and plants the same roles are performed by lytic vacuoles. Lysosomes digest excess or worn-out organelles, food particles and engulf viruses or bacteria. The membrane around a lysosome allows the digestive enzymes to work at the 4.5 pH they require. Lysosomes fuse with vacuoles and dispense their enzymes into the vacuoles, digesting their contents. They are created by the addition of hydrolytic enzymes to early endosomes from the Golgi apparatus. The name *lysosome* derives from the Greek words lysis, to separate and soma, body. They are frequently nicknamed suicide-bags or suicide-sacs by cell biologists due to their role in autolysis. Lysosomes were discovered by the Belgian cytologist Christian de Duve in the 1960s. The size of lysosomes varies from 0.1–1.2 ìm. At pH 4.8, the interior of the lysosomes is acidic compared to the slightly alkaline cytosol (pH 7.2). The lysosome maintains this pH differential by pumping protons (H^+ ions) from the cytosol across the membrane via proton pumps and chloride ion channels. The lysosomal membrane protects the cytosol and therefore the rest of the cell, from the degradative enzymes within the lysosome. The cell is additionally protected from any lysosomal acid hydrolases that drain into the cytosol, as these enzymes are not pH sensitive and function as well in alkaline environment of the cytosol.

Lysosomal Enzymes

Lysosomal enzymes are synthesized in the cytoplasm and the endoplasmic reticulum, where they receive a mannose-6-phosphate tag that targets them for the lysosome. Aberrant lysosomal targeting causes inclusion cell disease, whereby enzymes do not properly reach the lysosome, resulting in accumulation of waste within these organelles. Some important enzymes found within lysosomes include:

- Lipase, which digests lipids

- Amylase, which digests amylose, starch and maltodextrins

- Proteases, which digest proteins

- Nucleases, which digest nucleic acids

- Phosphoric acid monoesters.

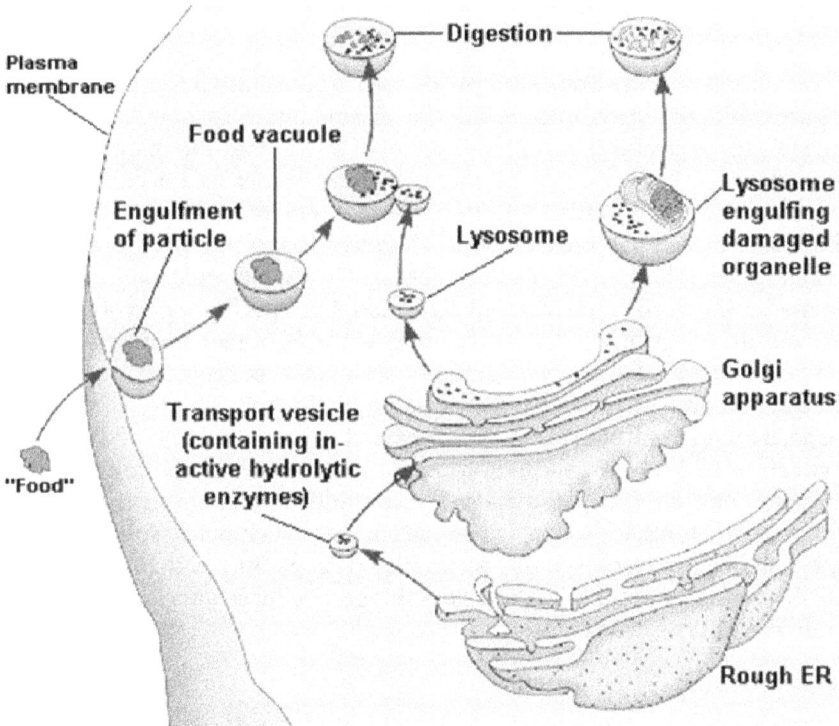

Figure 2.14: Function of bysomes

Functions of Lysosomes

Lysosomes are the cell's waste disposal system and can digest some compounds. They are used for the digestion of macromolecules from phagocytosis, ingestion of other dying cells or larger extracellular material, like foreign invading microbes, endocytosis where receptor proteins are recycled from the cell surface and autophagy where in old or unneeded organelles or proteins or microbes that have invaded the cytoplasm are delivered to the lysosome. Autophagy may also lead to autophagic cell death, a form of programmed self destruction or autolysis, of the cell, which means that the cell is digesting itself. Other functions include digesting foreign bacteria or other forms of waste that invade a cell and helping repair damage to the plasma membrane by serving as a membrane patch, sealing the wound. In the past, lysosomes were thought to kill cells that are no longer wanted, such as those in the tails of tadpoles or in the web from the fingers of a 3- to 6-month-old feotus. There are a number of lysosomal storage diseases that are caused by the malfunction of the lysosomes or one of their digestive proteins; examples include Niemann Pick Type C, Tay-Sachs disease and Pompe's disease. These diseases are caused by a defective or missing digestive protein, which leads to the accumulation of substrates within the cell, impairing metabolism. In the broad sense, these can be classified as mucopolysaccharidoses, GM_2 gangliosidoses, lipid storage disorders, glycoproteinoses, mucolipidoses or leukodystrophies.

Lysosomotropism

Weak bases with lipophilic properties accumulate in acidic intracellular compartments like lysosomes. While the plasma and lysosomal membranes are permeable for neutral and uncharged species of weak bases, the charged protonated species of weak bases do not permeate biomembranes and accumulate within lysosomes. The concentration within lysosomes may reach levels 100 to 1000 fold higher than extracellular concentrations. This phenomenon is called lysosomotropism or acid trapping. The amount of accumulation of lysosomotropic compounds may be estimated using a cell based mathematical model. A significant part of the clinically approved drugs are lipophilic weak bases with lysosomotropic properties. This explaines a number of pharmacological properties of these drugs, such as high tissue-to-blood concentration gradients or long tissue elimination half-lifes; these properties have been found for drugs such as haloperidol, levomepromazine and amantadine. However, in addition to lysosomotropism, high tissue concentrations and long elimination half-life is explained also by lipophilicity and absorption of drugs to fatty tissue structures. Important lysosomal enzymes, such as acid sphingomyelinase, may be inhibited by lysososomally accumulated drugs. Such compounds are termed FIASMAs, functional inhibitor of acid sphingomyelinase and include fluoxetine, sertraline or amitriptyline.

Peroxisomes

Mitochondria and chloroplasts are frequently found close to another membrane-bound organelle, the peroxisome. In human cells peroxisomes have a diameter of about 500 nm and their dense matrix contains a heterogeneous collection of proteins concerned with a variety of metabolic functions, some of which are only now beginning to be understood. Peroxisomes are so named because they are frequently responsible for the conversion of the highly reactive molecule hydrogen peroxide (H_2O_2), which is formed as a by-product of the reactions in the mitochondrion, into water:

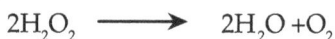

$$2H_2O_2 \longrightarrow 2H_2O + O_2$$

This reaction is carried out by a protein called catalase, which sometimes forms an obvious crystal within the peroxisome. Catalase is an enzyme a protein catalyst that increases the rate of a chemical reaction. In fact, it was one of the first enzymes to be discovered. In humans, peroxisomes are primarily associated with lipid metabolism. Understanding peroxisome function is important for a number of inherited human diseases such as X-linked adrenoleukodystrophy where peroxisome malfunction and the consequent inability to metabolise lipid properly typically leads to death in childhood or early adulthood unless dietary lipid is extremely restricted.

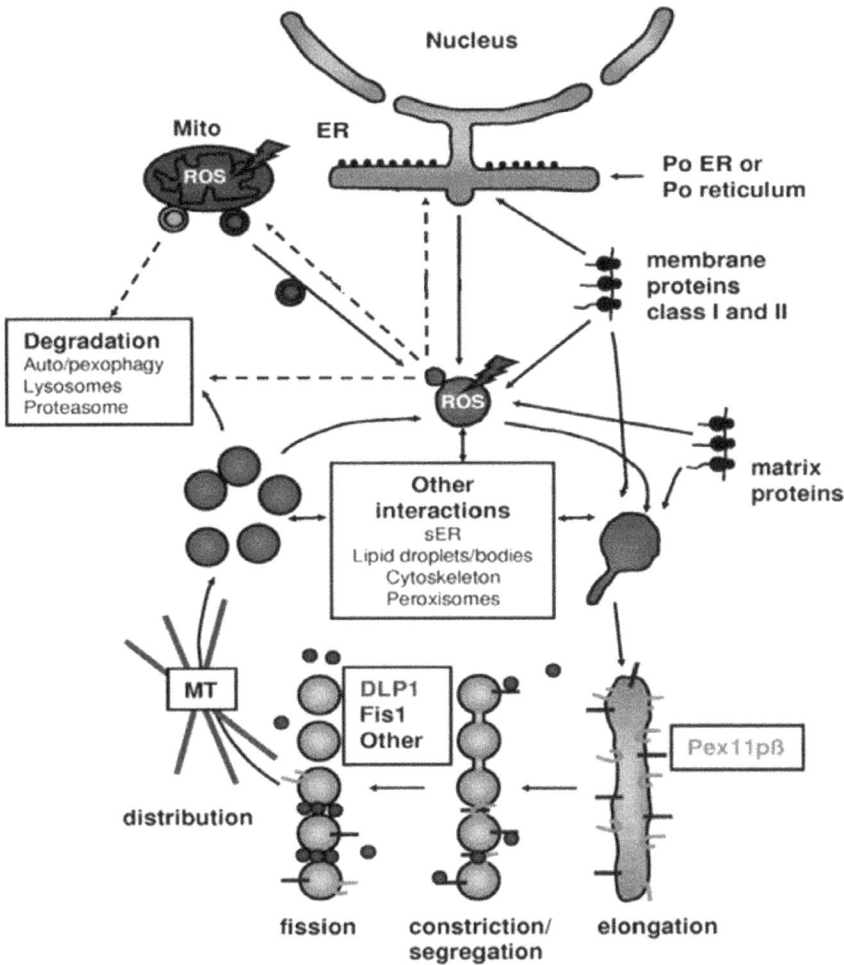

Figure 2.15: Molecular Mechanism of Peroxisom division

Mitochondria

The word mitochondrion comes from Greek word mitos meaning thread and chondrion meaning granule. Mitochondria are among the most easily recognizable organelles due to the extensive folding of their inner membrane to form shelf like projections named cristae. Mitochondria contain their own DNA termed mDNA and are thought to represent bacteria like organisms incorporated into eukaryotic cells over 700 million years ago. The mitochondrion (plural mitochondria) is a membrane enclosed organelle found in most eukaryotic cells. These organelles range from 0.5 to

10 micrometers (ìm) in diameter. Mitochondria are sometimes described as cellular power plants because they generate most of the cell's supply of adenosine triphosphate (ATP), used as a source of chemical energy. In addition to supplying cellular energy, mitochondria are involved in a range of other processes, such as signaling, cellular differentiation, cell death, as well as the control of the cell cycle and cell growth. Mitochondria have been implicated in several human diseases, including mitochondrial disorders and cardiac dysfunction and may play a role in the ageing process.

Several characteristics make mitochondria unique. The number of mitochondria in a cell varies widely by organism and tissue type. Many cells have only a single mitochondrion, whereas others can contain several thousand mitochondria. The organelle is composed of compartments that carry out specialized functions. These compartments or regions include the outer membrane, the intermembrane space, the inner membrane and the cristae and matrix. Mitochondrial proteins vary depending on the tissue and the species. In humans, 615 distinct types of proteins have been identified from cardiac mitochondria, whereas in Murinae (rats), 940 proteins encoded by distinct genes have been reported. The mitochondrial proteome is thought to be dynamically regulated. Although most of a cell's DNA is contained in the cell nucleus, the mitochondrion has its own independent genome. Further, its DNA shows substantial similarity to bacterial genomes. Mitochondrion was first identified as bioblasts by Richard Altmann, a German pathologist and histologist.

Structure of Mitochondria

A mitochondrion contains outer and inner membranes composed of phospholipid bilayers and proteins. The two membranes have different properties. Because of this double-membraned organization, there are five distinct compartments within the mitochondrion. There is the outer mitochondrial membrane, the intermembrane space, the space between the outer and inner membranes, the inner mitochondrial membrane, the cristae space formed by infoldings of the inner membrane and the matrix space within the inner membrane.

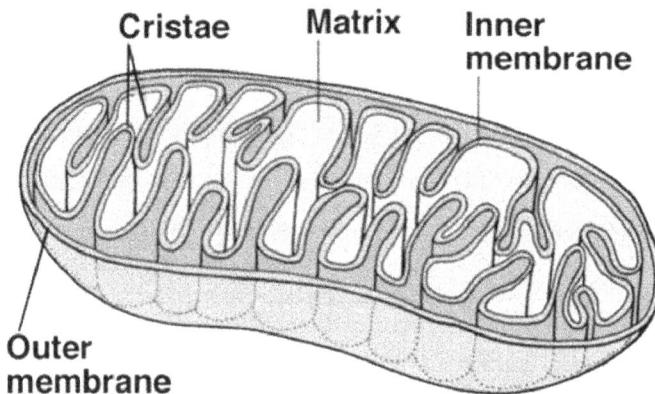

Figure 2.16: Structure of Mitochondria

Outermembrane: The outer mitochondrial membrane, which encloses the entire organelle, has a protein to phospholipid ratio similar to that of the eukaryotic plasma membrane about 1:1 by weight. It contains large numbers of integral proteins called porins. These porins form channels that allow molecules 5000 Daltons or less in molecular weight to freely diffuse from one side of the membrane to the other. Larger proteins can enter the mitochondrion if a signaling sequence at their N-terminus binds to a large multisubunit protein called translocase of the outer membrane, which then actively moves them across the membrane. Disruption of the outer membrane permits proteins in the intermembrane space to leak into the cytosol, leading to certain cell death. The mitochondrial outer membrane can associate with the endoplasmic reticulum (ER) membrane; in a structure called MAM (mitochondria associated ER-membrane). This is important in ER-mitochondria calcium signaling and involved in the transfer of lipids between the ER and mitochondria.

Intermembrane space: The intermembrane space is the space between the outer membrane and the inner membrane. Because the outer membrane is freely permeable to small molecules, the concentrations of small molecules such as ions and sugars in the intermembrane space are the same as the cytosol. However, large proteins must have a specific signaling sequence to be transported across the outer membrane, so the protein composition of this space is different from the protein composition of the cytosol. One protein that is localized to the intermembrane space in this way is cytochrome c. The inner mitochondrial membrane contains proteins with five types of functions:

i.   Those that perform the redox reactions of oxidative phosphorylation

ii. ATP synthase, which generates ATP in the matrix

iii. Specific transport proteins that regulate metabolite passage into and out of the matrix

iv. Protein import machinery.

v.   Mitochondria fusion and fission protein

It contains more than 151 different polypeptides and has a very high protein-to-phospholipid ratio more than 3:1 by weight, which is about 1 protein for 15 phospholipids. The inner membrane is home to around 1/5 of the total protein in a mitochondrion. In addition the inner membrane is rich in an unusual phospholipid *e.g.* cardiolipin. This phospholipid was originally discovered in cow hearts in 1942 and is usually characteristic of mitochondrial and bacterial plasma membranes. Cardiolipin contains four fatty acids rather than two and may help to make the inner membrane impermeable. Unlike the outer membrane, the inner membrane doesn't contain porins and is highly impermeable to all molecules. Almost all ions and molecules require special membrane transporters to enter or exit the matrix. Proteins are carried into the matrix via the translocase of the inner membrane (TIM) complex. In addition, there is a membrane potential across the inner membrane formed by the action of the enzymes of the electron transport chain.

Cristae: The inner mitochondrial membrane is compartmentalized into numerous cristae, which expand the surface area of the inner mitochondrial membrane, enhancing its ability to produce ATP. For typical liver mitochondria the area of the inner membrane is about five times greater than the outer membrane. This ratio is variable and mitochondria from cells that have a greater demand for ATP, such as muscle cells, contain even more cristae. These folds are studded with small round bodies known as F_1 particles or oxysomes. These are not simple random folds but rather invaginations of the inner membrane, which can affect overall chemiosmotic function. The optical properties of the cristae in filamentous mitochondria may affect the generation and propagation of light within the tissue.

Matrix: The matrix is the space enclosed by the inner membrane. It contains about 2/3 of the total protein in a mitochondrion. The matrix is important in the production of ATP with the aid of the ATP synthase contained in the inner membrane. The matrix contains a highly-concentrated mixture of hundreds of enzymes, special mitochondrial ribosomes, tRNA and several copies of the mitochondrial DNA genome. Of the enzymes, the major functions include oxidation of pyruvate and fatty acids and the citric acid cycle. Mitochondria have their own genetic material and the machinery to manufacture their own RNAs and proteins. A published human mitochondrial DNA sequence revealed 16569 base pairs encoding 37 total genes: 22 tRNA, 2 rRNA and 13 peptide genes. The 13 mitochondrial peptides in humans are integrated into the inner mitochondrial membrane along with proteins encoded by genes that reside in the host cell's nucleus.

Mitochondria-associated ER membrane (MAM): The mitochondria-associated ER membrane (MAM) is another structural element that is increasingly recognized for its critical role in cellular physiology and homeostasis. Once considered a technical snag in cell fractionation techniques, the alleged ER vesicle contaminants that invariably appeared in the mitochondrial fraction have been re-identified as membranous structures derived from the MAM, the interface between mitochondria and the ER. Physical coupling between these two organelles had previously been observed in electron micrographs and has more recently been probed with fluorescence microscopy. Such studies estimate that at the MAM which may comprise up to 20% of the mitochondrial outer membrane, ER and mitochondria are separated by a mere 10-25 nm and held together by protein tethering complexes. The purified MAM from subcellular fractionation has shown to be enriched in enzymes involved in phospholipid exchange, in addition to channels associated with Ca^{2+} signaling. These hints of a prominent role for the MAM in the regulation of cellular lipid stores and signal transduction have been borne out, with significant implications for mitochondrial-associated cellular phenomena. Not only has the MAM provided insight into the mechanistic basis underlying such physiological processes as intrinsic apoptosis and the propagation of calcium signaling, but it also favors a more refined view of the mitochondria.

Phospholipid Transfer: The MAM is enrichad in enzymes involved in lipid biosynthesis, such as phosphatidylserine synthase on the ER face and phosphatidylserine decarboxylase on the mitochondrial face. Because mitochondria are dynamic organelles constantly undergoing fission and fusion events, they require a constant and well-regulated supply of phospholipids for membrane integrity. But mitochondria are not only a destination for the phospholipids they finish synthesis of this organelle also plays a role in inter-organelle trafficking of the intermediates and products of phospholipid biosynthetic pathways, ceramide and cholesterol metabolism and glycosphingolipid anabolism. Such trafficking capacity depends on the MAM, which has been shown to facilitate transfer of lipid intermediates between organelles. In contrast to the standard vesicular mechanism of lipid transfer, evidence indicates that the physical proximity of the ER and mitochondrial membranes at the MAM allows for lipid flipping between apposed bilayers. Despite this unusual and seemingly energetically unfavorable mechanism, such transport does not require ATP. Instead, it has been shown to be dependent on a multiprotein tethering structure termed the ER-mitochondria encounter structure or ERMES, although it remains unclear whether this structure directly mediates lipid transfer or is required to keep the membranes in sufficiently close proximity to lower the energy barrier for lipid flipping. The MAM may also be part of the secretory pathway, in addition to its role in intracellular lipid trafficking. In particular, the MAM appears to be an intermediate destination between the rough ER and the Golgi in the pathway that leads to very-low-density lipoprotein or VLDL, assembly and secretion. The MAM thus serves as a critical metabolic and trafficking hub in lipid metabolism.

Calcium Signaling: A critical role for the ER in calcium signaling was acknowledged before such a role for the mitochondria was widely accepted, in part because the low affinity of Ca^{2+} channels localized to the outer mitochondrial membrane seemed to fly in the face of this organelle's purported responsiveness to changes in intracellular Ca^{2+} flux. But the presence of the MAM resolves this apparent contradiction: the close physical association between the two organelles results in Ca^{2+} microdomains at contact points that facilitate efficient Ca^{2+} transmission from the ER to the mitochondria. Transmission occurs in response to so called Ca^{2+} puffs generated by spontaneous clustering and activation of IP3R, a canonical ER membrane Ca^{2+} channel. The fate of these puffs in particular, whether they remain restricted to isolated locales or integrated into Ca^{2+} waves for propagation throughout the cell is determined in large part by MAM dynamics. Although reuptake of Ca^{2+} by the ER modulates the intensity of the puffs, thus insulating mitochondria to a certain degree from high Ca^{2+} exposure, the MAM often serves as a firewall that essentially buffers Ca^{2+} puffs by acting as a sink into which free ions released into the cytosol can be funneled. This Ca^{2+} tunneling occurs through the low-affinity Ca^{2+} receptor VDAC1, which recently has been shown to be physically tethered to the IP3R clusters on the ER membrane and enriched at the MAM. The ability of mitochondria to serve as a Ca^{2+} sink is a result of the electrochemical gradient generated during oxidative phosphorylation, which makes tunneling of the cation an exergonic process.

But transmission of Ca^{2+} is not unidirectional it is a two-way street. The properties of the Ca^{2+} pump SERCA and the channel IP3R present on the ER membrane facilitate feedback regulation coordinated by MAM function. In particular, clearance of Ca^{2+} by the MAM allows for spatio-temporal patterning of Ca^{2+} signaling because Ca^{2+} alters IP3R activity in a biphasic manner. SERCA is likewise affected by mitochondrial feedback; uptake of Ca^{2+} by the MAM stimulates ATP production, thus providing energy that enables SERCA to reload the ER with Ca^{2+} for continued Ca^{2+} efflux at the MAM. Thus the MAM is not a passive buffer for Ca^{2+} puffs; rather it helps modulate further Ca^{2+} signaling through feedback loops that affect ER dynamics. Regulating

ER release of Ca^{2+} at the MAM is especially critical because only a certain window of Ca^{2+} uptake sustains the mitochondria and consequently the cell at homeostasis. Sufficient intraorganelle Ca^{2+} signaling is required to stimulate metabolism by activating dehydrogenase enzymes critical to flux through the citric acid cycle. However once Ca^{2+} signaling in the mitochondria passes a certain threshold, it stimulates the intrinsic pathway of apoptosis in part by collapsing the mitochondrial membrane potential required for metabolism. Studies examining the role of pro- and anti-apoptotic factors support this model *e.g.* anti-apoptotic factor Bcl-2 has been shown to interact with IP3Rs to reduce Ca^{2+} filling of the ER, leading to reduced efflux at the MAM and preventing collapse of the mitochondrial membrane potential post-apoptotic stimuli. Given the need for such fine regulation of Ca^{2+} signaling, it is perhaps unsurprising that dysregulated mitochondrial Ca^{2+} has been implicated in several neurodegenerative diseases, while the catalogue of tumor suppressors includes a few that are enriched at the MAM.

Molecular Basis for Tethering: The scaffolding function of the molecular elements involved is secondary to other, non-structural functions. ERMES, a multiprotein complex of interacting ER and mitochondrial-resident membrane proteins, is required for lipid transfer at the MAM and exemplifies this principle. One of its components is also a constituent of the protein complex required for insertion of transmembrane beta-barrel proteins into the lipid bilayer. Other proteins implicated in scaffolding likewise have functions independent of structural tethering at the MAM, ER-resident and mitochondrial-resident mitofusins form heterocomplexes that regulate the number of inter-organelle contact sites, although mitofusins were first identified for their role in fission and fusion events between individual mitochondria. Glucose-related protein 75 (grp75) is another dual-function protein. In addition to the matrix pool of grp75, a portion serves as a chaperone that physically links the mitochondrial and ER Ca^{2+} channels VDAC and IP3R for efficient Ca^{2+} transmission at the MAM. Another prominent tether is Sigma-1R, another chaperone whose stabilization of ER-resident IP3R has been proposed to preserve communication at the MAM during the metabolic stress response. The MAM is a critical signaling, metabolic and trafficking hub in the cell that allows for the integration of ER and mitochondrial physiology. Coupling between these organelles is not simply structural but functional as well and critical for overall cellular physiology and homeostasis. The MAM thus offers a perspective on mitochondria that diverges from the traditional view of this organelle as a static, isolated unit appropriated for its metabolic capacity by the cell. Instead, this mitochondrial-ER interface emphasizes the integration of the mitochondria into diverse cellular processes.

Organization and Distribution of Mitochondria

Mitochondria are found in nearly all eukaryotes. They vary in number and location according to cell type. A single mitochondrion is often found in unicellular organisms. Conversely, numerous mitochondria are found in human liver cells, with about 1000–2000 mitochondria per cell making up 1/5 of the cell volume. The mitochondria can be found nestled between myofibrils of muscle or wrapped around the sperm flagellum. Often they form a complex 3D branching network inside the cell with the cytoskeleton. The association with the cytoskeleton determines mitochondrial shape, which can affect the function as well. Recent evidence suggests vimentin, one of the components of the cytoskeleton, is critical to the association with the cytoskeleton.

Functions of Mitochondria

The most prominent roles of mitochondria are to produce ATP *i.e.*, phosphorylation of ADP through respiration and to regulate cellular metabolism. The central set of reactions involved in ATP production is collectively known as the citric acid cycle or the Krebs cycle. However, the mitochondrion has many other functions in addition to the production of ATP.

Energy Conversion: A dominant role for the mitochondria is the production of ATP, as reflected by the large number of proteins in the inner membrane for this task. This is done by oxidizing the major products of glucose, pyruvate and NADH, which are produced in the cytosol. This process of cellular respiration, also known as aerobic respiration, is dependent on the presence of oxygen. When oxygen is limited, the glycolytic products will be metabolized by anaerobic respiration, a process that is independent of the mitochondria. The production of ATP from glucose has an approximately 13-fold higher yield during aerobic respiration compared to anaerobic respiration. Recently it has been shown that plant mitochondria can produce a limited amount of ATP without oxygen by using the alternate substrate nitrite.

Pyruvate and Citric Acid Cycle: Each pyruvate molecule produced by glycolysis is actively transported across the inner mitochondrial membrane and into the matrix where it is oxidized and combined with coenzyme A to form CO_2, acetyl-CoA and NADH. The acetyl-CoA is the primary substrate to enter the citric acid cycle also known as the tricarboxylic acid (TCA) cycle or Kreb's cycle. The enzymes of the citric acid cycle are located in the mitochondrial matrix, with the exception of succinate dehydrogenase, which is bound to the inner mitochondrial membrane as part of Complex II. The citric acid cycle oxidizes the acetyl-CoA to carbon dioxide and, in the process, produces reduced cofactors, three molecules of NADH and one molecule of $FADH_2$ that are a source of electrons for the electron transport chain and a molecule of GTP that is readily converted to an ATP.

Electron Transport Chain (NADH and $FADH_2$): The redox energy from NADH and $FADH_2$ is transferred to oxygen (O_2) in several steps via the electron transport chain. These energy-rich molecules are produced within the matrix via the citric acid cycle but are also produced in the cytoplasm by glycolysis. Reducing equivalents from the cytoplasm can be imported via the malate-aspartate shuttle system of antiporter proteins or feed into the electron transport chain using a glycerol phosphate shuttle. Protein complexes in the inner membrane (NADH dehydrogenase, cytochrome c reductase and cytochrome c oxidase) perform the transfer and the incremental release of energy is used to pump protons (H^+) into the intermembrane space. This process is efficient, but a small percentage of electrons may prematurely reduce oxygen, forming reactive oxygen species such as superoxide. This can cause oxidative stress in the mitochondria and may contribute to the decline in mitochondrial function associated with the aging process. As the proton concentration increases in the intermembrane space, a strong electrochemical gradient is established across the inner membrane. The protons can return to the matrix through the ATP synthase complex and their potential energy is used to synthesize ATP from ADP and inorganic phosphate (Pi). This process is called chemiosmosis and was first described by Peter Mitchell who was awarded the 1978 Nobel Prize in Chemistry for his work. Later, part of the 1997 Nobel Prize in Chemistry was awarded to Paul D. Boyer and John E. Walker for their clarification of the working mechanism of ATP synthase.

Heat Production: Under certain conditions, protons can re-enter the mitochondrial matrix without contributing to ATP synthesis. This process is known as proton leak or mitochondrial uncoupling and is due to the facilitated diffusion of protons into the matrix. The process results in the unharnessed potential energy of the proton electrochemical gradient being released as heat. The process is mediated by a proton channel called thermogenin or UCP1. Thermogenin is a 33kDa protein first discovered in 1973. Thermogenin is primarily found in brown adipose tissue or brown fat and is responsible for non-shivering thermogenesis. Brown adipose tissue is found in mammals and is at its highest levels in early life and in hibernating animals. In humans, brown adipose tissue is present at birth and decreases with age.

Storage of Calcium ions: The concentrations of free calcium in the cell can regulate an array of reactions and is important for signal transduction in the cell. Mitochondria can transiently store calcium, a contributing process for the cell's homeostasis of calcium. In fact, their ability to rapidly take in calcium for later release makes them very good cytosolic buffers for calcium. The endoplasmic reticulum (ER) is the most significant storage site of calcium and there is a significant interplay between the mitochondrion and ER with regard to calcium. The calcium is taken up into the matrix by a calcium uniporter on the inner mitochondrial membrane. It is primarily driven by the mitochondrial membrane potential. Release of this calcium back into the cell's interior can occur via a sodium-calcium exchange protein or via calcium-induced-calcium release pathways. This can initiate calcium spikes or calcium waves with large changes in the membrane potential. These can activate a series of second messenger system proteins that can coordinate processes such as neurotransmitter release in nerve cells and release of hormones in endocrine cells.

Some mitochondrial functions are performed only in specific types of cells. Mitochondria in liver cells contain enzymes that allow them to detoxify ammonia, a waste product of protein metabolism. A mutation in the genes regulating any of these functions can result in mitochondrial diseases. Mitochondria play a central role in many other metabolic tasks such as:

- Regulation of the membrane potential
- Apoptosis-programmed cell death
- Calcium signaling (including calcium-evoked apoptosis)
- Cellular proliferation regulation
- Regulation of cellular metabolism
- Certain heme synthesis reaction
- Steroid synthesis.

Origin of Mitochondria

Mitochondria have many features in common with prokaryotes. As a result, they are believed to be originally derived from endosymbiotic prokaryotes. A mitochondrion contains DNA which is organized as several copies of a single and circular chromosome. This mitochondrial chromosome contains genes for redox proteins such as those of the respiratory chain. The CoRR hypothesis proposes that this co-location is required for redox regulation. The mitochondrial genome codes for some RNAs of ribosomes and the twenty-two tRNA necessary for the translation of messenger RNAs into protein. The circular structure is also found in prokaryotes and the similarity is extended by the fact that mitochondrial DNA is organized with a variant genetic code similar to that of Proteobacteria. This suggests that their ancestor, the so-called proto-mitochondrion, was a member of the Proteobacteria. In particular, the proto-mitochondrion was probably closely related to the rickettsia. However, the exact relationship of the ancestor of mitochondria to the alpha-proteobacteria and whether the mitochondria were formed at the same time or after the nucleus remains controversial.

During the 1980s, Lynn Margulis proposed the theory of endosymbiosis to explain the origin of mitochondria and chloroplasts from permanent resident prokaryotes. According to this idea, a larger prokaryote or perhaps early eukaryote engulfed or surrounded a smaller prokaryote some 1.5 billion to 700 million years ago. Instead of digesting the smaller organisms the large one and the smaller one entered into a type of symbiosis known as mutualism, wherein both organisms benefit and neither is harmed. The larger organism gained excess ATP provided by the protomitochondrion and excess sugar provided by the protochloroplast, while providing a stable environment and the raw materials the endosymbionts required. This is so strong that eukaryotic cells cannot survive without mitochondria likewise photosynthetic eukaryotes cannot survive without chloroplasts and the endosymbionts cannot survive outside their hosts. Nearly all eukaryotes have mitochondria. The ribosomes coded for by the mitochondrial DNA are similar to those from bacteria in size and structure. They closely resemble the bacterial 70S ribosome and not the 80S cytoplasmic ribosomes, which are coded for by nuclear DNA. A few groups of unicellular eukaryotes lack mitochondria such as microsporidians, metamonads and archamoebae. These groups appear as the most primitive eukaryotes on phylogenetic trees constructed using rRNA information, which once suggested that they appeared before the origin of mitochondria. However, this is now known to be an artifact of long-branch attraction, they are derived groups and retain genes or organelles derived from mitochondria *e.g.* mitosomes and hydrogenosomes.

Genome of Mitochondria

The human mitochondrial genome is a circular DNA molecule of about 16 kilobases. It encodes 37 genes: 13 for subunits of respiratory complexes I, III, IV and V, 22 for mitochondrial tRNA, for the 20 standard amino acids, plus an extra gene for leucine and serine and 2 for rRNA. One mitochondrion can contain two to ten copies of its DNA. As in prokaryotes, there is a very high proportion of coding DNA and an absence of repeats. Mitochondrial genes are transcribed as multigenic transcripts, which are cleaved and polyadenylated to yield mature mRNAs. Not all proteins necessary for mitochondrial function are encoded by the mitochondrial genome; most are coded by genes in the cell nucleus and the corresponding proteins are imported into the mitochondrion. The exact number of genes encoded by the nucleus and the mitochondrial genome differs between species. The mitochondrial genomes are circular, although exceptions have been reported. In general, mitochondrial DNA lacks introns, as is the case in the human mitochondrial genome. However introns have been observed in some eukaryotic mitochondrial DNA such as that of yeast and protists including *Dictyostelium discoideum*. In animals the mitochondrial genome is typically a single circular chromosome that is approximately 16-kb long and has 37 genes. The genes while highly conserved may vary in location. Curiously this pattern is not found in the human body louse (*Pediculus humanus*). Instead this mitochondrial genome is arranged in 18 minicircular chromosomes each of which is 3–4 kb long and has one to three genes. This pattern is also found in other sucking lice but not in chewing lice. Recombination has been shown to occur between the mini chromosomes. The reason for this difference is not known. While slight variations on standard code had been predicted earlier, none was discovered until 1979, when researchers studying human mitochondrial genes determined that they used an alternative code. Many slight variants have been discovered since, including various alternative mitochondrial codes. Further, the AUA, AUC and AUU codons are all allowable start codons.

Table 10: Exceptions to the Universal Genetic code (UGC) in Mitochondria

S.No.	Organism	Codon	Standard	Novel
1.	Mammalian	AGA, AGG	Arginine	Stop codon
		AUA	Isoleucine	Methionine
		UGA	Stop codon	Tryptophan
2.	Invertebrates	AGA, AGG	Arginine	Serine
		AUA	Isoleucine	Methionine
		UGA	Stop codon	Tryptophan
3.	Fungi	AUA	Isoleucine	Methionine
		UGA	Stop codon	Tryptophan
		CUA	Leucine	Threonine

Some of these differences should be regarded as pseudo-changes in the genetic code due to the phenomenon of RNA editing which is common in mitochondria. In higher plants, it was thought that CGG encoded for tryptophan and not arginine. However the codon in the processed RNA was discovered to be the UGG codon, consistent with the universal genetic code for tryptophan. The arthropod mitochondrial genetic code has undergone parallel evolution within a phylum with some organisms uniquely translating AGG to lysine. Mitochondrial genomes have far fewer genes than the bacteria from which they are thought to be descended. Although some have been lost altogether, many have been transferred to the nucleus, such as the respiratory complex II protein subunits. This is thought to be relatively common over evolutionary time. A few organisms, such as the *Cryptosporidium*, actually have mitochondria that lack any DNA, presumably because all their genes have been lost or transferred. In *Cryptosporidium*, the mitochondria have an altered ATP generation system that renders the parasite resistant to many classical mitochondrial inhibitors such as cyanide, azide and atovaquone.

Mitochondrial Inheritance

Mitochondria divide by binary fission similar to bacterial cell division unlike bacteria however; mitochondria can also fuse with other mitochondria. The regulation of this division differs between eukaryotes. In many single celled eukaryotes, their growth and division is linked to the cell cycle. A single mitochondrion may divide synchronously with the nucleus. This division and segregation process must be tightly controlled so that each daughter cell receives at least one mitochondrion. In other eukaryotes mitochondria may replicate their DNA and divide mainly in response to the energy needs of the cell, rather than in phase with the cell cycle. When the energy needs of a cell are high, mitochondria grow and divide. When the energy use is low, mitochondria are destroyed or become inactive. In such examples and in contrast to the situation in many single celled eukaryotes, mitochondria are apparently randomly distributed to the daughter cells during the division of the cytoplasm. An individual's mitochondrial genes are not inherited by the same mechanism as nuclear genes. At fertilization of an egg cell by a sperm, the egg nucleus and sperm nucleus each contribute equally to the genetic makeup of the zygote nucleus. In contrast, the mitochondria and therefore the mitochondrial DNA come from the egg only. The sperm's mitochondria enter the egg but do not contribute genetic information to the embryo. Instead, paternal mitochondria are marked with ubiquitin to select them for later destruction inside the embryo. The egg cell contains relatively few mitochondria, but it is these mitochondria that survive and divide to populate the cells of the adult organism. Mitochondria are, therefore, in most cases inherited down the female line, known as maternal inheritance. This mode is seen in most organisms including all animals. However mitochondria in some species can sometimes be inherited paternally. This is the norm among certain coniferous plants, although not in pine trees and yew trees. It has been suggested that it occurs at a very low level in humans. Uniparental inheritance leads to little opportunity for genetic recombination between different lineages of mitochondria, although a single mitochondrion can contain 2–10 copies of its DNA. For this reason the mitochondrial DNA usually is thought to reproduce by binary fission. There are studies showing evidence of recombination in mitochondrial DNA. It is clear that the enzymes necessary for recombination are present in mammalian cells. Further evidence suggests that animal mitochondria can undergo recombination. The data are a bit more controversial in humans although indirect evidence of recombination exists. If recombination does not occur, the whole mitochondrial DNA sequence represents a single haplotype which makes it useful for studying the evolutionary history of populations.

The near absence of genetic recombination in mitochondrial DNA makes it a useful source of information for scientists involved in population genetics and evolutionary biology. Because the entire mitochondrial DNA is inherited as a single unit or haplotype, the relationships between mitochondrial DNA from different individuals can be represented as a gene tree. Patterns in these gene trees can be used to infer the evolutionary history of populations. The classic example of this is in human evolutionary genetics, where the molecular clock can be used to provide a recent date for mitochondrial Eve. This is interpreted as strong support for a recent modern human expansion out of Africa. Another human example is the sequencing of mitochondrial DNA from Neanderthal bones. The relatively large evolutionary distance between the mitochondrial DNA sequences of Neanderthals and living humans has been interpreted as evidence for lack of interbreeding between Neanderthals and anatomically-modern humans. However mitochondrial DNA reflects the history of only females in a population and so may not represent the history of the population as a whole. This can be partially overcome by the use of paternal genetic sequences, such as the non-recombining region of the Y-chromosome. In a broader sense, only studies that also include nuclear DNA can provide a comprehensive evolutionary history of a population.

Mitochondrial Diseases

With their central place in cell metabolism, damage and subsequent dysfunction in mitochondria is an important factor in a wide range of human diseases. Mitochondrial disorders often present themselves as neurological disorders but can manifest as myopathy, diabetes, multiple endocrinopathy or a variety of other systemic manifestations. Diseases caused by mutation in the mtDNA include Kearns-Sayre syndrome, MELAS syndrome and Leber's hereditary optic neuropathy. In the vast majority of cases, these diseases are transmitted by a female to her children as the zygote derives its mitochondria and hence its mtDNA from the ovum. Diseases such as Kearns-Sayre syndrome, Pearson's syndrome and progressive external ophthalmoplegia are thought to be due to large-scale mtDNA rearrangements, whereas other diseases such as MELAS syndrome, Leber's hereditary optic neuropathy, myoclonic epilepsy with ragged red fibers (MERRF) and others are due to point mutations in mtDNA. In other diseases, defects in nuclear genes lead to dysfunction of mitochondrial proteins. This is the case in Friedreich's ataxia, hereditary spastic paraplegia and Wilson's disease. These diseases are inherited in a dominance relationship, as applies to most other genetic diseases. A variety of disorders can be caused by nuclear mutations of oxidative phosphorylation enzymes, such as coenzyme Q10 deficiency and Barth syndrome. Environmental influences may interact with hereditary predispositions and cause mitochondrial disease. There may be a link between pesticide exposure and the later onset of Parkinson's disease. Other pathologies with etiology involving mitochondrial dysfunction include schizophrenia, bipolar disorder, dementia, Alzheimer's disease, Parkinson's disease, epilepsy, stroke, cardiovascular disease, retinitis pigmentosa and diabetes mellitus. A common thread thought to link these seemingly unrelated conditions is cellular damage causing oxidative stress. How exactly mitochondrial dysfunction fits into the etiology of these pathologies is yet to be elucidated.

The mitochondria works as powerhouse of cell, there may be some leakage of the high-energy electrons in the respiratory chain to form reactive oxygen species. This can result in significant oxidative stress in the mitochondria with high mutation rates of mitochondrial DNA. A vicious cycle is thought to occur, as oxidative stress leads to mitochondrial DNA mutations, which can lead to enzymatic abnormalities and further oxidative stress. A number of changes occur to mitochondria during the aging process. The tissues from elderly patients show a decrease in enzymatic activity of the proteins of the respiratory chain. Large deletions in the mitochondrial genome can lead to high levels of oxidative stress and neuronal death in Parkinson's disease. Hypothesized links between aging and oxidative stress are not new and were proposed over 50 years ago. However there is much debate over whether mitochondrial changes are causes of aging or merely characteristics of aging. One notable study in mice demonstrated shortened lifespan but no increase in reactive oxygen species despite increasing mitochondrial DNA mutations, suggesting that mitochondrial DNA mutations can cause lifespan shortening by other mechanisms. As a result the exact relationships between mitochondria, oxidative stress and ageing have not yet been settled.

Plastids

Plastids are also membrane-bound organelles that only occur in plants and photosynthetic eukaryotes like algae. Plastids are the site of manufacture and storage of important chemical compounds used by the cell. Plastids contain pigments used in photosynthesis and the types of pigments present can change or determine the cell's color. Leucoplasts, also known as amyloplasts store starch, as well as sometimes protein or oils. Chromoplasts store pigments associated with the bright colors of flowers and/or fruits. Chloroplasts are found only in photosynthetic protists and plant cells. Chloroplasts are the sites of photosynthesis in eukaryotes. They contain chlorophyll, the green pigment necessary for photosynthesis to occur and associated accessory pigments like carotenes and xanthophylls in photosystems embedded in membranous sacs, thylakoids (collectively a stack of thylakoids are a granum) floating in a fluid/matrix termed the stroma. The thylakoids contain the proteins and other molecules responsible for light capture. The dark reactions of photosynthesis take place in the matrix (stroma) which also contains the DNA and ribosomes.

Plastids in Plants

Plastids are responsible for photosynthesis, storage of products like starch and for the synthesis of many classes of molecules such as fatty acids and terpenes which are needed as cellular building blocks and/or for the function of the plant. Depending on their morphology and function, plastids have the ability to differentiate or redifferentiate, between these and other forms. All plastids are derived from proplastids (formerly eoplasts, eo-: dawn, early), which are present in the meristematic regions of the plant. Proplastids and young chloroplasts commonly divide but more mature chloroplasts also have this capacity.

In plants, plastids may differentiate into several forms, depending upon which function they need to play in the cell. Undifferentiated plastids (proplastids) may develop into any of the following plastids:

i.   Chloroplasts: For photosynthesis.

ii. Chromoplasts: For pigment synthesis and storage.

iii. Leucoplasts: For monoterpene synthesis; leucoplasts sometimes differentiate into more specialized plastids.

iv. Amyloplasts: For starch storage.

v.   Statoliths: For detecting gravity.

vi. Elaioplasts: For storing fat.

vii. Proteinoplasts: For storing and modifying protein.

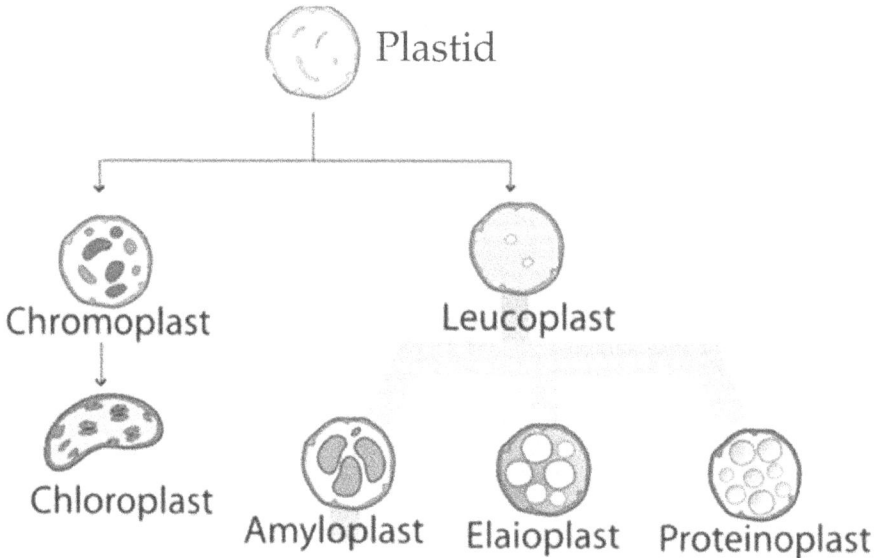

Figure 2.17: Different types of Plastids

Each plastid creates multiple copies of the circular 75-250 kilo bases plastome. The number of genome copies per plastid is flexible, ranging from more than 1000 in rapidly dividing cells, which generally contain few plastids to 100 or fewer in mature cells where plastid divisions has given rise to a large number of plastids. The plastome contains about 100 genes encoding ribosomal and transfer ribonucleic acids (rRNA and tRNA) as well as proteins involved in photosynthesis and plastid gene transcription and translation. However these proteins only represent a small fraction of the total protein set-up necessary to build and maintain the structure and function of a particular type of plastid. Nuclear genes encode the vast majority of plastid proteins and the expression of plastid genes and nuclear genes is tightly co-regulated to allow proper development of plastids in relation to cell differentiation.

Plastid DNA exists as large protein-DNA complexes associated with the inner envelope membrane and called plastid nucleoids. Each nucleoid particle may contain more than 10 copies of the plastid DNA. The proplastid contains a single nucleoid located in the centre of the plastid. The developing plastid has many nucleoids, localized at the periphery of the plastid, bound to the inner envelope membrane. During the development of proplastids to chloroplasts and when plastids convert from one type to another, nucleoids change in morphology, size and location within the organelle. The remodelling of nucleoids is believed to occur by modifications to the composition and abundance of nucleoid proteins. Many plastids, particularly those responsible for photosynthesis, possess numerous internal membrane layers. In plant cells, long thin protuberances called stromules sometimes form and extend from the main plastid body into the cytosol and interconnect several plastids. Proteins and presumably smaller molecules can move within stromules. Most cultured cells that are relatively large compared to other plant cells have very long and abundant stromules that extend to the cell periphery.

Plastids in Algae

In algae, the term leucoplast (leukoplast) is used for all unpigmented plastids. Their function differs from the leukoplasts in plants. Etioplast, amyloplast and chromoplast are plant-specific and do not occur in algae. Algal plastids may also differ from plant plastids in that they contain pyrenoids.

Inheritance of Plastids

Most plants inherit the plastids from only one parent. Angiosperms generally inherit plastids from the mother, while many gymnosperms inherit plastids from the father. Algae also inherit plastids from only one parent. The plastid DNA of the other parent is thus completely lost. In normal intraspecific crossings resulting in normal hybrids of one species, the inheritance of plastid DNA appears to be quite strictly 100% uniparental. In interspecific hybridisations, the inheritance of plastids appears to be more erratic. Although plastids inherit mainly maternally in interspecific hybridisations, there are many reports of hybrids of flowering plants that contain plastids of the father.

Origin of Plastids

Plastids are thought to have originated from endosymbiotic cyanobacteria. They developed around 1500 million years ago and allowed eukaryotes to carry out oxygenic photosynthesis. Due to a split-up into three evolutionary lineages, the plastids are named differently: chloroplasts in green algae and plants, rhodoplasts in red algae and cyanelles in the glaucophytes. The plastids differ by their pigmentation, but also in ultrastructure. The chloroplasts *e.g.* have lost all phycobilisomes, the light harvesting complexes found in cyanobacteria, red algae and glaucophytes, but only in plants and in closely related green algae - contain stroma and grana thylakoids. The glaucocystophycean plastid - in contrast to the chloroplasts and the rhodoplasts - is still surrounded by the remains of the cyanobacterial cell wall. All these primary plastids are surrounded by two membranes. Complex plastids start by secondary endosymbiosis when a eukaryote engulfs a red or green alga and retains the algal plastid which is typically surrounded by more than two membranes. In some cases these plastids may be reduced in their metabolic and/or photosynthetic capacity. Algae with complex plastids derived by secondary endosymbiosis of a red alga include the heterokonts, haptophytes, cryptomonads and most dinoflagellates (rhodoplasts). Those that endosymbiosed a green alga include the euglenids and chlorarachniophytes (chloroplasts). The Apicomplexa, a phylum of obligate parasitic protozoa including the causative agents of malaria (*Plasmodium* spp.), toxoplasmosis (*Toxoplasma gondii*) and many other human or animal diseases also harbor a complex plastid, although this organelle has been lost in some apicomplexans, such as *Cryptosporidium parvum*, which causes cryptosporidiosis. The apicoplast is no longer capable of photosynthesis but is an essential organelle and a promising target for antiparasitic drug development. Some dinoflagellates take up algae as food and keep the plastid of the digested alga to profit from the photosynthesis; after a while the plastids are also digested. These captured plastids are known as kleptoplastids.

Chloroplast

Chloroplasts are organelles found in plant cells and other eukaryotic organisms that conduct photosynthesis. Chloroplasts capture light energy to conserve free energy in the form of ATP and reduce NADP to NADPH through a complex set of processes called photosynthesis. The word chloroplast is derived from the Greek words chloros which means green and plast which means form or entity. Chloroplasts are members of a class of organelles known as plastids.

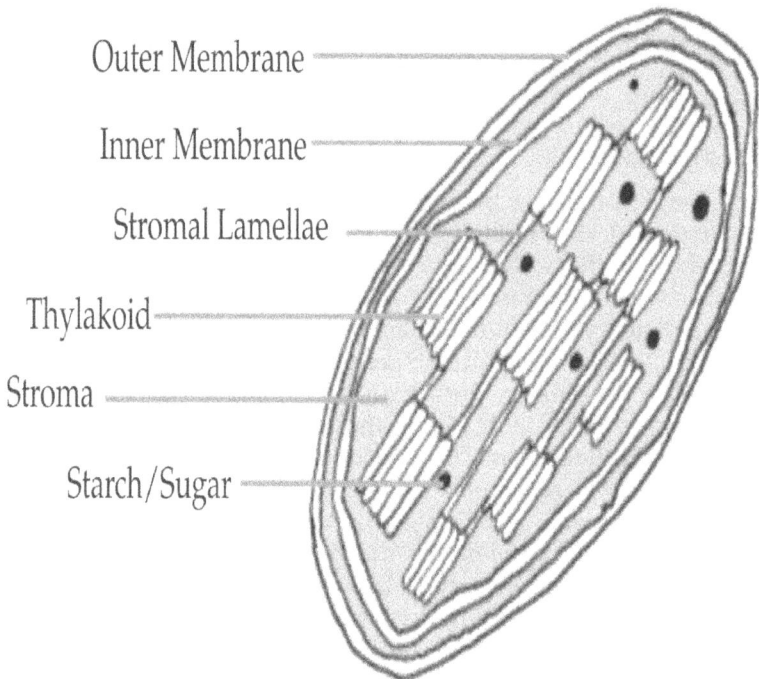

Outer Membrane
Inner Membrane
Stromal Lamellae
Thylakoid
Stroma
Starch/Sugar

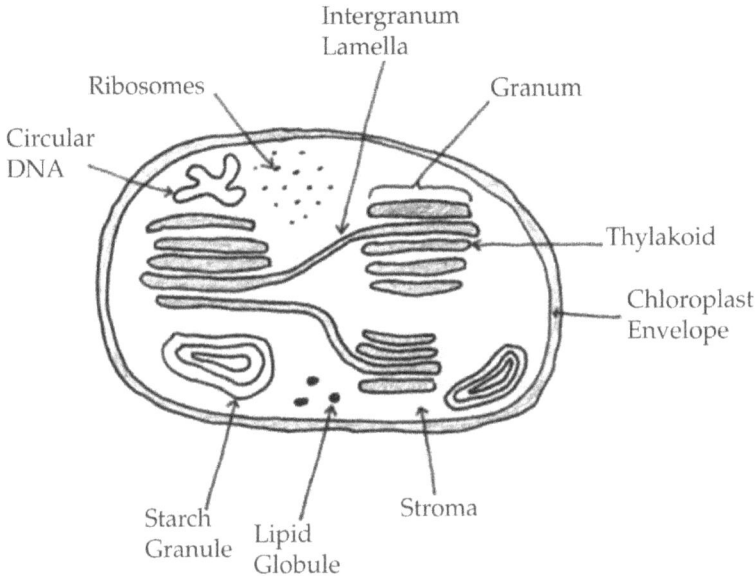

Figure 218: Chloroplast

Evolutionary Origin of Chloroplasts: Chloroplasts are one of the many different types of organelles in the cell. They are generally considered to have originated as endosymbiotic cyanobacteria *i.e.* blue-green algae. This was first suggested by Mereschkowsky in 1905 after an observation by Schimper in 1883 that chloroplasts closely resemble cyanobacteria. All chloroplasts are thought to derive directly or indirectly from a single endosymbiotic event in the Archaeplastida, except for *Paulinella chromatophora*, which has recently acquired a photosynthetic cyanobacterial endosymbiont which is not closely related to chloroplasts of other eukaryotes. In that they derive from an endosymbiotic event, chloroplasts are similar to mitochondria but chloroplasts are found only in plants and protista. The chloroplast is surrounded by a double-layered composite membrane with an intermembrane space; further, it has reticulations or many infoldings, filling the inner spaces. The chloroplast has its own DNA which codes for redox proteins involved in electron transport in photosynthesis. In green plants, chloroplasts are surrounded by two lipid-bilayer membranes. The inner membrane is now believed to correspond to the outer membrane of the ancestral cyanobacterium. Chloroplasts have their own genome, which is considerably reduced compared to that of free-living cyanobacteria, but the parts that are still present show clear similarities with the cyanobacterial genome. Plastids may contain 60-100 genes whereas cyanobacteria often contain more than 1500 genes. Many of the missing genes are encoded in the nuclear genome of the host. The transfer of nuclear information has been estimated in tobacco plants at one gene for every 16000 pollen grains.

In some algae such as the heterokonts and other protists such as Euglenozoa and Cercozoa, chloroplasts seem to have evolved through a secondary event of endosymbiosis, in which a eukaryotic cell engulfed a second eukaryotic cell containing chloroplasts, forming chloroplasts with three or four membrane layers. In some cases, such secondary endosymbionts may have themselves been engulfed by still other eukaryotes, thus forming tertiary endosymbionts. In the alga *Chlorella*, there is only one chloroplast, which is bell shaped. In some groups of mixotrophic protists such as the dinoflagellates, chloroplasts are separated from a captured alga or diatom and used temporarily. These klepto chloroplasts may only have a lifetime of a few days and are then replaced.

Structure of Chloroplast: Chloroplasts are observable morphologically as flat discs usually 2 to 10 micrometer in diameter and 1 micrometer thick. In land plants they are generally 5 ìm in diameter and 2.3 ìm thick. The chloroplast is contained by an envelope that consists of an inner and an outer phospholipid membrane. Between these two layers is the intermembrane space. A typical parenchyma cell contains about 10 to 100 chloroplasts. The material within the chloroplast is called the stroma, corresponding to the cytosol of the original bacterium and contains one or more molecules of small circular DNA. It also contains ribosomes, although most of its proteins are encoded by genes contained in the host cell nucleus, with the protein products transported to the chloroplast. Within the stroma are stacks of thylakoids, the sub-organelles which are the site of photosynthesis. The thylakoids are arranged in stacks called grana. A thylakoid has a flattened disk shape and inside it an empty area called the thylakoid space or lumen. Photosynthesis takes place on the thylakoid membrane; as in mitochondrial oxidative phosphorylation, it involves the coupling of cross-membrane fluxes with biosynthesis via the dissipation of a proton electrochemical gradient.

In the electron microscope, thylakoid membranes appear as alternating light-and-dark bands, each 0.01 ìm thick. Embedded in the thylakoid membrane is the antenna complex, which consists of the light-absorbing pigments, including chlorophyll and carotenoids and proteins which bind the chlorophyll. This complex both increases the surface area for light capture and allows capture of photons with a wider range of wavelengths. The energy of the incident photons is absorbed by the pigments and funneled to the reaction centre of this complex through resonance energy transfer. Two chlorophyll molecules are then ionised, producing an excited electron which then passes onto the photochemical reaction centre. Recent studies have shown that chloroplasts can be interconnected by tubular bridges called stromules, formed as extensions of their outer membranes. Chloroplasts appear to be able to exchange proteins via stromules and thus function as a network.

Transplastomic Plants: In most flowering plants, chloroplasts are not inherited from the male parent, although in plants such as pines, chloroplasts are inherited from males. Where chloroplasts are inherited only from the female, transgenes in these plastids cannot be disseminated by pollen. This makes plastid transformation a valuable tool for the creation and cultivation of genetically modified plants that are biologically contained, thus posing significantly lower environmental risks. This biological containment strategy is therefore suitable for establishing the coexistence of conventional and organic agriculture.

Chromoplasts

Chromoplasts are plastids responsible for pigment synthesis and storage. Like all other plastids including chloroplasts and leucoplasts, the chromoplasts are organelles found in specific photosynthetic eukaryotic species. Chromoplasts in the traditional sense are found in coloured organs of plants such as fruit and floral petals, to which they give their distinctive colors. This is always associated with a massive increase in the accumulation of carotenoid pigments. The conversion of chloroplasts to chromoplasts in ripening tomato fruit is a classic example. Chromoplasts synthesize and store pigments such as orange carotene, yellow xanthophylls and various other red pigments; as such, their color varies depending on what pigment they contain. The probable main evolutionary role of chromoplasts is to act as an attractant for pollinating animals *e.g.* insects or for seed dispersal via the eating of coloured fruits. They allow the accumulation of large quantities of water insoluble compounds in otherwise watery parts of plants. In chloroplasts, some carotenoids are also used as accessory pigments in photosynthesis, where they act to increase the efficiency of chlorophyll in harvesting light energy. When leaves change color in autumn, it is due to the loss of green chlorophyll unmasking these carotenoids that are already present in the leaf. In this case, relatively little new carotenoids are produced. Therefore, the change in plastid pigments associated with leaf senescence is somewhat different from the active conversion to chromoplasts observed in fruit and flowers. The term chromoplast is occasionally utilized to include any plastid that has pigment, mostly to emphasize the contrast with the various types of leucoplasts, which are those plastids that have no pigments. In this sense, chloroplasts are a specific type of chromoplast. Still, chromoplast is more often used to denote those plastids with pigments other than chlorophyll.

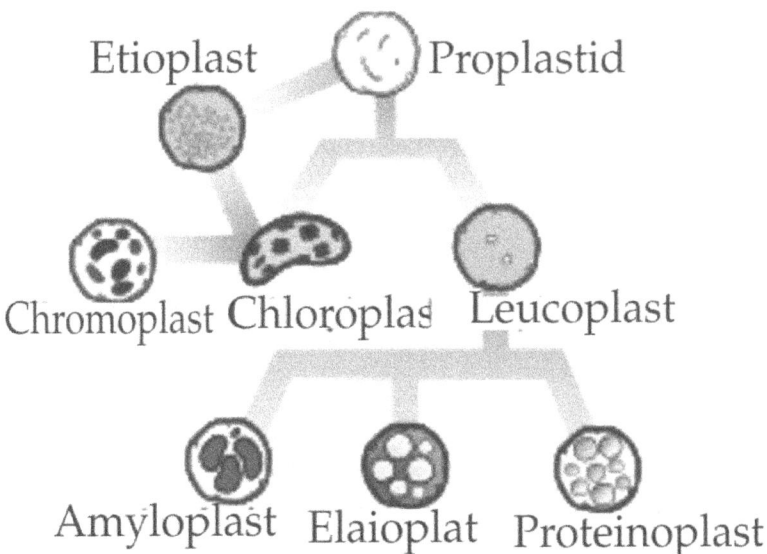

Etioplast · Proplastid · Chromoplast · Chloroplast · Leucoplast · Amyloplast · Elaioplat · Proteinoplast

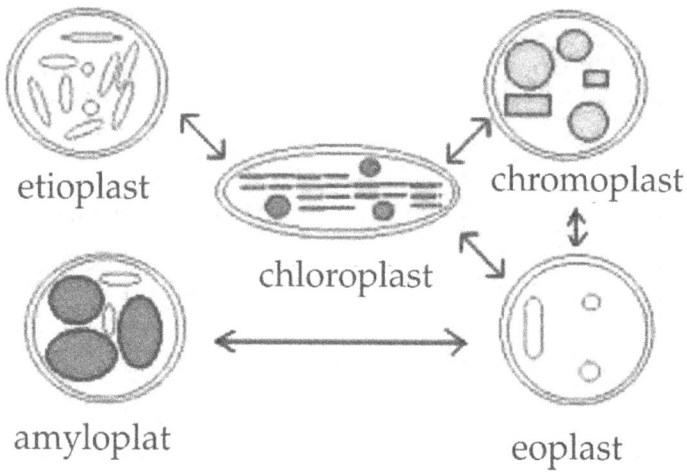

etioplast   chromoplast

chloroplast

amyloplat   eoplast

Figure 2.19:

Leucoplast

Leucoplasts are a category of plastid and as such are organelles found in plant cells. They are non-pigmented, in contrast to other plastids such as the chloroplast. Lacking pigments, leucoplasts are not green so they are predictably located in roots and non-photosynthetic tissues of plants. They may become specialized for bulk storage of starch, lipid or protein and are then known as amyloplasts, elaioplasts or proteinoplasts respectively. However, in many cell types, leucoplasts do not have a major storage function and are present to provide a wide range of essential biosynthetic functions, including the synthesis of fatty acids, many amino acids and tetrapyrrole compounds such as haem. In general, leucoplasts are much smaller than chloroplasts and have a variable morphology, often described as amoeboid. Extensive networks of stromules interconnecting leucoplasts have been observed in epidermal cells of roots, hypocotyls and petals and in callus and suspension culture cells of tobacco. In some cell types at certain stages of development, leucoplasts are clustered around the nucleus with stromules extending to the cell periphery, as observed for proplastids in the root meristem. Etioplasts, which are pre-granal, immature chloroplasts but can also be chloroplasts that have been deprived of light, lack active pigment and can be considered leucoplasts. After several minutes of exposure to light, etioplasts begin to transform into functioning chloroplasts and cease being leucoplasts.

Plasmodesmata

Plasmodesmata are microscopic channels which traverse the cell walls of plant cells and some algal cells, enabling transport and communication between them. Species that have plasmodesmata include members of the Charophyceae, Charales and Coleochaetales which are all algae as well as all embryophytes better known as

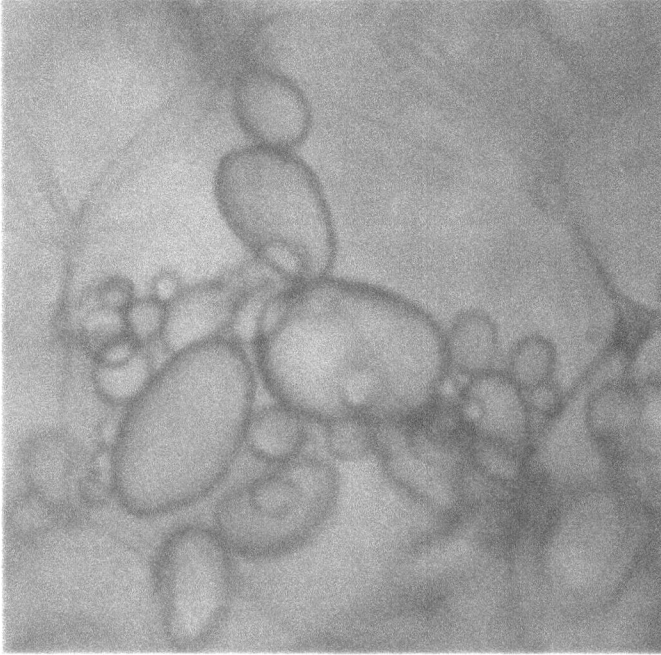

Figure 2.20 : Leucoplasts

land plants. Unlike animal cells, every plant cell is surrounded by a polysaccharide cell wall. Neighbouring plant cells are therefore separated by a pair of cell walls and the intervening lamella, forming an extracellular domain known as the apoplast. Although cell walls are permeable to small soluble proteins and other solutes, plasmodesmata enable direct, regulated, symplastic intercellular transport of substances between cells. There are two forms of plasmodesmata: primary ones are formed during cell division and secondary ones can form between mature cells. Plasmodesma allows molecules to travel between plant cells through the symplastic pathway. Similar structures, called gap junctions and membrane nanotubes, interconnect animal cells and stromules form between plastids in plant cells.

Plasmodesmata are formed when portions of the endoplasmic reticulum are trapped across the middle lamella as new cell wall is laid down between two newly divided plant cells and these eventually become the cytoplasmic connections between cells (primary plasmodesmata). Here the wall is not thickened further and depressions or thin areas known as pits are formed in the walls. Pits normally pair up between adjacent cells. Alternatively, plasmodesmata can be inserted into existing cell walls between non-dividing cells known as secondary plasmodesmata.

Plasmodesmatal Plasma Membrane: A typical plant cell may have between 10^3 and 10^5 plasmodesmata connecting it with adjacent cells equating to between 1 and 10 per μm^2. Plasmodesmata are approximately 50-60 nm in diameter at the mid-point and are constructed of three main layers, the plasma membrane, the cytoplasmic sleeve and the desmotubule. They can transverse cell walls that are up to 90 nm thick.The plasma membrane portion of the plasmodesma is a continuous extension of the cell membrane or plasmalemma. It is similar in structure to the cellular phospholipid bilayers.

Cytoplasmic sleeve: The cytoplasmic sleeve is a fluid-filled space enclosed by the plasmalemma and a continuous extension of the cytosol. Trafficking of molecules and ions through plasmodesmata occurs through this passage. Smaller molecules *e.g.* sugars and amino acids and ions can easily pass through plasmodesmata by diffusion without the need for additional chemical energy. Proteins can also pass through the cytoplasmic sleeve *e.g.* Green fluorescent protein. It is not yet known how the selective transport of larger molecules, such as proteins, occurs. One hypothesis is that the polysaccharide callose accumulates around the neck region of plasmodesmata to form a collar, reducing their diameter and thereby controlling permeability to substances in the cytoplasm.

Desmotubule: The desmotubule is a tube of appressed endoplasmic reticulum that runs between two adjacent cells. Some molecules are known to be transported through this channel, but it is not thought to be the main route for plasmodesmatal transport. Around the desmotubule and the plasma membrane areas of an electron dense material have been seen, often joined together by spoke-like structures that seem to split the plasmodesma into smaller channels. These structures may be composed of myosin and actin, which are part of the cell's cytoskeleton. If this is the case these proteins could be used in the selective transport of large molecules between the two cells.

Transport: Plasmodesmata have been shown to transport proteins (including transcription factors), short interfering RNA, messenger RNA and viral genomes from cell to cell. One example of viral movement proteins is the tobacco mosaic virus MP-30. MP-30 is thought to bind to the virus's own genome and shuttle it from infected cells to uninfected cells through plasmodesmata. The size of molecules that can pass through plasmodesmata is determined by the size exclusion limit. This limit is highly variable and can is subject to active modification. MP-30 is able to increase the size exclusion limit from 700 Daltons to 9400 Daltons thereby aiding its movement through a plant. Several models for possible active transport through plasmodesmata exist. It has been suggested that such transport is mediated by interactions with proteins localized on the desmotubule and/or by chaperones partially unfolding proteins, allowing them to fit through the narrow passage. A similar mechanism may be involved in transporting viral nucleic acids through the plasmodesmata

Cytoskeleton

The cytoskeleton is cellular scaffolding or skeleton contained within a cell's cytoplasm and is made out of protein. The cytoskeleton is present in all cells. It has structures such as flagella, cilia and lamellipodia and plays important roles in both intracellular transport *e.g.* movement of vesicles and organelles and cellular division. In 1903 Nikolai K. Koltsov proposed that the shape of cells was determined by a network of tubules which he termed the cytoskeleton. The concept of a protein mosaic that dynamically coordinated cytoplasmic biochemistry was proposed by Rudolph

Peters in 1929 while the term (cytosquelette in French) was first introduced by French embryologist Paul Wintrebert in 1931.

Eukaryotic Cytoskeleton

Eukaryotic cells contain three main kinds of cytoskeletal filaments, which are microfilaments, intermediate filaments and microtubules. The cytoskeleton provides the cell with structure and shape and by excluding macromolecules from some of the cytosol it adds to the level of macromolecular crowding in this compartment. Cytoskeletal elements interact extensively and intimately with cellular membranes.

Microfilaments (Actin Filaments): These are the thinnest filaments of the cytoskeleton. They are composed of linear polymers of actin subunits and generate force by elongation at one end of the filament coupled with shrinkage at the other, causing net movement of the intervening strand. They also act as tracks for the movement of myosin molecules that attach to the microfilament and walk along them.

Intermediate Filaments: These filaments, around 10 nanometers in diameter, are more stable (strongly bound) than actin filaments and heterogeneous constituents of the cytoskeleton. Like actin filaments, they function in the maintenance of cell-shape by bearing tension (microtubules, by contrast, resist compression. It may be useful to think of micro- and intermediate filaments as cables and of microtubules as cellular support beams). Intermediate filaments organize the internal tridimensional structure of the cell, anchoring organelles and serving as structural components of the nuclear lamina and sarcomeres. They also participate in some cell-cell and cell-matrix junctions.

Different intermediate filaments are:

* Made of vimentins, being the common structural support of many cells.

* Made of keratin, found in skin cells, hair and nails.

* Neurofilaments of neural cells.

* Made of lamin, giving structural support to the nuclear envelope.

Microtubules : Microtubules are hollow cylinders about 23 nm in diameter (lumen = approximately 15 nm in diameter), most commonly comprising 13 protofilaments which, in turn, are polymers of alpha and beta tubulin. They have a very dynamic behaviour, binding GTP for polymerization. They are commonly organized by the centrosome. In nine triplet sets (star-shaped), they form the centrioles and in nine doublets oriented about two additional microtubules (wheel-shaped) they form cilia and flagella. The latter formation is commonly referred to as a 9+2 arrangement, wherein each doublet is connected to another by the protein dynein. As both flagella and cilia are structural components of the cell and are maintained by microtubules, they can be considered part of the cytoskeleton. They play key roles in:

* Intracellular transport (associated with dyneins and kinesins, they transport organelles like mitochondria or vesicles).

* The axoneme of cilia and flagella.

- The mitotic spindle.

- Synthesis of the cell wall in plants.

Table 11: Comparison of Cytoskeleton Type

S. No.	Cytoskeleton type	Diameter (nm)	Structure	Subunit examples
1.	Microfilaments	6	double helix	actin
2.	Intermediate filaments	10	two anti-parallel helices/ dimers, forming tetramers	• vimentin (mesenchyme) · • glial fibrillary acidic protein (glial cells) · • neurofilament proteins (neuronal processes) · • keratins (epithelial cells) • nuclear lamins
3.	Microtubules	23	protofilaments, in turn consisting of tubulin subunits	a- and B-tubulin

Prokaryotic Cytoskeleton

The cytoskeleton was previously thought to be a feature only of eukaryotic cells, but homologues to all the major proteins of the eukaryotic cytoskeleton have recently been found in prokaryotes. Although the evolutionary relationships are so distant that they are not obvious from protein sequence comparisons alone, the similarity of their three dimensional structures and similar functions in maintaining cell shape and polarity provides strong evidence that the eukaryotic and prokaryotic cytoskeletons are truly homologous.

FtsZ: FtsZ was the first protein of the prokaryotic cytoskeleton to be identified. Like tubulin, FtsZ forms filaments in the presence of GTP, but these filaments do not group into tubules. During cell division, FtsZ is the first protein to move to the division site and is essential for recruiting other proteins that synthesize the new cell wall between the dividing cells.

MreB and ParM: Prokaryotic actin-like proteins, such as MreB, are involved in the maintenance of cell shape. All non-spherical bacteria have genes encoding actin-like proteins and these proteins form a helical network beneath the cell membrane that guides the proteins involved in cell wall biosynthesis. Some plasmids encode a partitioning system that involves an actin-like protein ParM. Filaments of ParM exhibit dynamic instability and may partition plasmid DNA into the dividing daughter cells by a mechanism analogous to that used by microtubules during eukaryotic mitosis.

Crescentin: The bacterium *Caulobacter crescentus* contains a third 3rd protein crescentin that is related to the intermediate filaments of eukaryotic cells. Crescentin is also involved in maintaining cell shape, such as helical and vibrioid forms of bacteria, but the mechanism by which it does this is currently unclear.

Microtrabeculae: A fourth eukaryotic cytoskeletal element microtrabeculae was proposed by Keith Porter based on images obtained from high-voltage electron microscopy of whole cells in the 1970s. The images showed short, filamentous structures of unknown molecular composition associated with known cytoplasmic structures. Porter proposed that this microtrabecular structure represented a novel filamentous network distinct from microtubules, filamentous actin or intermediate filaments. It is now generally accepted that microtrabeculae are nothing more than an artifact of certain types of fixation treatment, although we have yet to fully understand the complexity of the cell's cytoskeleton.

Cell Movement

Cell movement referred to as cytoplasmic streaming and external referred to as motility. Internal movements of organelles are governed by actin filaments and other components of the cytoskeleton. These filaments make an area in which organelles such as chloroplasts can move. Internal movement is known as cytoplasmic streaming. External movement of cells is determined by special organelles for locomotion. The cytoskeleton is a network of connected filaments and tubules. It extends from the nucleus to the plasma membrane. Electron microscopic studies showed the presence of an organized cytoplasm. Immunofluorescence microscopy identifies protein fibers as a major part of this cellular feature. The cytoskeleton components maintain cell shape and allow the cell and its organelles to move. Actin filaments are long, thin fibers approximately seven nm in diameter. These filaments occur in bundles or meshlike networks. These filaments are polar, meaning there are differences between the ends of the strand. An actin filament consists of two chains of globular actin monomers twisted to form a helix. Actin filaments play a structural role, forming a dense complex web just under the plasma membrane. Actin filaments in microvilli of intestinal cells act to shorten the cell and thus to pull it out of the intestinal lumen. Likewise, the filaments can extend the cell into intestine when food is to be absorbed. In plant cells, actin filaments form tracts along which chloroplasts circulate.

Actin filaments move by interacting with myosin, the myosin combines with and splits ATP, thus binding to actin and changing the configuration to pull the actin filament forward. Similar action accounts for pinching off cells during cell division and for amoeboid movement. Intermediate filaments are between eight and eleven nm in diameter. They are between actin filaments and microtubules in size. The intermediate fibers are rope-like assemblies of fibrous polypeptides. Some of them support the nuclear envelope, while others support the plasma membrane, form cell to cell junctions. Microtubules are small hollow cylinders of 25 nm in diameter and from 200 nm-25 µm in length. These microtubules are composed of a globular protein tubulin. Assembly brings the two types of tubulin (alpha and beta) together as dimers, which arrange themselves in rows. In animal cells and most protists, a structure known as a centrosome occurs. The centrosome contains two centrioles lying at right angles to each other. Centrioles are short cylinders with a 9 + 0 pattern of microtubule triplets. Centrioles serve as basal bodies for cilia and flagella. Plant and fungal cells have a structure equivalent to a centrosome, although it does not contain centrioles. Cilia are short usually numerous, hairlike projections that can move in an undulating fashion *e.g.* the protzoan Paramecium, the cells lining the human upper respiratory tract. Flagella are longer, usually fewer in number, projections that move in whip-like fashion *e.g.* sperm cells. Cilia and flagella are similar except for length, cilia being much shorter. They both have the characteristic 9 + 2 arrangement of microtubules. Cilia and flagella move when the microtubules slide past one another. Both oif these locomotion structures have a basal body at base with thesame arrangement of microtubule triples as centrioles. Cilia and flagella grow by the addition of tubulin dimers to their tips.

Cell Junction

In multicellular organisms and particularly in epithelia, it is often necessary for neighboring cells within a tissue to be connected together. This function is provided by cell junctions. In animal cells there are three types of junctions. Those that form a tight seal between adjacent cells are known as tight junctions; those that allow communication between cells are known as gap junctions. A third class of cell junction that anchors cells together, allowing the tissue to be stretched without tearing, are called anchoring junctions. Plant cells do not have tight junctions, gap junctions or anchoring junctions but do contain a unique class of communicating junction known as plasmodesmata. Tight junctions are found wherever flow of extracellular medium is to be restricted and are particularly common in epithelial cells such as those lining the small intestine. The plasma membranes of adjacent cells are pressed together so tightly that no intercellular space exists between them. Tight junctions between the epithelial cells of the intestine ensure that the only way that molecules can get from the lumen of the intestine to the blood supply that lies beneath is by passing through the cells, a route that can be selective. Gap junctions are specialized structures that allow cell-to-cell communication in animals. When two cells form a gap junction, ions and small molecules can pass directly from the cytosol of one cell to the cytosol of the other cell without going into the extracellular fluid. Since ions can move through the junction, changes in electrical voltage are also rapidly transmitted from cell to cell by this route. The structure that makes this possible is the gap junction channel. Channels are water-filled holes through membranes. When two gap junction channels or connexons meet, they form a water-filled tube that runs all the way through the plasma membrane of the first cell, across the small gap between the cells and through the plasma membrane of the second cell. In the middle of the channel is a continuous hole about 1.5 nm in diameter. This hole is large enough to allow small ions through and therefore to pass electrical current together with amino acids and nucleotides, but it is too small for proteins or nucleic acids. Gap junctions are especially important in the heart, where they allow an electrical signal to pass rapidly between all the cardiac muscle cells, ensuring that they all contract at the proper time. Each gap junction channel is composed of six protein subunits that can twist against each other to open and close the central channel in a process called gating that allows the cell to control the degree to which it shares solute with its neighbor. The plasmodesmata that perforate the cell walls of many plant tissues serve much the same purpose as the gap junctions of animal cells but are much bigger and cannot shut quickly. Some plant viruses use plasmodesmata to spread from cell to cell.

Table 2.6: Summary of Organelles

S.No.	Organelle		Properties
1.	Chromosomes	i.	Usually in the form of chromatin
		ii.	Contains genetic information
		iii.	Composed of DNA
		iv.	Thicken for cellular divisionv. Set number per species (*i.e.* 23 pairs for human)
2..	Nuclear membrane	i.	Surrounds nucleus
		ii.	Composed of two layers
		iii.	Numerous openings for nuclear traffic
3.	Nucleolus	i.	Spherical shape
		ii.	Visible when cell is not dividing
		iii.	Contains RNA for protein manufacture
4.	Centrioles	i.	Paired cylindrical organelles near nucleus
		ii.	Composed of nine tubes, each with three tubules
		iii.	Involved in cellular divisioniv. Lie at right angles to each other
5.	Chloroplasts	i.	A plastid usually found in plant cells
		ii.	Contain green chlorophyll where photosynthesis takes place
6.	Cytoskeleton	i.	Composed of microtubules
		ii.	Supports cell and provides shape
		iii.	Aids movement of materials in and out of cells
7.	Endoplasmic reticulum	i.	Tubular network fused to nuclear membrane
		ii.	Goes through cytoplasm onto cell membrane
		iii.	Stores, separates and serves as cell's transport systemiv.Smooth type: lacks ribosomes
		v.	Rough type: ribosomes embedded in surface
8.	Golgi apparatus	i.	Protein packaging plant
		ii.	A membrane structure found near nucleus
		iii.	Composed of numerous layers forming a sac
9.	Lysosome	i.	Digestive 'plant' for proteins, lipids and carbohydrates
		ii.	Transports undigested material to cell membrane for removal
		iii.	Vary in shape depending on process being carried outi
		v.	Cell breaks down if lysosome explodes
10.	Mitochondria	i.	Second largest organelle with unique genetic structure

Contd....

Table 2.6 : Contd...

S.No.	Organelle		Properties
		ii.	Double-layered outer membrane with inner folds called cristae
		iii.	Energy-producing chemical reactions take place on cristaei
		v.	Controls level of water and other materials in cellv. Recycles and decomposes proteins, fats and carbohydrates and forms urea
11.	Ribosomes	i.	Each cell contains thousands
		ii.	Miniature protein factories
		iii.	Composes 25% of cell's mass
		iv.	Stationary type: embedded in rough endoplasmic reticulum
		v.	Mobile type: injects proteins directly into cytoplasm
12.	Vacuoles	i.	Membrane-bound sacs for storage, digestion and waste remova
		Lii.	Contains water solution
		iii.	Contractile vacuoles for water removal (in unicellular organisms)
13.	Cell wall	i.	Most commonly found in plant cells
		ii.	Controls turgity
		iii.	Extracellular structure surrounding plasma membrane
		iv.	Primary cell wall: extremely elastic
		v.	Secondary cell wall: forms around primary cell wall after growth is complete
14.	Plasma membrane	i.	Outer membrane of cell that controls cellular traffic
		ii.	Contains proteins that span through the membrane and allow passage of materials
		iii.	Proteins are surrounded by a phospholipid bi-layer.

Summary

1. A plasma membrane and ribosomes are the only two structural features common to cells of all three groups.

2. Organelles are found only in eukaryotic cells, where they play indispensable roles in the compartmentalization of function.

3. Bacterial and archaeal cells are relatively small and structurally less complex than eukaryotic cells, lacking the internal membrane systems and organelles of eukaryotes.

4. Cells are bounded by membranes while cell functions are compartmentalized into membrane bound organelles. Membranes are made of phospholipids and protein.

5. Besides the plasma membrane and ribosomes common to all cells, eukaryotic cells have a nucleus that houses most of the cell's DNA, a variety of organelles

and the cytosol with its cytoskeleton of microtubules, microfilaments and intermediate filaments.

6. The plant cells have a rigid cell wall and animal cells are usually surrounded by a strong but flexible extracellular matrix of collagen and proteoglycans.

7. The nucleus contains the cell's DNA complexed with protein in the form of chromatin, which condenses during cell division to form the visible structures we call chromosomes. The nucleus is surrounded by a double membrane called the nuclear envelope, which has pores that allow the regulated exchange of macromolecules with the cytoplasm.

8. Solutes with a significant solubility in hydrophobic solvents can pass across biological membranes by simple diffusion.

9. The extracellular matrix is found on the outside of animal cells. A cellulose-based cell wall is found outside plant cells.

10. Turgor pressure gives nonlignified plant tissue its stiffness.

11. Tight junctions prevent the passage of extracellular water or solute between the cells of an epithelium.

12. Gap junctions allow solute and electrical current to pass from the cytosol of one cell to the cytosol of its neighbor.

13. The nucleus, mitochondrion and chloroplast are bounded by double-membrane envelopes. In the case of the nucleus, this is perforated by nuclear pores. All three organelles contain DNA.

14. Mitochondria, which are surrounded by a double membrane, oxidize food molecules to provide the energy used to make ATP. Mitochondria also contain ribosomes and their own circular DNA molecules.

15. Chloroplasts trap solar energy and use it to fix carbon dioxide into organic form and convert it to sugar.

16. Chloroplasts are surrounded by a double membrane and have an extensive system of internal membranes called the thylakoids, in which most of the components involved in ATP generation are found.

17. Chloroplasts also contain ribosomes and circular DNA molecules.

18. The endoplasmic reticulum is an extensive network of membranes that are known as either rough ER or smooth ER.

19. Rough ER is studded with ribosomes and is responsible for the synthesis of secretory and membrane proteins, whereas smooth ER is involved in lipid synthesis and drug detoxification.

20. Proteins synthesized on the rough ER are further processed and packaged in the Golgi complex and are then transported either to membranes or to the surface of the cell via secretory vesicles.

21. Lysosomes contain hydrolytic enzymes and are involved in cellular digestion. They were the first organelles to be discovered on the basis of their function rather than their morphology. Because of their close functional relationships,

the ER, Golgi complex, secretory vesicles and lysosomes are collectively called the endomembrane system.

22. Peroxisomes are about the same size as lysosomes and both generate and degrade hydrogen peroxide.

23. Animal peroxisomes play an important role in catabolizing long chain fatty acids. In plants, specialized peroxisomes known as glyoxysomes are involved in the process of photorespiration and in converting stored fat into carbohydrate during seed germination.

24. Ribosomes are sites of protein synthesis in all cells. The striking similarities between mitochondrial and chloroplast ribosomes and those of bacteria and cyanobacteria, respectively, lend strong support to the endosymbiont theory that these organelles are of bacterial origin.

25. The cytoskeleton is an extensive network of microtubules, microfilaments and intermediate filaments that gives eukaryotic cells their distinctive shapes.

26. The cytoskeleton is also important in cellular motility and the intracellular movement of cellular structures and materials.

Chapter 3
Biomolecules

Introduction

The scientific study of heredity is called genetics. The modern approach to genetics can be traced to the mid-nineteenth century with Gregor Mendel's careful analyses of inheritance in peas. Mendel's experiments were simple and direct and brought forth the most significant principles that determine how traits are passed from one generation to the next. Mendel's experiments which occupied most of genetic research until the middle of 20th century are called transmission genetics. Some people have called it formal genetics, because the subject can be understood and the rules clearly seen without any reference to the biochemical nature of genes or gene products. Beginning about 1900, geneticists began to wonder about a subject molecular genetics. Is the gene a known kind of molecule? How can genetic information be encoded in a molecule? How is the genetic information transmitted from one generation to the next? In what way is the genetic information changed in a mutant organism? At that time, there was no logical starting point for such an investigation, no experimental handle. In the 1940s, critical observations were made that implicated the molecule deoxyribonucleic acid (DNA), first discovered in 1869 by F. Mischer. Since the early 1970s, genetics has undergone another revolution: the development of recombinant DNA technology. This technology is a collection of methods that enable genes to be transferred, at the will of the molecular geneticist, from one organism to another. This branch of genetics is known as genetic engineering.

The members of any biological species are similar in some characteristics but different in others *e.g.* all human beings share a set of observable characteristics or traits that define as a species. Man has a backbone and a spinal cord; these traits are among those that define us as a type of vertebrate. Human are warm blooded and feed our young with milk from mammary glands; these traits are among those that define us as a type of mammal. Human beings are a type of primate that habitually stands upright and has long legs, relatively little body hair, a large brain, a flat face with a prominent nose, jutting chin, distinct lips and small teeth. These traits set us apart from other primates, such as chimpanzees and gorillas. The biological characteristics that define us as a species are inherited, but they do not differ from one person to the next. Within the human species, however, there is also much variation. Traits such as hair color, eye color, skin color, height, weight and personality characteristics are tremendously variable from one person to the next. There is also variation in health related traits, such as predisposition to high blood pressure, diabetes, chemical dependence, mental depression and the Alzheimer disease. Some of these traits are inherited biologically, others are inherited culturally. Eye color results from biological inheritance. Many traits are influenced jointly by biological inheritance and environmental factors. The weight is determined in part by inheritance but also in part by eating habits and level of physical activity. The study of biologically inherited traits is genetics. Among the traits studied in genetics are those that are influenced in part by the environment. The fundamental concept of genetics is Inherited traits are determined by elements of heredity called genes that are transmitted from parents to offspring in reproduction. The elements of heredity and some basic rules governing their transmission from generation to generation were discovered by Gregor Mendel in experiments with garden peas. His results were published in 1866. Mendel's experiments are among the most beautifully designed, carefully executed and elegantly interpreted in the history of experimental science. Mendel interpreted his data in terms of a few abstract rules by which hereditary elements are transmitted from parents to offspring. Three years later, in 1869, Friedrich Miescher discovered a new type of weakly acid substance, abundant in the nuclei of salmon sperm and white blood cells. At the time he had no way of knowing that it would turn out to be the chemical substance of which genes are made. Miescher's weak acid, the chemical substance of the gene, is now called deoxyribonucleic acid (DNA). However, the connection between DNA and heredity was not demonstrated until about the middle of the twentieth century.

DNA: Genetic Material

The importance of the cell nucleus in inheritance became apparent in 1870s with the observation that the nuclei of male and female reproductive cells fuse in the process of fertilization. This observation suggested that there was something inside the sperm and egg nucleus that was responsible for inherited characteristics. The next major advance was the discovery of thread like objects inside the nucleus that become visible in the light microscope when stained with certain dyes; these threads were called chromosomes. By 1900 it had become clear that the number of chromosomes is constant within each species but differs among species. The characteristics of chromosomes made it seem likely that they were the carriers of the genes. By the 1920s, more and more evidence suggested a close relationship between DNA and the genetic material. Studies using special stains showed that DNA, in addition to certain proteins, is present in chromosomes. Furthermore, investigations disclosed that almost all cells of a given species contain a constant amount of DNA, whereas the amount and kinds of proteins and other molecules differ greatly in different cell types. The indirect evidence that genes are DNA was rejected because crude chemical analyses of DNA had suggested that it lacks the chemical diversity needed for a genetic substance. In contrast, proteins were known to be an exceedingly diverse collection of molecules. And so, on the basis of incorrect data, it became widely accepted that proteins were the genetic material and that DNA merely provided the structural framework of chromosomes. Against the prevailing opinion that genes are proteins, experiments purporting to demonstrate that DNA is the genetic material had also to demonstrate that proteins are not the genetic material.

Experimental Proof of Genetic Function of DNA

An important first step was taken by Frederick Griffith in 1928 when he demonstrated that a physical trait can be passed from one cell to another. He was working with two strains of the bacterium *Streptococcus pneumoniae* identified as S and R. When a bacterial cell is grown on solid medium, it undergoes repeated cell divisions to form a visible clump of cells called a colony. The S type of *S. pneumoniae* synthesizes a gelatinous capsule composed of complex carbohydrate (polysaccharide). The enveloping capsule makes each colony large and gives it a glistening or smooth (S) appearance. This capsule also enables the bacterium to cause pneumonia by protecting it from the defense mechanisms of an infected animal. The R strains of *S. pneumonia* are unable to synthesize the capsular polysaccharide; they form small colonies that have a rough (R) surface. This strain of the bacterium does not cause pneumonia, because without the capsule the bacteria are inactivated by the immune system of the host. Both types of bacteria breed true in the sense that the progeny formed by cell division have the capsular type of the parent, either S or R. Mice injected with living S cells get pneumonia. Mice injected either with living R cells or with heat-killed S cells remain healthy. Here is Griffith's critical finding: mice injected with a mixture of living R cells and heat-killed S cells contract the disease they often die of pneumonia. Bacteria isolated from blood samples of these dead mice produce S cultures with a capsule typical of the injected S cells, even though the injected S cells had been killed by heat. Evidently, the injected material from the dead S cells includes a substance that can be transferred to living R cells and confers the ability to resist the immunological system of the mouse and cause pneumonia. In other words, the R bacteria can be changed or undergo transformation into S bacteria.

The new characteristics are inherited by descendants of the transformed bacteria. Transformation in *Streptococcus* was originally discovered in 1928, but it was not until 1944 that the chemical substance responsible for changing the R cells into S cells was identified. In a milestone experiment, Oswald Avery, Colin MacLeod and Maclyn McCarty showed that the substance causing the transformation of R cells into S cells was DNA. In doing these experiments, they first had to develop chemical procedures for isolating almost pure DNA from cells, which had never been done before. When they added DNA isolated from S cells to growing cultures of R cells, they observed transformation: A few cells of type S cells were produced. Although the DNA preparations contained traces of protein and RNA, the transforming activity was not altered by treatments that destroyed either protein or RNA. However, treatments that destroyed DNA eliminated the transforming activity. These experiments

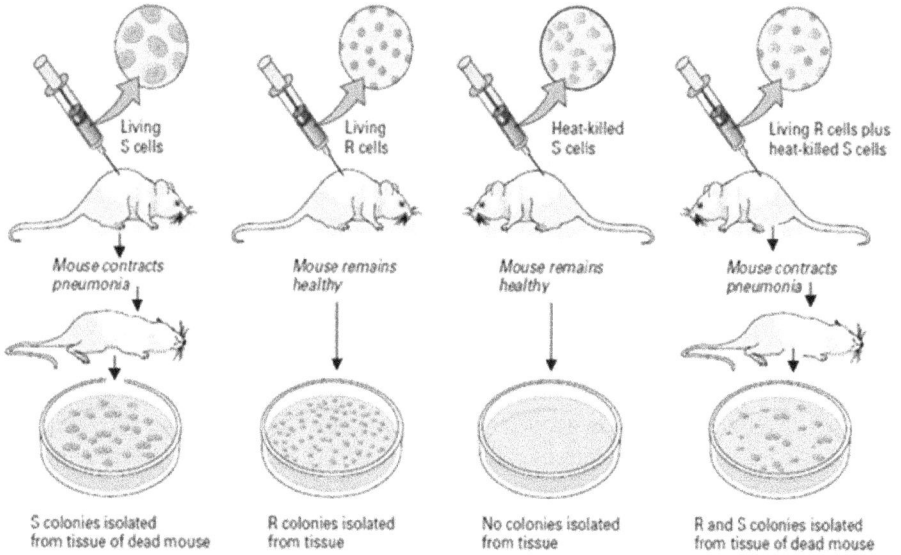

Figure 3.1: Transformation Experiment of Griffith

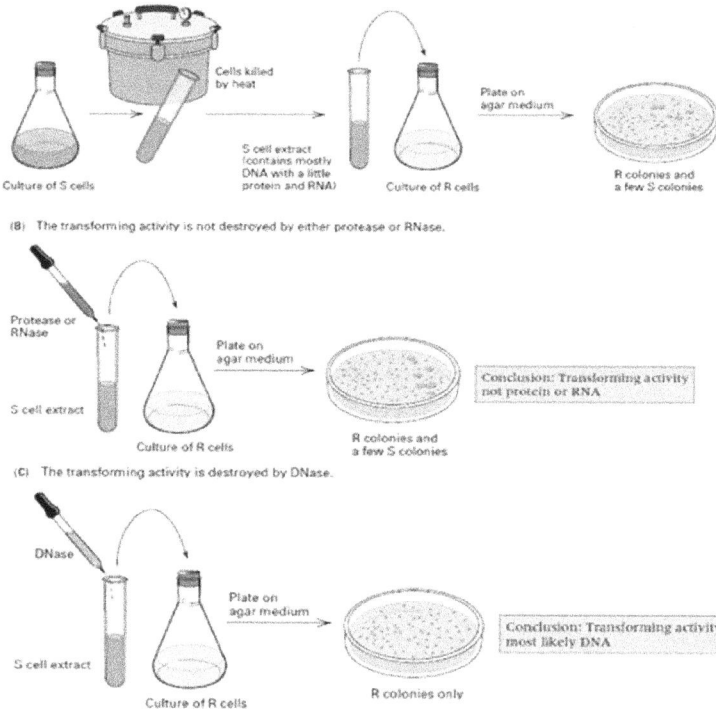

Figure 3.2: Transformation Experiment of Avery, MacLeod and McCarty

implied that the substance responsible for genetic transformation was the DNA of the cell; hence the DNA is the genetic material and play vital role in heredity.

Chromosome Structure

A chromosome is a long strand of DNA that contains certain genes. These genes are portions of the DNA strand and carry the genetic information of the cell. In a eukaryotic cell there are multiple chromosomes and each of these is part of a pair. Both of the chromosomes in a pair contain the genes for the same trait. However, a prockaryotic cell has a long circular chromosome that contains all of the genes of the cell. Cells in the human body are eukaryotic and contain twenty-three pairs of chromosomes. Other organisms have a different chromosome count. Each chromosome of a pair stands for the same traits as its counterpart.

All essential bacterial genes are found in a single, circular, double stranded DNA chromosome located in the nucleoid region of the cytoplasm. The bacterial chromosome is believed to be attached to the plasma membrane and specifies between 1,000 and 5,000 proteins. It is highly condensed and consists of DNA, RNA and protein. In addition, there may be one or more plasmids. Plasmids are small circular pieces of extra chromosomal DNA which may encode 20-100 proteins. The genes of eukaryotes are distributed among a number of linear chromosomes that vary in size and number. Eukaryotic chromosomes are condensed by packing the DNA to different degrees. Nucleosomes consist of DNA wound twice around an octet of proteins called histones (two each of H2a, H2b, H3 and H4). Approximately 200 base pairs (bp) of the DNA are wound around the spherical bodies formed by the histones and about 50 bp of DNA connect the nucleosomes.

Further compaction may be accomplished by histone H1 binding, which induces the nucleosomes to associate into a ring of six nucleosomes and the rings to associate into a cylinder called a solenoid. Phosphorylation of histone H1 results in the dissociation of the solenoid into an extended nucleosome form. The so lenoid is the form in which most of the cell's DNA exists during interphase. However, further packing can occur by certain proteins binding the solenoid and stimulating it to loop back and forth from a central core of proteins called a scaffold. Dephosphorylation of topoisomerase II and other proteins causes dissociation of the scaffold and results in the decondensation of the chromosomes to the solenoid form. In some eukaryotes, 18 loops of the solenoid form a disklike structure and the chromosome condenses as hundreds of disks stack together. This is the form that is predominant during nuclear division.

Heterochromatin is highly condensed DNA that remains in the solenoid form throughout the cell cyle except during DNA replication, when it decondenses. Most of the genes associated with heterochromatin are not expressed because of the DNA's condensed state. In contrast, euchromatin is decondensed DNA that exists in the solenoid form or in an extended nucleosome form. A centromere is a highly constricted region of a mitotic or meiotic chromosome where the spindle fibers attach. Complex sequences of DNA constitute centromeres. If the centromere is in the middle of the chromosome, the chromosome is said to be metacentric. If the centromere is near the tip, it is called telocentric. The short and long arms of the chromosome with respect to

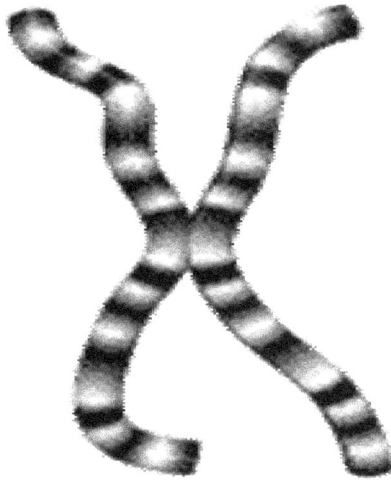

Figure 3.3: Chromosome Structure

the centromere are designated as p and q respectively. Each chromosome has a specific pattern of dark and light regions called bands. Homologous chromosomes have the same banding pattern. Protein complexes associated with the centromeric regions are called kinetochores. Kinetochores bind microtubules of the spindle bundle and function to distribute chromosomes as cells proliferate. Propagation and maintenance of any piece of DNA requires the presence of one or more origin of replication sites (*OriR*) and special ends called telomeres. Origin of replication sites are special sequences where DNA replication initiates. Telomeres protect the ends of linear chromosomes from cellular enzymes that degrade nucleic acids from their ends. Chromosomes can be aligned with their pairs into a karyotype. The arrangement of pair of chromosomes by their size, shape and bands or centromere is called Karyotyping.

Table 3.1: Number of Chromosomes

S. No.	Organism	No. of Chromosome Pairs
1.	Tomato	12 Pairs
2.	Mouse	20 Pairs
3.	Human	23 Pairs
4.	Dog	39 Pairs

Deoxyribo Nucleic Acid (DNA)

Deoxyribonucleic acid is an extremely long polymer made from units called deoxyribonucleotides which are simply called nucleotides. Deoxyribo nucleic acid is a nucleic acid that contains the genetic instructions used in the development and functioning of all known living organisms with the exception of RNA viruses. The DNA segments that carry this genetic information are called genes but other DNA sequences have structural purposes or are involved in regulating the use of this genetic information. Along with RNA and proteins, DNA is one of the three major macromolecules that are essential for all known forms of life. DNA consists of two long polymers of simple units called nucleotides, with backbones made of sugars and phosphate groups joined by ester bonds. These two strands run in opposite directions to each other and are therefore anti parallel. Attached to each sugar is one of four types of molecules called nucleobases (bases). It is the sequence of these four nucleobases along the backbone that encodes information. This information is read using the genetic code, which specifies the sequence of the amino acids within proteins. The code is read by copying stretches of DNA into the related nucleic acid RNA in a process called transcription. Within cells DNA is organized into long structures called chromosomes. During cell division these chromosomes are duplicated in the process of DNA replication, providing each cell its own complete set of chromosomes. Eukaryotic organisms store most of their DNA inside the cell nucleus and some of their DNA in organelles, such as mitochondria or chloroplasts. In contrast, prokaryotes (bacteria and archaea) store their DNA only in the cytoplasm. Within the chromosomes, chromatin proteins such as histones compact and organize DNA. These compact structures guide the interactions between DNA and other proteins, helping control which parts of the DNA are transcribed.

Structure of DNA

DNA is a long polymer made from repeating units called nucleotides. As first discovered by James D. Watson and Francis Crick, the structure of DNA of all species comprises two helical chains each coiled round the same axis and each with a pitch of 34 Å (3.4 nanometres) and a radius of 10 Å (1.0 nanometres). According to another study, when measured in a particular solution, the DNA chain measured 22 to 26 Å wide (2.2 to 2.6 nanometres) and one nucleotide unit measured 3.3 Å (0.33 nm) long. Although each individual repeating unit is very small, DNA polymers can be very large molecules containing millions of nucleotides. For instance, the largest human chromosome, chromosome number 1, is approximately 220 million base pairs long. In living organisms DNA does not usually exist as a single molecule, but instead as a pair of molecules that are held tightly together. These two long strands entwine like vines, in the shape of a double helix. The nucleotide repeats contain both the segment of the backbone of the molecule, which holds the chain together and a nucleobase, which interacts with the other DNA strand in the helix. A nucleobase linked to a sugar is called a nucleoside and a base linked to a sugar and one or more phosphate groups is called a nucleotide. Polymers comprising multiple linked nucleotides are called a polynucleotide.

The backbone of the DNA strand is made from alternating phosphate and sugar residues. The sugar in DNA is 2-deoxyribose, which is a pentose (five-carbon) sugar. The sugars are joined together by phosphate groups that form phosphodiester bonds between the third and fifth carbon atoms of adjacent sugar rings. These asymmetric bonds mean a strand of DNA has a direction. In a double helix the direction of the nucleotides in one strand is opposite to their direction in the other strand: the strands are antiparallel. The asymmetric ends of DNA strands are called the 52 (five prime) and 32 (three prime) ends, with the 5' end having a terminal phosphate group and

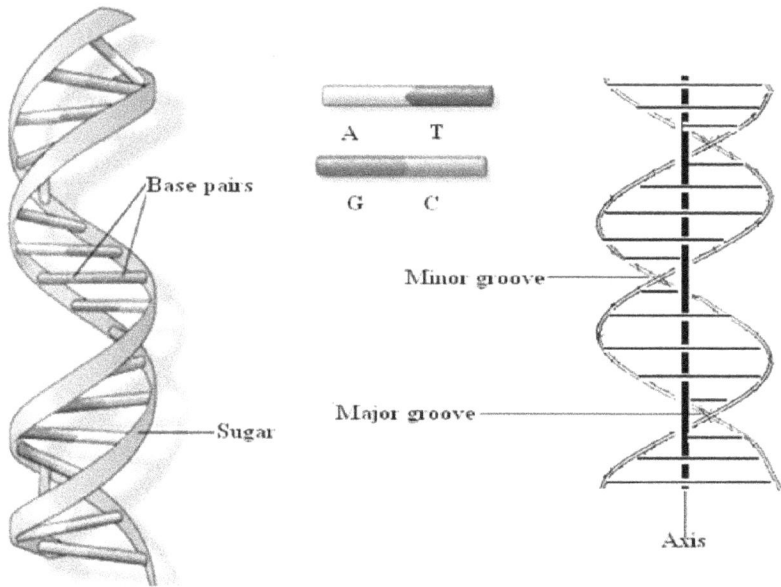

Figure 3.4: Double Helix Struture of DNA (B DNA)

the 3' end a terminal hydroxyl group. One major difference between DNA and RNA is the sugar, with the 2-deoxyribose in DNA being replaced by the alternative pentose sugar ribose in RNA. The DNA double helix is stabilized primarily by two forces: hydrogen bonds between nucleotides and base-stacking interactions among the aromatic nucleobases. In the aqueous environment of the cell, the conjugated δ bonds of nucleotide bases align perpendicular to the axis of the DNA molecule, minimizing their interaction with the solvation shell and therefore, the Gibbs free energy. The four bases found in DNA are adenine (abbreviated A), cytosine (C), guanine (G) and thymine (T). These four bases are attached to the sugar/phosphate to form the complete nucleotide, as shown for adenosine monophosphate.

The nucleobases are classified into two types: the purines, A and G, being fused five and six membered heterocyclic compounds and the pyrimidines, the six membered rings C and T. A fifth pyrimidine nucleobase, uracil (U), usually takes the place of thymine in RNA and differs from thymine by lacking a methyl group on its ring. Uracil is not usually found in DNA, occurring only as a breakdown product of cytosine. Apart from adenosine (A), cytidine (C), guanosine (G), thymidine (T) and uridine (U), DNA and RNA also contain bases that have been modified after the nucleic acid chain has been formed. In DNA, the most common modified base is 5-methylcytidine (m5C). In RNA, there are many modified bases, including pseudouridine (Ø), dihydrouridine (D), inosine (I), ribothymidine (rT) and 7-methylguanosine (m7G). Hypoxanthine and xanthine are two of the many bases created through mutagen presence, both of them through deamination *i.e.* replacement of amine group with a carbonyl group. Hypoxanthine is produced from adenine, xanthine from guanine. Similarly, deamination of cytosine results in uracil.

Types of Bases

a. Main Bases

These are incorporated into the growing chain during RNA and/or DNA synthesis.

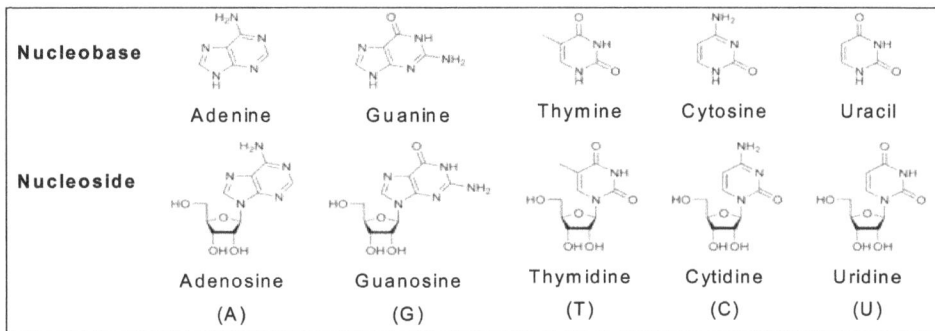

Nucleobase	Adenine	Guanine	Thymine	Cytosine	Uracil
Nucleoside	Adenosine (A)	Guanosine (G)	Thymidine (T)	Cytidine (C)	Uridine (U)

Figure 3.5a: Main Bases of DNA and RNA

b. Modified purine bases

These are examples of modified adenosine or guanosine.

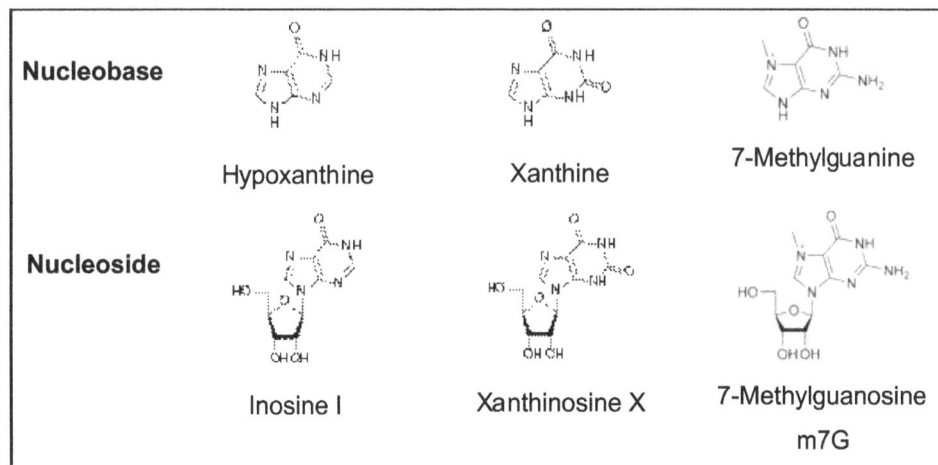

Nucleobase	Hypoxanthine	Xanthine	7-Methylguanine
Nucleoside	Inosine I	Xanthinosine X	7-Methylguanosine m7G

Figure 3.5b: Modified Purine Bases

c. Modified pyrimidine bases

These are examples of modified cytidine, thymidine or uridine.

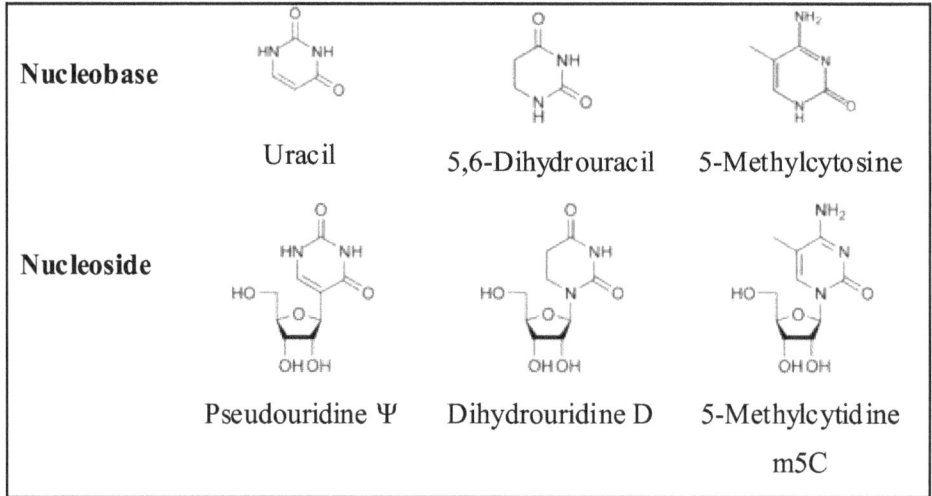

Nucleobase		
Uracil	5,6-Dihydrouracil	5-Methylcytosine
Nucleoside		
Pseudouridine Ψ	Dihydrouridine D	5-Methylcytidine m5C

Figure 3.5c: Modified Pyrimidine Base

d. Novel Bases

A vast number of nucleobase analogues exist. The most common applications are used as fluorescent probes, either directly or indirectly, such as Aminoallyl nucleotide which is used to label cRNA or cDNA in microarrays. Several groups are working on alternative extra base pairs to extend the genetic code, such as isoguanine and isocytosine or the fluorescent 2-amino-6-(2-thienyl) purine and pyrrole-2-carbaldehyde. In medicine, several nucleoside analogues are used as anticancer and antiviral agents. The viral polymerase incorporates these compounds with non-canon bases. These compounds are activated in the cells by being converted into nucleotides; they are administered as nuclosides as charged nucleotides cannot easily cross cell membranes.

Base Pairing: In a DNA double helix, each type of nucleobase on one strand normally interacts with just one type of nucleobase on the other strand. This is called complementary base pairing. At this point, purines form hydrogen bonds to pyrimidines, with A bonding only to T and C bonding only to G. This arrangement of two nucleotides binding together across the double helix is called a base pair. As hydrogen bonds are not covalent, they can be broken and rejoined relatively easily. The two strands of DNA in a double helix can therefore be pulled apart like a zipper, either by a mechanical force or high temperature. As a result of this complementarity, all the information in the double-stranded sequence of a DNA helix is duplicated on each strand, which is vital in DNA replication. Indeed, this reversible and specific interaction between complementary base pairs is critical for all the functions of DNA in living organisms. The two types of base pairs form different numbers of hydrogen bonds, AT forming two hydrogen bonds and GC forming three hydrogen bonds. DNA with high GC-content is more stable than DNA with low GC-content. Although it is often stated that this is due to the added stability of an additional hydrogen bond, this is incorrect. DNA with high GC-content is more stable due to intra-strand base stacking interactions.

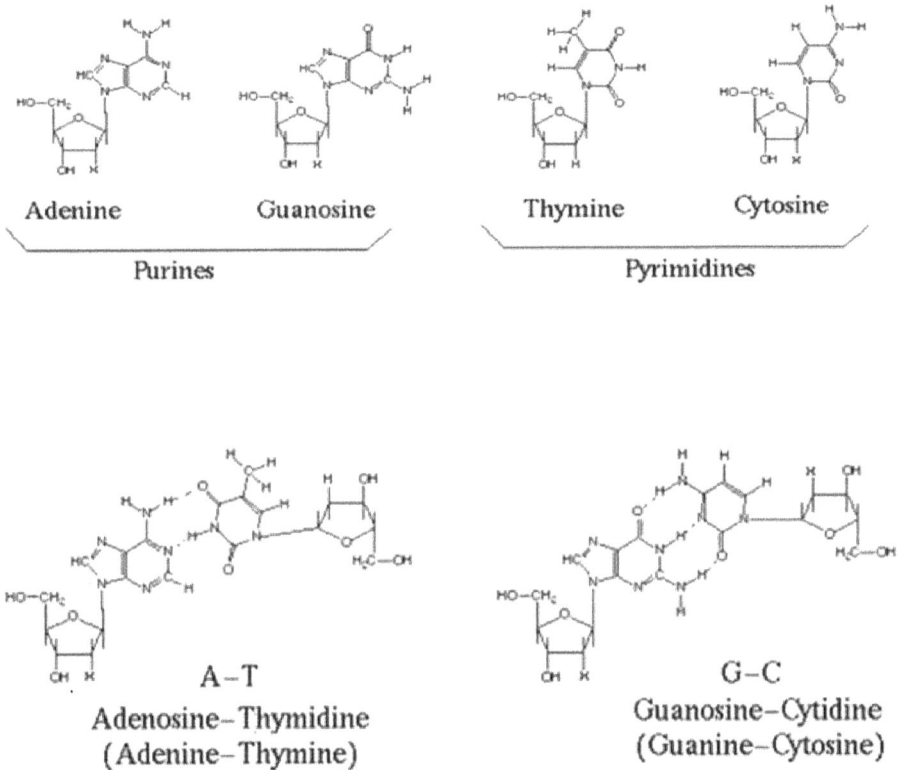

| Adenine | Guanosine | Thymine | Cytosine |

Purines   Pyrimidines

A–T
Adenosine–Thymidine
(Adenine–Thymine)

G–C
Guanosine–Cytidine
(Guanine–Cytosine)

Figure 3.6: Base Pairing

Most DNA molecules are actually two polymer strands, bound together in a helical fashion by noncovalent bonds; this double stranded structure (dsDNA) is maintained largely by the intrastrand base stacking interactions, which are strongest for G, C stacks. The two strands can come apart, a process known as melting, to form two ss DNA molecules. Melting occurs when conditions favor ssDNA; such conditions are high temperature, low salt and high pH. The low pH also melts DNA since DNA is unstable due to acid depurination; therefore low pH is rarely used. The stability of the dsDNA form depends not only on the GC-content (% G and C basepairs) but also on sequence and also length as longer molecules are more stable. The stability can be measured in various ways; a common way is the melting temperature, which is the temperature at which 50% of the ds molecules are converted to ss molecules; melting temperature is dependent on ionic strength and the concentration of DNA. As a result, it is both the percentage of GC base pairs and the overall length of a DNA double helix that determine the strength of the association between the two strands of DNA. Long DNA helices with a high GC content have stronger interacting strands while short helices with high AT content have weaker interacting strands. The parts of the DNA double helix that need to separate easily, such as the TATAAT Pribnow box in some promoters, tend to have a high AT content, making the strands easier to pull apart. The strength of this interaction can be measured by finding the temperature required to break the hydrogen bonds, their melting temperature also called T_m value. When all the base pairs in a DNA double helix melt, the strands separate and exist in solution as two entirely independent molecules. These single-stranded DNA molecules (ssDNA) have no single common shape, but some conformations are more stable than others.

Grooves : Twin helical strands form the DNA backbone. Another double helix may be found by tracing the spaces or grooves, between the strands. These voids are adjacent to the base pairs and may provide a binding site. As the strands are not directly opposite each other, the grooves are unequally sized. One groove, the major groove, is 22 Å wide and the other, the minor groove, is 12 Å wide. The narrowness of the minor groove means that the edges of the bases are more accessible in the major groove. As a result, proteins like transcription factors that can bind to specific sequences in double-stranded DNA usually make contacts to the sides of the bases exposed in the major groove. This situation varies in unusual conformations of DNA within the cell, but the major and minor grooves are always named to reflect the differences in size that would be seen if the DNA is twisted back into the ordinary B form.

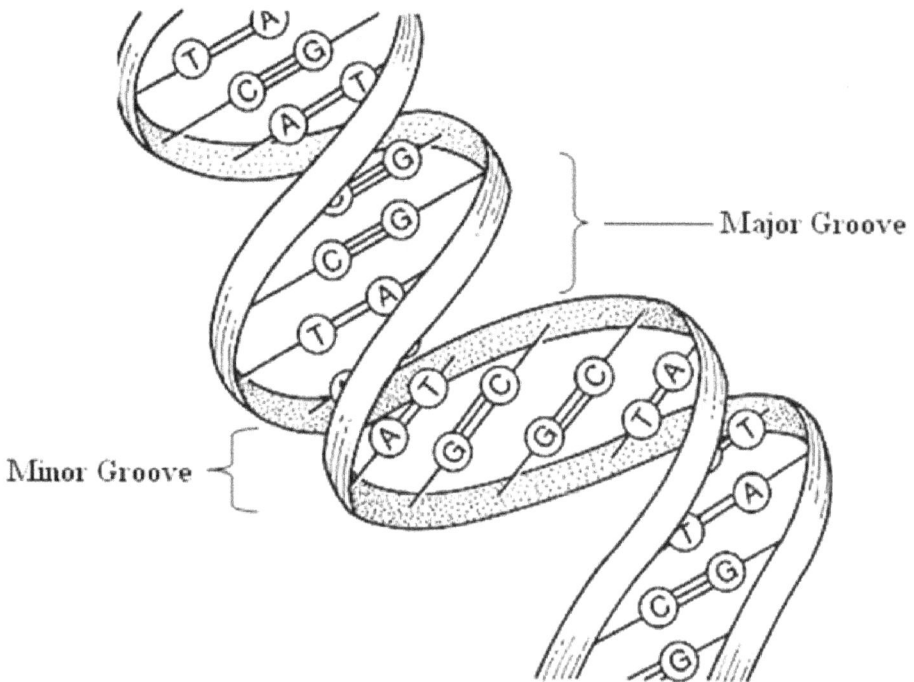

Figure 3.7: Major and Minor Grooves

Sense and Antisense: The DNA sequence is called sense if its sequence is the same as that of a messenger RNA copy that is translated into protein. The sequence on the opposite strand is called the antisense sequence. Both sense and antisense sequences can exist on different parts of the same strand of DNA *i.e.* both strands contain both sense and antisense sequences. In both prokaryotes and eukaryotes, antisense RNA sequences are produced, but the functions of these RNAs are not entirely clear. One proposal is that antisense RNAs are involved in regulating gene expression through RNA-RNA base pairing. A few DNA sequences in prokaryotes and eukaryotes and more in plasmids and viruses, blur the distinction between sense and antisense strands by having overlapping genes. In these cases, some DNA sequences do double duty, encoding one protein when read along one strand and a second protein when read in the opposite direction along the other strand. In bacteria, this overlap may be involved in the regulation of gene transcription, while in viruses, overlapping genes increase the amount of information that can be encoded within the small viral genome.

DNA Supercoiling : DNA super coiling refers to the over or under winding of a DNA strand and is an expression of the strain on the polymer. Supercoiling is important in a number of biological processes, such as compacting DNA. Additionally, certain enzymes such as topoisomerases are able to change DNA topology to facilitate functions such as DNA replication or transcription. Mathematical expressions are used to describe supercoiling by comparing different coiled states to relaxed B-form DNA. With DNA in its relaxed state, a strand usually circles the axis of the double helix once every 10.4 base pairs, but if the DNA is twisted the strands become more tightly or more loosely wound. If the DNA is twisted in the direction of the helix, this is positive supercoiling and the bases are held more tightly together. If they are twisted in the opposite direction, this is negative supercoiling and the bases come apart more easily. In nature, most DNA has slight negative supercoiling that is introduced by enzymes called topoisomerases. These enzymes are also needed to relieve the twisting stresses introduced into DNA strands during processes such as transcription and DNA replication.

Role of Supercoiling : In a relaxed double helical segment of B-DNA, the two strands twist around the helical axis once every 10.4-10.5 base pairs of sequence. Adding or subtracting twists, as some enzymes can do, imposes strain. If a DNA segment under twist strain were closed into a circle by joining its two ends and then allowed to move freely, the circular DNA would contort into a new shape such as a simple figure eight (8). Such a contortion is a supercoil. The simple figure eight is the simplest supercoil and is the shape a circular DNA assumes to accommodate one too many or one too few helical twists. The two lobes of the figure eight will appear rotated either clockwise or counterclockwise with respect to one another, depending on whether the helix is over or underwound. For each additional helical twist being accommodated, the lobes will show one more rotation about their axis. The noun form supercoil is rarely used in the context of DNA topology. Instead, global contortions of a circular DNA such as the rotation of figure eight (8) lobes are referred to as writhe. The above example illustrates that twist and writhe are interconvertible. Supercoiling is an abstract mathematical property representing the sum of twist and writhe. The twist is the number of helical turns in the DNA and the writhe is the number of times the double helix crosses over on itself. Extra helical twists are positive and lead to positive supercoiling, while subtractive twisting causes negative supercoiling. Many topoisomerase enzymes sense supercoiling and either generate or dissipate it as they change DNA topology. DNA of most organisms is negatively supercoiled.

In part because chromosomes may be very large, segments in the middle may act as if their ends are anchored. As a result, they may be unable to distribute excess twist to the rest of the chromosome or to absorb twist to recover from underwinding; the segments may become supercoiled. In response to supercoiling, they will assume an amount of writhe, just as if their ends were joined. Supercoiled DNA forms two structures; a plectoneme or a toroid or a combination of both. A negatively supercoiled DNA molecule will produce a one-start left handed helix, the toroid or a two-start right handed helix with terminal loops, the plectoneme. Plectonemes are typically more common in nature and this is the shape most bacterial plasmids will take. For larger molecules it is common for hybrid structures to form - a loop on a toroid can extend into a plectoneme. If all the loops on a toroid extend then it becomes a branch point in the plectonemic structure.

Occurrence of DNA supercoiling

DNA super coiling is important for DNA packaging within all cells. Because the length of DNA can be thousands of times that of a cell, packaging this genetic material into the cell or nucleus (in eukaryotes) is a difficult feat. Supercoiling of DNA reduces the space and allows for much more DNA to be packaged. In prokaryotes, plectonemic supercoils are predominant, because of the circular chromosome and relatively small amount of genetic material. In eukaryotes, DNA supercoiling exists on many levels of both plectonemic and solenoidal supercoils, with the solenoidal supercoiling proving most effective in compacting the DNA. Solenoidal supercoiling is achieved with histones to form a 10 nm fiber. This fiber is further coiled into a 30 nm fiber and further coiled upon itself numerous times more. DNA packaging is greatly increased during nuclear division events such as mitosis or meiosis, where DNA must be compacted and segregated to daughter cells. Condensins and cohesins are structural maintenance of chromosome proteins that aid in the condensation of sister chromatids and the linkage of the centromere in sister chromatids. These SMC proteins induce positive supercoils. Supercoiling is also required for DNA/RNA synthesis. Because DNA must be unwound for DNA/RNA polymerase action, supercoils will result. The region ahead of the polymerase complex will be unwound; this stress is compensated with positive supercoils ahead of the complex. Behind the complex, DNA is rewound and there will be compensatory negative supercoils. It is important to note that topoisomerases such as DNA gyrase (Type II Topoisomerase) play a role in relieving some of the stress during DNA/RNA synthesis.

Modeling Using Mathematics

DNA supercoiling can be described numerically by changes in the linking number (Lk). The linking number is the most descriptive property of supercoiled DNA. Lk_o, the number of turns in the relaxed (B type) DNA plasmid/molecule, is determined by dividing the total base pairs of the molecule by the relaxed bp/turn which, depending on reference is 10.4-10.5.

$Lk_o = bp \,/\, 10.4$

Lk is merely the number of crosses a single strand makes across the other in a planar projection. The topology of the DNA is described by the equation below in which the linking number is equivalent to the sum of TW, which is the number of twists or turns of the double helix and Wr which is the number of coils or 'writhes'. If there is a closed DNA molecule, the sum of TW and Wr or the linking number, does not change. However, there may be complementary changes in TW and Wr without changing their sum.

$Lk = Tw + Wr$

The change in the linking number, ÄLk, is the actual number of turns in the plasmid/molecule, Lk, minus the number of turns in the relaxed plasmid/molecule Lk_o.

$ÄLk = Lk \,''\, Lk_o$

If the DNA is negatively supercoiled ÄLk < 0. The negative supercoiling implies that the DNA is underwound. A standard expression independent of the molecule size is the specific linking difference or superhelical density denoted ó. ó represents the number of turns added or removed relative to the total number of turns in the relaxed molecule/plasmid, indicating the level of supercoiling.

$ó = ÄLk \,/\, Lk_o$

The Gibbs free energy associated with the coiling is given by the equation below

$ÄG \,/\, N = 10RTó^2$

Examples

Since the linking number L of supercoiled DNA is the number of times the two strands are intertwined (and both strands remain covalently intact), L cannot change. The reference state (or parameter) L_o of a circular DNA duplex is its relaxed state. In this state, its writhe $W = 0$. Since $L = T + W$, in a relaxed state $T = L$. Thus, if we have a 400 bp relaxed circular DNA duplex, $L \sim 40$ (assuming ~10 bp per turn in B-DNA).

Then $T \sim 40$.

Positively supercoiling:

T = 0, W = 0, then L = 0

T = +3, W = 0, then L = +3

T = +2, W = +1, then L = +3

Negatively supercoiling:

T = 0, W = 0, then L = 0

T = -3, W = 0, then L = -3

T = -2, W = -1, then L = -3

Negative supercoils favor local unwinding of the DNA, allowing processes such as transcription, DNA replication and recombination. Negative supercoiling is also thought to favour the transition between B-DNA and Z-DNA and moderate the interactions of DNA binding proteins involved in gene regulation.

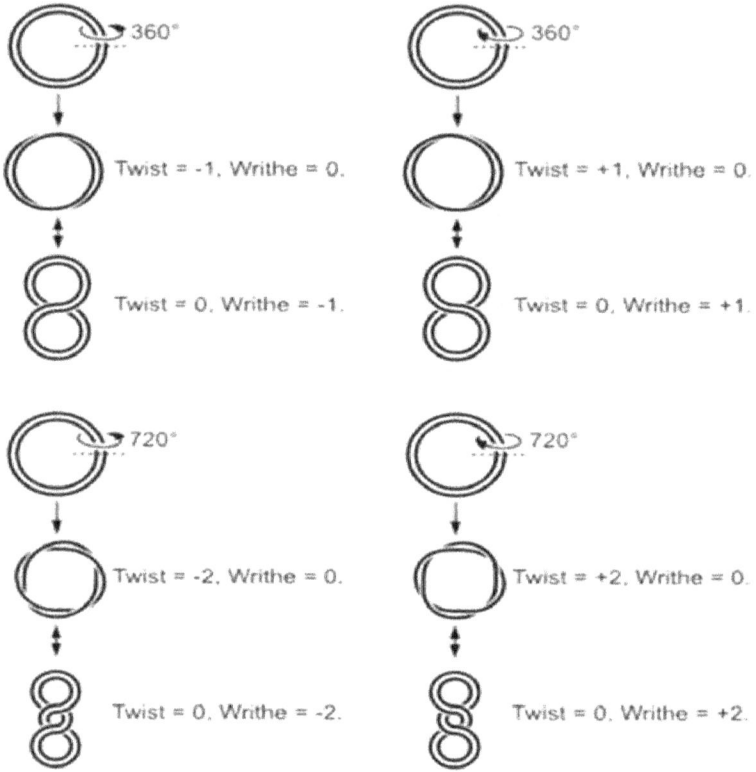

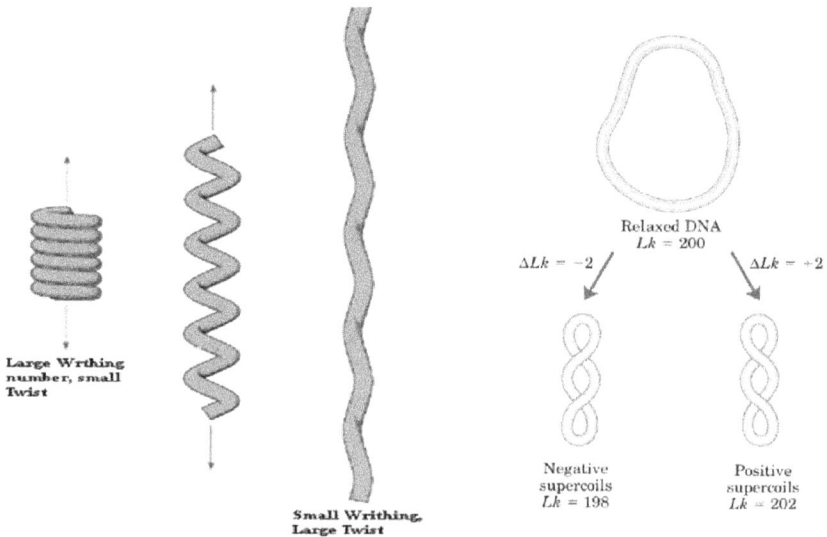

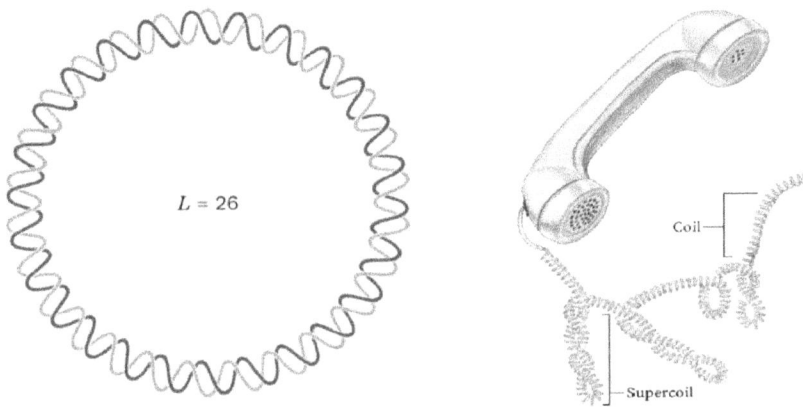

Figure 3.8: Supercoiling

Alternate DNA Structures

DNA exists in many possible conformations that include A-DNA, B-DNA and Z-DNA forms, although only B-DNA and Z-DNA have been directly observed in functional organisms. The conformation that DNA adopts depends on the hydration level, DNA sequence, the amount and direction of supercoiling, chemical modifications of the bases, the type and concentration of metal ions, as well as the presence of polyamines in solution. An alternate analysis was proposed by Wilkins in 1953, for the *in vivo* B-DNA X-ray diffraction/scattering patterns of highly hydrated DNA fibers in terms of squares of Bessel functions. In the same journal, James D. Watson and Francis Crick presented their molecular modeling analysis of the DNA X-ray diffraction patterns to suggest that the structure was a double helix. Although the B-DNA form is most common under the conditions found in cells, it is not a well defined conformation but a family of related DNA conformations that occur at the high hydration levels present in living cells. Their corresponding X-ray diffraction and scattering patterns are characteristic of molecular paracrystals with a significant degree of disorder. Compared to B-DNA, the A-DNA form is a wider right-handed spiral, with a shallow, wide minor groove and a narrower, deeper major groove. The A form occurs under non-physiological conditions in partially dehydrated samples of DNA, while in the cell it may be produced in hybrid pairings of DNA and RNA strands, as well as in enzyme-DNA complexes. Segments of DNA where the bases have been chemically modified by methylation may undergo a larger change in conformation and adopt the Z form. Here, the strands turn about the helical axis in a left handed spiral, the opposite of the more common B form. These unusual structures can be recognized by specific Z-DNA binding proteins and may be involved in the regulation of transcription.

Quadruplex Structures

At the ends of the linear chromosomes are specialized regions of DNA called telomeres. The main function of these regions is to allow the cell to replicate chromosome ends using the enzyme telomerase, as the enzymes that normally replicate

DNA cannot copy the extreme 32 ends of chromosomes. These specialized chromosome caps also help protect the DNA ends and stop the DNA repair systems in the cell from treating them as damage to be corrected. In human cells, telomeres are usually lengths of single-stranded DNA containing several thousand repeats of a simple TTAGGG sequence. DNA quadruplex formed by telomere repeats. The looped conformation of the DNA backbone is very different from the typical DNA helix. These guanine-rich sequences may stabilize chromosome ends by forming structures of stacked sets of four base units, rather than the usual base pairs found in other DNA molecules. Here, four guanine bases form a flat plate and these flat four base units then stack on top of each other, to form a stable G-quadruplex structure. These structures are stabilized by hydrogen bonding between the edges of the bases and chelation of a metal ion in the centre of each four-base unit. Other structures can also be formed, with the central set of four bases coming from either a single strand folded around the bases or several different parallel strands, each contributing one base to the central structure. In addition to these stacked structures, telomeres also form large loop structures called telomere loops or T-loops. Here, the single-stranded DNA curls around in a long circle stabilized by telomere-binding proteins. At the very end of T-loop, the single stranded telomere DNA is held onto a region of double-stranded DNA by the telomere strand disrupting the double helical DNA and base pairing to one of the two strands. This triple stranded structure is called a displacement loop or D-loop.

Branched DNA

In DNA fraying occurs when non-complementary regions exist at the end of an otherwise complementary double-strand of DNA. However, branched DNA can occur if a third strand of DNA is introduced and contains adjoining regions able to hybridize with the frayed regions of the pre-existing double strand. Although the simplest example of branched DNA involves only three strands of DNA, complexes involving additional strands and multiple branches are also possible.

A-DNA

A DNA is one of the many possible double helical structures of DNA. A-DNA is thought to be one of three biologically active double helical structures along with B- and Z-DNA. It is a right-handed double helix fairly similar to the more common and well-known B-DNA form, but with a shorter more compact helical structure. It appears likely that it occurs only in dehydrated samples of DNA, such as those used in crystallographic experiments and possibly is also assumed by DNA-RNA hybrid helices and by regions of double stranded RNA. A DNA is fairly similar to B-DNA given that it is a right handed double helix with major and minor grooves. However, there is a slight increase in the number of base pairs per rotation resulting in a tighter rotation angle and smaller rise/turn. This results in a deepening of the major groove and a shallowing of the minor. An algorithm for predicting the propensity of a sequence to flip from B-DNA to A-DNA was developed by Beth Basham, Gary Schroth and P. Shing Ho at Oregon State University.

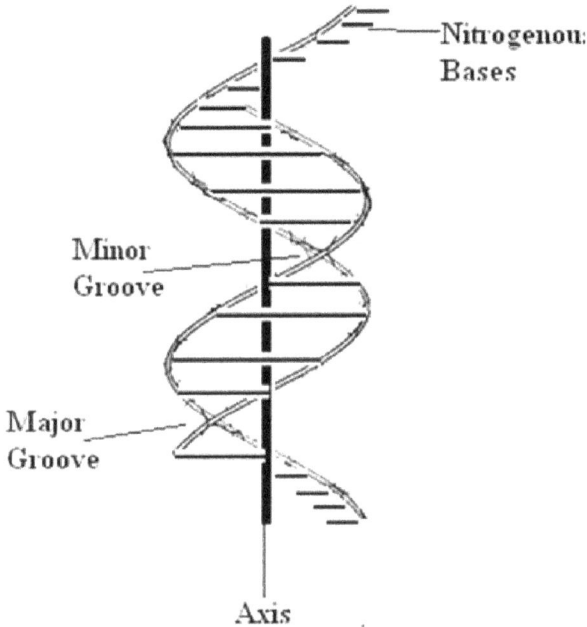

Figure 3.9: A-DNA

Z-DNA

Z-DNA is one of the many possible double helical structures of DNA. It is a left handed double helical structure in which the double helix winds to the left in a zig zag pattern instead of to the right, like the more common B-DNA form. Z-DNA is thought to be one of three biologically active double helical structures along with A- and B-DNA. Z-DNA is quite different from the right handed forms. In fact, Z-DNA is compared against B-DNA in order to illustrate the major differences. The Z-DNA helix is left-handed and has a structure that repeats every 2 base pairs. The major and minor grooves, unlike A and B DNA, show little difference in width. Formation of structure is generally unfavourable, although certain conditions can promote it; such as alternating purine-pyrimidine sequence especially poly $(dGC)_2$, negative DNA supercoiling or low salt and some cations, all at physiological temperature, 37°C and pH 7.3-7.4. Z-DNA can form a junction with B-DNA in a structure which involves the extrusion of a base pair. The Z-DNA conformation has been difficult to study because it does not exist as a stable feature of the double helix. Instead, it is a transient structure that is occasionally induced by biological activity and then quickly disappears.

It is possible to predict the likelihood of a DNA sequence forming a Z-DNA structure. An algorithm Z Hunt, for predicting the propensity of DNA to flip from the B-form to Z-form, was written by Dr. P. Shing Ho in 1984 at MIT. This algorithm was later developed by Tracy Camp, P. Christoph Champ, Sandor Maurice and Jeffrey M. Vargason for genome-wide mapping of Z-DNA with P. Shing Ho as the principal investigator.

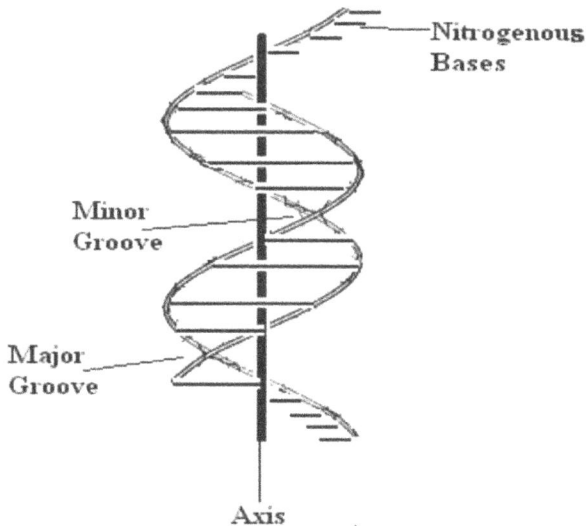

Figure 3.10: Z-DNA

Biological Significance of Z DNA

While no definitive biological significance of Z-DNA has been found, it is commonly believed to provide torsional strain relief (supercoiling) while DNA transcription occurs. The potential to form a Z-DNA structure also correlates with regions of active transcription. A comparison of regions with a high sequence dependent, predicted propensity to form Z-DNA in human chromosome 22 with a selected set of known gene transcription sites suggests there is a correlation. Biophysicist Alexander Rich of the Massachusetts Institute of Technology in Cambridge never doubted the relevance of Z-DNA, which he and colleagues unveiled in 1979 using X-ray crystallography. In 2003, noticed that a poxvirus virulence factor called E3L, mimicked a mammalian protein that binds Z-DNA. In 2005, Rich and his colleagues pinned down what E3L does for the poxvirus. When expressed in human cells, E3L increases by five to 10 fold the production of several genes that block a cell's ability to self destruct in response to infection.

In 2005, A. Rich hypothesizes that Z-DNA is necessary for transcription and that E3L stabilizes the Z-DNA, thus prolonging expression of the anti-apoptotic genes. He suggests that a small molecule that interferes with E3L binding to Z-DNA could prevent the activation of these genes and help protect people from pox infections.

Table 3.2: Difference between A, B and Z DNA

S No.	Geometry Attribute	A-form	B-form	Z-form
1.	Helix sense	right-handed	right-handed	left-handed
2.	Repeating unit	1 bp	1 bp	2 bp
3.	Rotation/bp	32.7°	35.9°	60°/2
4.	bp/turn	11	10.5	12
5.	Inclination of bp to axis	+19°	"1.2°	"9°
6.	Rise/bp along axis	2.3 Å (0.23 nm)	3.32 Å (0.332 nm)	3.8 Å (0.38 nm)
7.	Pitch/turn of helix	28.2 Å (2.82 nm)	33.2 Å (3.32 nm)	45.6 Å (4.56 nm)
8.	Mean propeller twist	+18°	+16°	0°
9.	Glycosyl angle	anti	anti	C: anti,G: syn
10.	Sugar pucker	C3'-endo	C2'-endo	C: C2'-endo,G: C2'-exo
11.	Diameter	23 Å (2.3 nm)	20 Å (2.0 nm)	18 Å (1.8 nm)

Nucleosides, Phosphate and Nucleotides

The nucleoside composed of ribose coupled to a nitrogen-rich compound called bases. The numbers on the sugar 1', 2' and so on are the same numbering system; the symbol ' ('or -) is pronounced prime and is there to indicate that atoms of the sugar, not the atoms of the adenine. The name nucleoside reflects the fact that phosphorylated nucleosides are the building blocks of the nucleic acids that form the genetic material in the nucleus. However, nucleosides also play important roles in other places inside and outside the cell. Seven different compounds can be used to generate nucleosides. All seven contain many nitrogen atoms and one or more ring structures. They are the three purines called adenine, guanine and hypoxanthine, the three pyrimidines called cytosine, thymine and uracil and an odd man out called nicotinamide. These ring compounds are called bases. They will exchange an H^+ with water. The roots of the name are now forgotten by most molecular biologists, which now use the word base to mean a purine, a pyrimidine or nicotinamide. In general, a nucleoside is formed by attaching one of these bases to the 1'-carbon atom of ribose. Phosphorous, although by weight a relatively minor fraction of the whole cell, plays a number of critical roles. In solution phosphorous is mainly found as a phosphate ion with a single hydrogen atom still attached, HPO_4^{2-}. The phosphate ions indicated with the symbol Pi, meaning inorganic phosphate. Phosphate can substitute into any C-OH group with the loss of a water molecule. The equilibrium in the reaction shown lies far to the left, but cells have other strategies for attaching phosphate groups to organic molecules. Once one phosphate group has been added, more can be added to form a chain. Once again, the equilibrium in the reaction shown lies far to the left, but cells can achieve this result using other strategies.

Chemical Modifications of DNA

Base Modifications: The expression of genes is influenced by how the DNA is packaged in chromosomes, in a structure called chromatin. Base modifications can be involved in packaging, with regions that have low or no gene expression usually containing high levels of methylation of cytosine bases. Cytosine methylation produces 5-methylcytosine which is important for X-chromosome inactivation. The average level of methylation varies between organisms *e.g.* worm *Caenorhabditis elegans* lacks cytosine methylation, while vertebrates have higher levels with up to 1% of their DNA containing 5-methylcytosine. Despite the importance of 5-methylcytosine, it can deaminate to leave a thymine base, so methylated cytosines are particularly prone to mutations. Other base modifications include adenine methylation in bacteria, the presence of 5-hydroxymethylcytosine in brain and glycosylation of uracil to produce J-base in kinetoplastids.

Biological Functions

DNA usually occurs as linear chromosomes in eukaryotes and circular chromosomes in prokaryotes. The set of chromosomes in a cell makes up its genome; the human genome has approximately 3 billion base pairs of DNA arranged into 46 chromosomes. The information carried by DNA is held in the sequence of pieces of DNA called genes. Transmission of genetic information in genes is achieved via complementary base pairing *e.g.* in transcription when a cell uses the information in a gene, DNA sequence is copied into a complementary RNA sequence through the attraction between the DNA and the correct RNA nucleotides. This RNA copy is used to make a matching protein sequence in a process called translation which depends on the same interaction between RNA nucleotides. In alternative fashion, a cell may simply copy its genetic information in a process called DNA replication.

Genes and Genomes : Genomic DNA is tightly and orderly packed in the process called DNA condensation to fit the small available volumes of the cell. In eukaryotes, DNA is located in the cell nucleus, as well as small amounts in mitochondria and chloroplasts. In prokaryotes, the DNA is held within an irregularly shaped body in the cytoplasm called the nucleoid. The genetic information in a genome is held within genes and the complete set of this information in an organism is called its genotype. A gene is a unit of heredity and is a region of DNA that influences a particular characteristic in an organism. Genes contain an open reading frame that can be transcribed, as well as regulatory sequences such as promoters and enhancers, which control the transcription of the open reading frame. In many species, only a small fraction of the total sequence of the genome encodes protein. Only about 1.5% of the human genome consists of protein-coding exons, with over 50% of human DNA consisting of non-coding repetitive sequences. The reasons for the presence of so much noncoding DNA in eukaryotic genomes and the extraordinary differences in genome size or C-value, among species represent a long-standing puzzle known as C-value enigma or C-value paradox. However, DNA sequences that do not code protein may still encode functional non-coding RNA molecules which are involved in the regulation of gene expression. A gene is a sequence of DNA that contains genetic information and can influence the phenotype of an organism. Within a gene, the sequence of bases along a DNA strand defines a messenger RNA sequence which defines one or more protein sequences. The relationship between the nucleotide sequences of genes and the amino-acid sequences of proteins is determined by the rules of translation known as the genetic code. The genetic code consists of three-letter words called codons formed from a sequence of three nucleotides *e.g.* ACT, CAG, TTT etc.

Interactions with Proteins: All the functions of DNA depend on interactions with proteins. These protein interactions can be non-specific or the protein can bind specifically to a single DNA sequence. Enzymes can also bind to DNA and of these, the polymerases that copy the DNA base sequence in transcription and DNA replication are particularly important.

DNA-binding Proteins : Structural proteins that bind DNA are well understood examples of non-specific DNA-protein interactions. Within chromosomes, DNA is held in complexes with structural proteins. These proteins organize the DNA into a compact structure called chromatin. In eukaryotes this structure involves DNA binding to a complex of small basic proteins called histones, while in prokaryotes multiple types of proteins are involved. The histones form a disk shaped complex called a nucleosome which contains two complete turns of double stranded DNA wrapped around its surface. These non-specific interactions are formed through basic residues in the histones making ionic bonds to the acidic sugar phosphate backbone of the DNA and are therefore largely independent of the base sequence. Chemical modifications of these basic amino acid residues include methylation, phosphorylation and acetylation. These chemical changes alter the strength of the interaction between the DNA and the histones, making the DNA more or less accessible to transcription factors and changing the rate of transcription. Other non-specific DNA-binding proteins in chromatin include the high mobility group proteins, which bind to bent or distorted DNA. These proteins are important in bending arrays of nucleosomes and arranging them into the larger structures that make up chromosomes. A distinct group of DNA-binding proteins are the DNA-binding proteins that specifically bind single-stranded DNA. In humans, replication protein A is the best understood member of this family and is used in processes where the double helix is separated, including DNA replication, recombination and DNA repair. These binding proteins seem to stabilize single-stranded DNA and protect it from forming stem-loops or being degraded by nucleases. The lambda repressor helix turn helix transcription factor bound to its DNA target.

In contrast, other proteins have evolved to bind to particular DNA sequences. The most intensively studied of these are the various transcription factors, which are proteins that regulate transcription. Each transcription factor binds to one particular set of DNA sequences and activates or inhibits the transcription of genes that have these sequences close to their promoters. The transcription factors do this in two ways. Firstly, they can bind the RNA polymerase responsible for transcription, either directly or through other mediator proteins; this locates the polymerase at the promoter and allows it to begin transcription. Alternatively, transcription factors can bind enzymes that modify the histones at the promoter; this will change the accessibility of the DNA template to the polymerase.

As these DNA targets can occur throughout an organism's genome and changes in the activity of one type of transcription factor can affect thousands of genes. Consequently, these proteins are the targets of the signal transduction processes that control responses to environmental changes or cellular differentiation and development. The specificity of these transcription factors' interactions with DNA come from the proteins making multiple contacts to the edges of the DNA bases, allowing them to read the DNA sequence. Most of these base-interactions are made in the major groove, where the bases are most accessible.

Uses of DNA in Technology

Genetic Engineering : Discoveries in molecular biology have allowed scientists to duplicate natural genetic transfer phenomena in the laboratory and to develop methods to introduce almost any type of genetic information into an organism. Genetic engineering is the creation of new DNA, usually by linking DNA from different organisms together by artificial means using enzymes known as restriction enzymes. Cloning is the production of many copies of the newly engineered DNA. The amplification of a specific cloned gene or genes, coupled with a marked increase in production of their protein products, makes it relatively easy to extract and purify these proteins in the laboratory. A suitable plasmid (vector) is selected in which to insert a desired gene (donor DNA). Both donor DNA and vector are digested with the same restriction enzyme and then incubated together with ligase to join the donor DNA fragments with the plasmid. The result is a recombinant plasmid that contains the desired DNA fragment. The recombinant plasmid is then used to transform a host bacterial cell, creating a new genetic strain of bacteria that stably maintains the recombinant plasmid. The goal of cloning is to isolate a desired gene or segment of DNA from an organism and introduce it into a suitable host cell to obtain large quantities of the DNA. Generally, this donor DNA is used for the large-scale production of important proteins, but the DNA may also be used in the detection of infectious agents or abnormal cells. Usually, donor DNA is a small portion of the genome of a cell and it is present as one or two copies in each cell. Therefore, before donor DNA can be extracted, a sufficient number of cells containing the desired DNA must be obtained, either from a small segment of tissue or by culturing the cells. Then cells must be disrupted and the genetic material either in chromosomes or in plasmids extracted.

Nucleic Acid Hybridizatio: From developments in the area of genetic engineering and molecular biology, a powerful tool known as DNA hybridization has emerged. This technique is used to detect the presence of DNA from pathogens in clinical specimens and to locate specific genes in cells. DNA hybridization takes advantage of the ability of nucleic acids to form stable, double stranded molecules when two single strands with complementary bases are brought together under favorable conditions. In DNA hybridization assays, DNA from a virus or cell is denatured with alkali to separate the strands. The single strands of DNA are then attached to a solid support such as a nitrocellulose or nylon membrane so that the strands do not reanneal. The DNA is attached to the membrane by its sugar-phosphate backbone with the nitrogenous bases projecting outward. To characterize or identify the target DNA, a single-stranded DNA or RNA molecule of known origin, called a probe, is added to the membrane in a buffered solution. This allows the formation of hydrogen bonds between complementary bases. The probe, so called because it is used to seek or probe for DNA sequences, is labeled with a reporter group, which may be a radioactive atom or an enzyme whose presence can be easily detected. The probe is allowed to react with the target DNA; then any unreacted probe is removed by washing in buffered solutions. After the washes, all that remains on the nitrocellulose are the target DNA and any probe molecules that have attached to complementary sequences in the target DNA, forming stable hybrids. Hybridization of target and probe DNAs is detected by assaying for the probe's reporter group. If the reporter group is detected, hybridization has taken place. If no reporter group is detected, it can be assumed that the target molecule does not have sequences that are complementary to those of the probe and hence, the gene or DNA segment sought is not present in the sample.

Three common formats are used in solid phase hybridization assays; dot blot, Southern blotting and *in situ* hybridization. In the dot blot assay, a specified volume of sample or specimen is spotted onto a small area of nitrocellulose membrane. Southern hybridization assays involve restriction enzyme digestion and agarose gel electrophoresis of the target DNA prior to the hybridization assay. The different bands on the agarose gel are transferred by capillary action onto a nitrocellulose or nylon membrane in a blotting apparatus. During the transfer, each of the DNA bands is transferred onto the membrane in the same relative position that it had in the gel. After the transfer, the target DNA is probed and detected, as in the dot blot assay. *In situ* hybridization assays involve the probing of intact cells or tissue sections affixed to a microscope slide. This type of solid-phase assay has the advantage that one cannot only detect the presence of target DNA in intact cells but also determine the location of such target DNA within a tissue. An important application of *in situ* hybridization is for the detection of viruses and certain types of bacteria within infected cells.

Polymerase Chain Reaction : The replication of genetic material is carried out by enzymes called DNA polymerases. These enzymes initiate the synthesis of DNA starting from a primer bound to a template. The primers are generally 9 to 25 bases in length and establish the site where DNA replication begins. With the polymerase chain reaction (PCR), any particular stretch of genetic material can be pinpointed and replicated numerous times simply by selecting a pair of primers that flank the desired stretch of DNA. The PCR is predicated on the annealing of two oligonucleotides (primers) of known composition to a target sequence of interest and the extension of the oligonucleotides with a DNA polymerase. Each reaction is repeated subsequent to a denaturation step, thus allowing for exponential amplification. The PCR involves three temperature incubations or steps that are repeated 20-50 times. One repetition of three steps is called a cycle. In the first step called denaturation, the two strands of the target DNA molecule are separated (denatured) by heating the DNA to 94°C to break the hydrogen bonds between bases, yielding two separate strands. In the second step, called annealing, two primers hybridize to complementary sequences in the single strands. The primers are short (20–30 bases in length); synthetic stretches of single-stranded DNA. They are selected so that one primer is complementary to one end of the gene of interest on one strand, while the second primer is complementary to the opposite end on the other strand. The primers form hydrogen bonds with anneal to their complementary sequences, forming stable, doublestranded molecules. Annealing temperatures range between 37 and 60°C. During the third step, extension or elongation, the primers are extended by a thermostable DNA polymerase at 72°C. To study the effects of mutations on gene expression, a technique known as site directed mutagenesis which introduces point mutations at specific sites has been developed. One of the most commonly used strategies takes advantage of primer-directed amplification of DNA to introduce mutations. One of the primers is designed with a sequence complementary to the region in the target DNA, but with the desired substitution, insertion or deletion. The mutagenic sequence within the primer must be either at 5 end of the primer or internal to the primer, but never at the 3 end of the mutagenic primer. The 3 end of the mutagenic primer at least 6–10 bp long must be totally complementary to the target DNA to permit full annealing of the primer to its target and allow the polymerase to extend the primer. The PCR is carried out initially (first 5–10 cycles) under low stringency conditions, to allow the mismatch to occur. Once a few mutagenized templates are produced during the PCR, these will serve as targets and will be fully complementary to the primer. The end products will contain the mutation at the desired site.

Nucleic Acid Sequencing : Nucleic acid sequencing reveals the genetic code of a DNA molecule. It may be carried out using one of two methods, each of which results in the production of DNA fragments of various lengths, differing from each other by a single base and from which one can infer the nucleic acid sequence of the molecule. This is accomplished using denaturing polyacrylamide gels. Whereas agarose gels can separate DNA molecules differing in length by 30–50 bases, polyacrylamide gels can discriminate among DNA molecules differing in length by a single base. Denaturing gels cause the DNA molecule to become single stranded and remain that way throughout the entire process of electrophoresis. Denaturing gels contain urea and are run at elevated temperatures, both of which promote the separation of the two strands of the DNA molecule. Again, the DNA must be labeled in order to be visualized. The most common form of labeling is with radioactive isotopes, in particular, 32P, 33P or 35S. After electrophoresis, the gel is dried and placed next to a sheet of X-ray film in a dark place. During this time the radioactive particles emitted from the isotope in each DNA molecule expose the film and after development, a dark band is seen on the film at the position where the DNA band was located in the gel. This picture, called an auto- radiograph, is a mirror image of the position of the DNA bands in the gel.

There are two methods that can be used to sequence DNA molecules. The Maxam-Gilbert method is based on cleavage of DNA at specific sites by chemicals rather than enzymes. However, this method is seldom used anymore; the Sanger method is preferred. In the Sanger method, the enzymatic synthesis of DNA takes place by the sequential formation of a phosphodiester bond between the free 5 phosphate group of an incoming nucleotide and the 3' OH group of the growing chain. This process takes place throughout the length of the DNA molecule. Dideoxynucleotides lack a 3 OH group and have a 3H group instead. In the presence of a dideoxynucleotide, the synthesis of DNA stalls because the diphosphate bond cannot be formed. The chain growth terminates at that point and the last base on the 3 end of the chain is a dideoxy terminator. This modification of Sanger's method of DNA sequencing is known as dideoxy termination sequencing. In the Sanger sequencing technique, four different reaction mixtures are used to sequence a DNA fragment. Each reaction mixture contains the template DNA molecule to be sequenced, radioactively labeled primers, all four deoxynucleotides, DNA polymerase and a different dideoxy terminator (ddATP, ddCTP, ddGTP or ddTTP). When one of these terminators is incorporated in the newly synthesized DNA strand, it will stop further synthesis of that strand; the result is that all the strands of various lengths in the reaction mixture end in the same base. The radioactive products are separated by electrophoresis and visualized by autoradiography. Reading from the bottom of the gel (shortest fragments terminated closest to the 5 end) upward reveals the base sequence complementary to that of the template strand.

Forensics: Forensic scientists can use DNA in blood, semen, skin, saliva or hair found at a crime scene to identify a matching DNA of an individual, such as a perpetrator. This process is formally termed DNA profiling, but may also be called genetic fingerprinting. In DNA profiling, the lengths of variable sections of repetitive DNA, such as short tandem repeats and minisatellites, are compared between people. This method is usually an extremely reliable technique for identifying a matching DNA. However, identification can be complicated if the scene is contaminated with DNA from several people. DNA profiling was developed in 1984 by British geneticist Sir Alec Jeffreys and first used in forensic science to convict Colin Pitchfork in the 1988 Enderby murders case. People convicted of certain types of crimes may be required to provide a sample of DNA for a database. This has helped investigators solve old cases where only a DNA sample was obtained from the scene. DNA profiling can also be used to identify victims of mass casualty incidents. On the other hand, many convicted people have been released from prison on the basis of DNA techniques, which were not available when a crime had originally been committed.

Bioinformatics: Bioinformatics involves the manipulation, searching and data mining of biological data and this includes DNA sequence data. The development of techniques to store and search DNA sequences have led to widely applied advances in computer science, especially string searching algorithms, machine learning and database theory. String searching or matching algorithms, which find an occurrence of a sequence of letters inside a larger sequence of letters, were developed to search for specific sequences of nucleotides. The DNA sequenced may be aligned with other DNA sequences to identify homologous sequences and locate the specific mutations that make them distinct. These techniques, especially multiple sequence alignment, are used in studying phylogenetic relationships and protein function. Data sets representing entire genomes' worth of DNA sequences, such as those produced by the Human Genome Project, are difficult to use without the annotations that identify the locations of genes and regulatory elements on each chromosome. Regions of DNA sequence that have the characteristic patterns associated with protein or RNA coding genes can be identified by gene finding algorithms, which allow to predict the presence of particular gene products and their possible functions in an organism even before they have been isolated experimentally. Entire genomes may also be compared which can shed light on the evolutionary history of particular organism and permit the examination of complex evolutionary events.

DNA Nanotechnology : DNA nanotechnology uses the unique molecular recognition properties of DNA and other nucleic acids to create self assembling branched DNA complexes with useful properties. DNA is thus used as a structural material rather than as a carrier of biological information. This has led to the creation of two-dimensional periodic lattices as well as three-dimensional structures in the shapes of polyhedra. Nanomechanical devices and algorithmic self-assembly have also been demonstrated and these DNA structures have been used to template the arrangement of other molecules such as gold nanoparticles and streptavidin proteins.

History and Anthropology : Beca use DNA collects mutations over time, which is then inherited, it contains historical information and, by comparing DNA sequences, geneticists can infer the evolutionary history of organisms, their phylogeny. This field of phylogenetics is a powerful tool in evolutionary biology. If DNA sequences within a species are compared, population geneticists can learn the history of particular populations. This can be used in studies ranging from ecological genetics to anthropology. DNA has also been used to look at modern family relationships, such as establishing family relationships between the descendants of Sally Hemings and Thomas Jefferson. This usage is closely related to the use of DNA in criminal investigations detailed above. Indeed, some criminal investigations have been solved when DNA from crime scenes has matched relatives of the guilty individual.

Watson and Crick Model of DNA

DNA is found in cells, the smallest living units in our body or the smallest separate living organisms. DNA is the material that codes for the many physical characteristics of every living creature. The cells use different codes to determine what functions to carry out. In 1953, James Watson and Francis Crick proposed a structure for DNA that not only accounts for this pairing of bases but also explains how relatively simply the system of storing and transferring genetic information is. According to the Watson -Crick Model, a DNA molecule consists of two polynucleotide strands coiled around each other in a helical twisted ladder structure. The sugar phosphate backbone is on the outside of the double helix and the bases are on the inside, so that a base on one strand points directly toward a base on the second strand. When using the twisted ladder analogy, think of the sugar phosphate backbones as the two sides of the ladder and the bases in the middle as the rungs of the ladder. In effect, each strand of DNA is one-half of the double helix. The two halves come together to form the double helix structure. The two strands of the DNA double helix run in opposite directions, one in the 5' to 3' direction, the other in the 3' to 5' direction. The term that describes how the two strands relate to each other is known as antiparallel. The strands are held together by hydrogen bonds between the nitrogenous bases. In the double helix, adenine and thymine form two hydrogen bonds to each other but not to cytosine or guanine. Similarly, cytosine and guanine form three hydrogen bonds to each other in the double helix, but not to adenine or thymine.

Hydrogen bonds occur only between a Hydrogen atom on one base and either an oxygen or nitrogen atom on the other base. This explains why only two hydrogen bonds can form between A's and T's and three can form between G's and C's, because a hydrogen bond can only form where a H atom comes in close proximity to an Oxygen or Nitrogen atom of a base on the opposite strand. The every base pair contains one purine and one pyrimidine. Again, this is related to the structure of each base and how a proper fit, both in base size and chemical makeup, allows the DNA helix to exist in a physically and chemically stable structure. This type of base pairing is called complementary rather than identical. Identical base pairing would mean that A's bond with A's, G's with G's and so on.

Features of Watson-Crick base pair

i.   The permitted hydrogen bonds are: adenine with thymine (2 bonds); and cytosine with guanine (3 bonds).

ii. The dimensions of the 2 permitted base-pairs are similar, *i.e.* C1'-C1' distance is nearly identical in both cases.

iii. The beta-glycosidic bond is attached on the same edge of the base pair. This has implications for the structure of B-DNA, in particular.

iv. Although some of the atoms in the purine and pyrimidine bases are involved in hydrogen bonds, there is still potential for further hydrogen bonding. This potential is particularly important for sequence specific protein binding.

v.   The Watson-Crick base-pair is a planar structure.

vi. The beta glycosidic bonds point in opposite directions. As a result, both chains can contain both purines and pyrimidines and the backbones of the two chains run in opposite directions.

Features of Watson-Crick model of B-DNA

i.   It is an antiparallel double helix.

ii.   It is a right handed helix.

iii. The base pairs are perpendicular to the axis of the helix. Actually, they are very slightly tilted at an angle of 4 degrees.

iv.   The axis of the helix passes through the centre of the base pairs.

v.   Each base pair is rotated by 36 degrees from the adjacent base pair.

vi.   The base-pairs are stacked 0.34 nm apart from one another.

vii. The double helix repeats every 3.4 nm, *i.e.* the pitch of the double helix is 3.4 nm.

viii. B-DNA has two distinct grooves: a MAJOR groove and, a MINOR groove. These grooves form as a consequence of the fact that the beta-glycosidic bonds of the two bases in each base pair are attached on the same edge. However, because the axis of the helix passes through the centre of the base pairs, both grooves are similar in depth.

Real Structure of B-DNA

Watson and Crick's structure was a just a model. However, it took nearly 30 years before the structures of DNA were resolved at atomic resolution. In 1980, Richard Dickerson and Horace Drew explained the structure of 12-mer double stranded self complementary oligonucleotide with the following sequence:

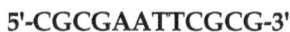

5'-CGCGAATTCGCG-3'

Their results showed that crystals of B-DNA had a structure very similar to that proposed by Watson and Crick. Although there were numerous small variations, the overall structure was as expected.

- The molecule was a right handed double helix.

- The backbone chains were antiparallel.

- The base pairs were very nearly perpendicular to the helix axis.

- The base pairs were centred on the helix axis.

- On average each base pair was rotated 35.6 degrees from the adjacent base pair. However, the individual measured rotations (twist) varied from as little as 28 degrees to as much as 42 degrees.

- On average the rise per base pair *i.e.* the distance between adjacent base pairs was 0.34 nm. However, the rise between individual base pairs varied from 0.274 nm to 0.435 nm.

One of the most striking features of the structure solved by Dickerson and Drew was that there is considerable variation in the structure of individual base pairs. Many were not exactly planar but were slightly twisted (propellor twist). This feature, as well as the variations in the twist angles and the rise between base pairs can be explained or understood as resulting from the complex interplay of attractive and repulsive forces due to the different chemical properties of the four distinct bases within a DNA double helix. The detailed structure of a DNA molecule is actually influenced by the sequence.

History of DNA Research

DNA was first isolated by the Swiss physician Friedrich Miescher in 1869, who discovered a microscopic substance in the pus of discarded surgical bandages. As it resided in the nuclei of cells, he called it nuclein. In 1878, Albrecht Kossel isolated the non-protein component of nuclein, nucleic acid and later isolated its five primary nucleobases. In 1919, Phoebus Levene identified the base, sugar and phosphate nucleotide unit. Levene suggested that DNA consisted of a string of nucleotide units linked together through the phosphate groups. However, Levene thought the chain was short and the bases repeated in a fixed order. In 1937 William Astbury produced the first X-ray diffraction patterns that showed that DNA had a regular structure.

Important Contributors to the Field of DNA

i.   **Gregor Mendel** : Gregor Mendel, who was a monk, played a very important role in the discovery of genes and heredity. He is known as the father of genetics with his famous experiment about peapods that explained the patterns of inheritance. Mendel originally hypothesized that in every generation, a plant inherits two units of information. They were called units at that time because genes had not yet been established for a trait, one from each parent. He crossed-fertilized two true breeding pea plants, one with purple flowers and one with white flowers and observed the offspring's characteristics, they both had purple flowers. Then he let the offspring self fertilize and he saw that some flowers were white but mainly they were still purple. He continued to let the pea plants self-fertilize and he eventually saw that his hypothesis was correct. Both units of information from each parent

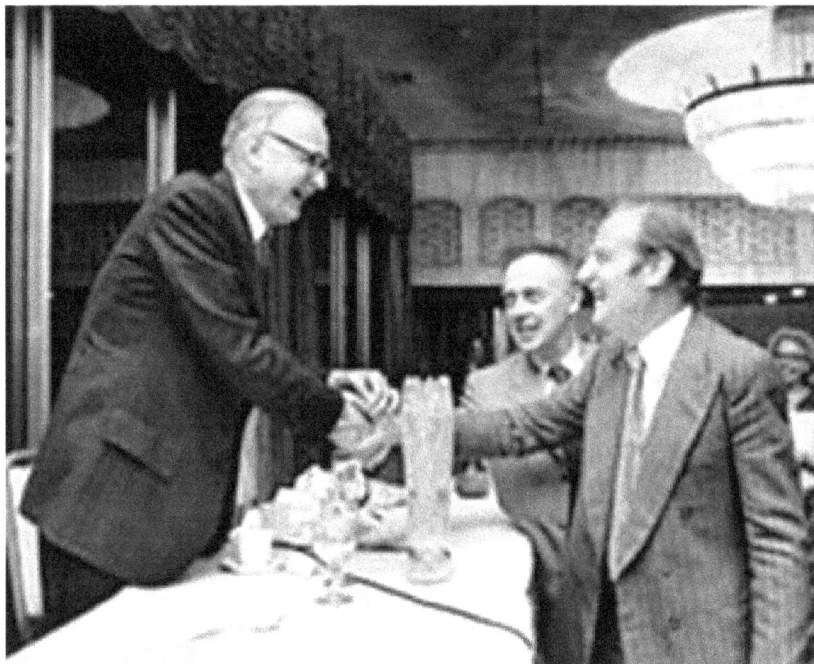

Figure 3.11: James D. Watson and Francis Crick (right), co-originators of the double-helix model, with Maclyn McCarty (left).

flower existed and one trait was dominant (purple) because it covered the other trait (white). Though this is very far from what DNA actually is, without this information about inheritance, the idea of heredity would never have developed and without the idea of heredity, nobody would know about DNA.

ii.   **Frederick Griffith** : In 1928 an army medical officer named Frederick Griffith was trying to find a vaccine against *Streptococcus pneumoniae*, but instead made a breakthrough in world of heredity. He did four experiments in which he injected strands of bacteria into mice, one strand that was harmless (R) and one that was harmful (S).

   i.   In his first experiment, he injected the live R bacteria cells into the mice and the mice lived.

   ii.   In his second experiment, he injected the live S bacteria cells into the mice and mice died.

   iii.   In his third experiment, he killed the harmful S cells with extreme heat and then injected the dead S cells into mice and mice lived.

   iv.   In his last experiment, he added live R cell (which are harmless) to the already dead heat-killed S cells and then injected it into the mice, but the mice died.

Griffith found from this experiment that even though he had killed the S cells, he hadn't destroyed their hereditary material, which was the one part that caused the disease! When some more experiments had been done, it had been discovered that the harmless R cells, had used the information from the hereditary material of the dead S cells and became harmful; this he called, hereditary transformation.

iii. **Oswald Avery** : Oswald Avery was interested by what Frederick Griffith had discovered so he and his colleagues found a way to extract the heat-killed disease carrying cells. In 1944, they had reported that DNA, not proteins (which was believed at the time), was the hereditary substance in these extracts. They backed there report up by the results of an experiment in which they added protein digesting enzymes to some of the extracts and the cells were still transformed, but when the added an enzyme that broke the DNA but not the protein, the hereditary transformation was blocked.

iv. **Erwin Chargaff** : Erwin Chargaff was a biochemist who first figured out the equation for the different bases. Here is what he concluded: the amount of Adenine will always equal the amount of Thymine and the amount of Guanine will always equal the amount of Cytosine.

v. **Maurice Wilkins and Rosalind Franklin** : Maurice Wilkins and Rosalind Franklin were the first to obtain very good X-ray diffration images of the DNA fibers. At that time, little was known about the structure of DNA; though these photos didn't show the structure of the DNA, there were patterns on those images that could be used to determine the position of the DNA molecule's atoms. From these photos, Franklin determined that the DNA molecule must be long and thin.

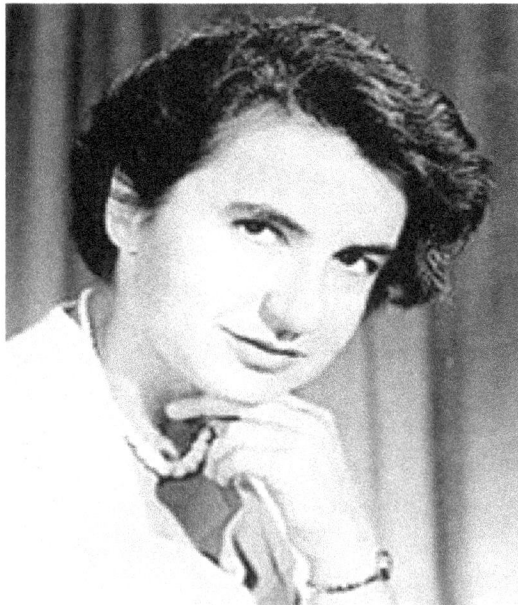

Figure 3.12: Rosalind Franklin: She used X-ray crystallography to help visualize the structure of DNA

vi. James Watson and Francis Crick : In 1951 James Watson and Francis Crick began to examine the DNA's structure. Using previous X-ray diffraction photos of DNA fibers taken by Maurice Wilkins and Rosalind Franklin, they discovered that it showed an X shape, which is also the characteristic of a helix. In April of 1953, using this information, they came up with the double helix, the structure that is almost always associated with DNA. By using the picture of the crystallized DNA, Watson and Crick were able to put together the model of DNA. Some have speculated that they did not give Rosalind Franklin enough credit for her work; she had certainly made history. Watson and Crick did use the new information very quickly as it is shown by the fact that their paper showing the model of DNA was published in the same issue of *Nature* as Franklin's picture. Watson and Crick did use this new information and information from Avery, Chargaff, Griffith and others. They simply pieced together the puzzle. The Nobel Prize was awarded a few years after the presentation of the model to Watson, Crick and Maurice Wilkins. Rosalind Franklin did not receive the prize because she had died of cancer by this time. Maurice Wilkins was able to share the prize with Watson and Crick, though, because of his work with Franklin.

BOX-3.1

X-RAY CRYSTALLOGRAPHY AND WATSON AND CRICK

In 1951, 23-year old biologist James Watson traveled from the United States to work with Francis Crick, an English physicist at the University of Cambridge. Crick was already using the process of X-ray crystallography to study the structure of protein molecules. Together, Watson and Crick used X-ray crystallography data, produced by Rosalind Franklin and Maurice Wilkins at King's College in London, to decipher DNA's structure. This is what they already knew from the work of many scientists, about the DNA molecule:

1. DNA is made up of subunits which scientists called nucleotides.

2. Each nucleotide is made up of a sugar, a phosphate and a base.

3. There are 4 different bases in a DNA molecule: adenine (a purine) cytosine (a pyrimidine) guanine (a purine) thymine (a pyrimidine).

4. The number of purine bases equals the number of pyrimidine bases.

5. The number of adenine bases equals the number of thymine bases.

6. The number of guanine bases equals the number of cytosine bases.

7. The basic structure of the DNA molecule is helical, with the bases being stacked on top of each other.

Working with nucleotide models made of wire, Watson and Crick attempted to put together the puzzle of DNA structure in such a way that their model would account for the variety of facts that they knew described the molecule. Once satisfied with their model, they published their hypothesis, entitled "Molecular Structure of Nucleic Acids: A Structure for Deoxyribose Nucleic Acid" in the British Journal Nature (April 25, 1953. volume 171:737-738).

Ribonucleic Acid

Ribonucleic acid (RNA) is a type of molecule that consists of a long chain of nucleotide units. Each nucleotide consists of a nitrogenous base, a ribose sugar and a phosphate. RNA is very similar to DNA, but differs in a few important structural details: in the cell, RNA is usually single-stranded, while DNA is usually double-stranded; RNA nucleotides contain ribose while DNA contains deoxyribose and RNA has the base uracil rather than thymine that is present in DNA. RNA is transcribed from DNA by enzymes called RNA polymerases and is generally further processed by other enzymes. RNA is central to the synthesis of proteins. Here, a type of RNA called messenger RNA carries information from DNA to structures called ribosomes. These ribosomes are made from proteins and ribosomal RNAs, which come together to form a molecular machine that can read messenger RNAs and translate the information they carry into proteins. There are many RNAs with other roles, in particular regulating which genes are expressed, but also as the genomes of most viruses.

Each nucleotide in RNA contains a ribose sugar, with carbons numbered 1' through 5'. A base is attached to the 1' position, generally adenine (A), cytosine (C), guanine (G) or uracil (U). Adenine and guanine are purines, cytosine and uracil are pyrimidines. A phosphate group is attached to the 3' position of one ribose and the 5' position of the next. The phosphate groups have a negative charge each at physiological pH, making RNA a charged molecule (polyanion). The bases may form hydrogen bonds between cytosine and guanine, between adenine and uracil and between guanine and uracil. However other interactions are possible, such as a group of adenine bases binding to each other in a bulge or the GNRA tetraloop that has a guanine-adenine base pair.

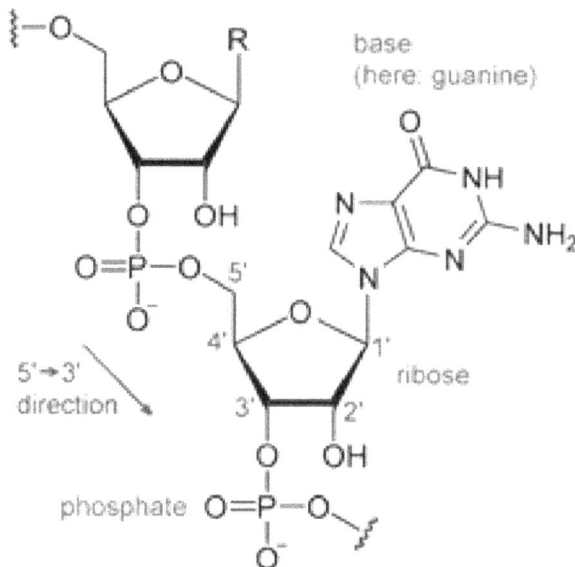

Figure 33: Chemical Structure of RNA Nucleotide

An important structural feature of RNA that distinguishes it from DNA is the presence of a hydroxyl group at the 2' position of the ribose sugar. The presence of this functional group causes the helix to adopt A-form geometry rather than the B-form most commonly observed in DNA. This results in a very deep and narrow major groove and a shallow and wide minor groove. A second consequence of the presence of the 2'-hydroxyl group is that in conformationally flexible regions of an RNA molecule (that is, not involved in formation of a double helix), it can chemically attack the adjacent phosphodiester bond to cleave the backbone. RNA is transcribed with only four bases (adenine, cytosine, guanine and uracil), but there are numerous modified bases and sugars in mature RNAs. Pseudouridine (Ø), in which the linkage between uracil and ribose is changed from a C–N bond to a C–C bond and ribothymidine (T), are found in various places (most notably in the TØC loop of tRNA). Another notable modified base is hypoxanthine, a deaminated adenine base whose nucleoside is called inosine (I). Inosine plays a key role in the wobble hypothesis of the genetic code. There are nearly 100 other naturally occurring modified nucleosides, of which pseudouridine and nucleosides with 2'-O-methylribose are the most common. The specific roles of many of these modifications in RNA are not fully understood. However, it is notable that in ribosomal RNA, many of the post-transcriptional modifications occur in highly functional regions, such as the peptidyl transferase center and the subunit interface, implying that they are important for normal function. The functional form of single stranded RNA molecules, just like proteins, frequently requires a specific tertiary structure. The scaffold for this structure is provided by secondary structural elements which are hydrogen bonds within the molecule. This leads to several recognizable domains of secondary structure like hairpin loops, bulges and internal loops. Since RNA is charged, metal ions such as Mg^{2+} are needed to stabilise many secondary structures.

Discovery of RNA

The role of RNA in protein synthesis was suspected already in 1939. Severo Ochoa won the 1959 Nobel Prize in Medicine after he discovered how RNA is synthesized. The sequence of the 77 nucleotides of yeast tRNA was found by Robert W. Holley in 1965, winning Holley the 1968 Nobel Prize in Medicine. In 1967, Carl Woese realized RNA can be catalytic and proposed that the earliest forms of life relied on RNA both to carry genetic information and to catalyze biochemical reactions, an RNA world. In 1976, Walter Fiers and his team determined the first complete nucleotide sequence of an RNA virus genome, that of bacteriophage MS2. In 1990 it was found in petunia that introduced genes can silence similar genes of the plant's own, now known to be a result of RNA interference. At about the same time, 22 nt long RNA, now called microRNAs, were found to have a role in the development of *C. elegans*. The discovery of gene regulatory RNAs has led to attempts to develop drugs made of RNA, such as siRNA, to silence genes.

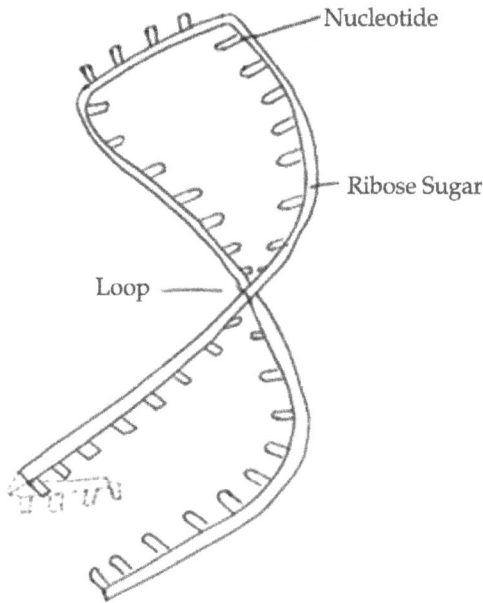

Figure 3.14: Pre-mRNA with Hairpin Loop

Type of RNA

i.   **Ribosomal RNAs**-exist outside the nucleus in the cytoplasm of a cell in structures called ribosomes. Ribosomes are small, granular structures where protein synthesis takes place. Each ribosome is a complex consisting of about 60% ribosomal RNA (rRNA) and 40% protein.

ii. **Messenger RNAs**-are the nucleic acids that record information from DNA in the cell nucleus and carry it to the ribosomes and are known as messenger RNAs (mRNA).

iii. **Transfer RNAs**-The function of transfer RNAs (tRNA) is to deliver amino acids one by one to protein chains growing at ribosomes.

Ribosomal RNA (rRNA) : Ribosomal RNA (rRNA) is the central component of the ribosome, the protein manufacturing machinery of all living cells. The function of the rRNA is to provide a mechanism for decoding mRNA into amino acids and to interact with the tRNA during translation by providing peptidyl transferase activity. The tRNA is sandwiched between the small and large subunits and the ribosome catalyzes the formation of a peptide bond between the 2 amino acids that are contained in the rRNA. The ribosome also has 3 binding sites called A, P and E. The A site in the ribosome binds to an aminoacyl-tRNA (a tRNA bound to an amino acid). The NH_2 group of the aminoacyl-tRNA which contains the new amino acid, attacks the carboxyl group of peptidyl-tRNA (contained within the P site) which contains the last amino acid of the growing chain called peptidyl transferase reaction. The tRNA that was holding on the last amino acid is moved to the E site and what used to be the aminoacyl-tRNA is now the peptidyl-tRNA. A single mRNA can be translated simultaneously by multiple ribosomes.

Prokaryotes vs. Eukaryotes

Both prokaryotic and eukaryotic can be broken down into two subunits 70S and 80S. The S units of the subunits cannot simply be added because they represent measures of sedimentation rate rather than of mass. The sedimentation rate of each subunit is affected by its shape, as well as by its mass.

Table 15: Sizes of Ribosome

S.No.	Type	Size	Large subunit	Small subunit
1.	Prokaryotic	70S	50S (5S, 23S)	30S (16S)
2.	Eukaryotic	80S	60S (5S, 5.8S, 28S)	40S (18S)

Prokaryotes

i.   In prokaryotes a small 30S ribosomal subunit contains the 16S rRNA.

ii. The large 50S ribosomal subunit contains two rRNA species (the 5S and 23S rRNAs).

iii. Bacterial 16S, 23S and 5S rRNA genes are typically organized as a co-transcribed operon.

iv. There may be one or more copies of the operon dispersed in the genome *e.g.* *E.coli* has seven.

v.   Archaea contains either a single rDNA operon or multiple copies of the operon.

vi. The 3' end of the 16S rRNA (in a ribosome) binds to a sequence on the 5' end of mRNA called the Shine-Dalgarno sequence.

Eukaryotes

i)   In contrast, eukaryotes generally have many copies of the rRNA genes organized in tandem repeats; in humans approximately 300–400 rDNA repeats are present in five clusters (on chromosomes 13, 14, 15, 21 and 22).

ii) The 18S rRNA in most eukaryotes is in the small ribosomal subunit and the large subunit contains three rRNA species (the 5S, 5.8S and 28S rRNAs).

iii) Mammalian cells have 2 mitochondrial (12S and 16S) rRNA molecules and 4 types of cytoplasmic rRNA (28S, 5.8S, 5S (large ribosome subunit) and 18S (small subunit). 28S, 5.8S and 18S rRNAs are encoded by a single transcription unit (45S) separated by 2 internally transcribed spacers. The 45S rDNA organized into 5 clusters (each has 30-40 repeats) on chromosomes 13, 14, 15, 21 and 22. These are transcribed by RNA polymerase I. 5S occurs in tandem arrays (~200-300 true 5S genes and many dispersed pseudogenes), the largest one on the chromosome 1q41-42. 5S rRNA is transcribed by RNA polymerase III.

iv) The tertiary structure of the small subunit ribosomal RNA (SSU rRNA) has been resolved by X-ray crystallography. The secondary structure of SSU rRNA contains 4 distinct domains, the 5', central, 3' major and 3' minor domains.

Importance of rRNA

Ribosomal RNA characteristics are important in medicine and in evolution. The rRNA is the target of several clinically relevant antibiotics: chloramphenicol, erythromycin, kasugamycin, micrococcin, paromomycin, ricin, sarcin, spectinomycin, streptomycin and thiostrepton. The rRNA is the most conserved (least variable) gene in all cells. For this reason, genes that encode the rRNA (rDNA) are sequenced to identify an organism's taxonomic group, calculate related groups and estimate rates of species divergence. For this reason many thousands of rRNA sequences are known and stored in specialized databases such as RDP-II and the European SSU database.

MESSENGER RNA (mRNA)

Messenger ribonucleic acid (mRNA) is a molecule of RNA encoding a chemical blueprint for a protein product. The mRNA is transcribed from a DNA template and carries coding information to the sites of protein synthesis: the ribosomes. Here, the nucleic acid polymer is translated into a polymer of amino acids: a protein. In mRNA as in DNA, genetic information is encoded in the sequence of nucleotides arranged into codons consisting of three bases each. Each codon encodes for a specific amino acid, except the stop codons that terminate protein synthesis. This process requires two other types of RNA: transfer RNA (tRNA) mediates recognition of the codon and provides the corresponding amino acid, while ribosomal RNA (rRNA) is the central component of the ribosome's protein manufacturing machinery.

Synthesis, Processing and Function

The brief existence of an mRNA molecule begins with transcription and ultimately ends in degradation. During its life, an mRNA molecule may also be processed, edited and transported prior to translation. Eukaryotic mRNA molecules often require extensive processing and transport, while prokaryotic molecules do not.

Transcription

During transcription, RNA polymerase makes a copy of a gene from the DNA to mRNA as needed. This process is similar in eukaryotes and prokaryotes. One notable difference, however, is that eukaryotic RNA polymerase associates with mRNA processing enzymes during transcription so that processing can proceed quickly after the start of transcription. The short-lived, unprocessed or partially processed, product is termed pre-mRNA; once completely processed, it is termed mature mRNA.

Eukaryotic pre-mRNA Processing

Processing of mRNA differs greatly among eukaryotes, bacteria and archea. Non-eukaryotic mRNA is essentially mature upon transcription and requires no processing, except in rare cases. Eukaryotic pre-mRNA requires extensive processing.

i. **5' cap addition:** A 5' cap is a modified guanine nucleotide that has been added to the front or 5' end of a eukaryotic messenger RNA shortly after the start of transcription. The 5' cap consists of a terminal 7-methylguanosine residue which is linked through a 5'-5'-triphosphate bond to the first transcribed nucleotide. Its presence is critical for recognition by the ribosome and protection from RNases. Cap addition is coupled to transcription and occurs co-transcriptionally, such that each influences the other. Shortly after the start of transcription, the 5' end of the mRNA being synthesized is bound by a cap-synthesizing complex associated with RNA polymerase. This enzymatic complex catalyzes the chemical reactions that are required for mRNA capping. Synthesis proceeds as a multi-step biochemical reaction.

ii. **Splicing:** Splicing is the process by which pre-mRNA is modified to remove certain stretches of non-coding sequences called introns; the stretches that remain include protein-coding sequences and are called exons. Sometimes pre-mRNA messages may be spliced in several different ways, allowing a single gene to encode multiple proteins. This process is called alternative splicing. Splicing is usually performed by an RNA-protein complex called the spliceosome, but some RNA molecules are also capable of catalyzing their own splicing.

iii. **Editing:** In some instances, an mRNA will be edited, changing the nucleotide composition of that mRNA. An example in humans is the apolipoprotein B mRNA, which is edited in some tissues, but not others. The editing creates an early stop codon, which upon translation, produces a shorter protein.

iv. **Polyadenylation:** Polyadenylation is the covalent linkage of a polyadenylyl moiety to a messenger RNA molecule. In eukaryotic organisms, most messenger RNA molecules are polyadenylated at the 3' end. The poly (A) tail and the protein bound to it aid in protecting mRNA from degradation by exonucleases. Polyadenylation is also important for transcription termination, export of the mRNA from the nucleus and translation. The mRNA can also be polyadenylated in prokaryotic organisms, where poly (A) tails acts to facilitate, rather than impede, exonucleolytic degradation. Polyadenylation occurs during and immediately after transcription of DNA into RNA. After transcription has been terminated, the mRNA chain is cleaved through the action of an endonuclease complex associated with RNA polymerase. After the mRNA has been cleaved, around 250 adenosine residues are added to the free 3' end at the cleavage site. This reaction is catalyzed by polyadenylate polymerase. Just as in alternative splicing, there can be more than one polyadenylation variant of an mRNA.

v. **Transport:** Another difference between eukaryotes and prokaryotes is mRNA transport. Because eukaryotic transcription and translation is compartmentally separated, eukaryotic mRNAs must be exported from the nucleus to the cytoplasm. Mature mRNAs are recognized by their processed modifications and then exported through the nuclear pore. In neurons mRNA must be transported from the soma to the dendrites where local translation occurs in response to external stimuli. Many messages are marked with so-called zip codes which targets their transport to a specific location.

vi. Translation: Because prokaryotic mRNA does not need to be processed or transported, translation by the ribosome can begin immediately after the end of transcription. Therefore, it can be said that prokaryotic translation is coupled to transcription and occurs co-transcriptionally. Eukaryotic mRNA that has been processed and transported to the cytoplasm *i.e.* mature mRNA can then be translated by the ribosome. Translation may occur at ribosomes free-floating in the cytoplasm or directed to the endoplasmic reticulum by the signal recognition particle. Therefore, unlike prokaryotes, eukaryotic translation is not directly coupled to transcription.

Structure of mRNA

5' cap: The 5' cap is a modified guanine nucleotide added to the front (5' end) of the pre-mRNA using a 5'-5'-triphosphate linkage. This modification is critical for recognition and proper attachment of mRNA to the ribosome, as well as protection from 5' exonucleases. It may also be important for other essential processes, such as splicing and transport.

Coding regions: Coding regions are composed of codons, which are decoded and translated into one (mostly eukaryotes) or several (mostly prokaryotes) proteins by the ribosome. Coding regions begin with the start codon and end with a stop codon. Generally, the start codon is an AUG triplet and the stop codon is UAA, UAG or UGA. The coding regions tend to be stabilised by internal base pairs, this impedes degradation. In addition to being protein-coding, portions of coding regions may serve as regulatory sequences in the pre-mRNA as exonic splicing enhancers or exonic splicing silencers.

Untranslated regions: Untranslated regions (UTRs) are sections of the mRNA before the start codon and after the stop codon that are not translated, termed the five prime untranslated region (5' UTR) and three prime untranslated region (3' UTR), respectively. These regions are transcribed with the coding region and thus are exonic as they are present in the mature mRNA. Several roles in gene expression have been attributed to the untranslated regions, including mRNA stability, mRNA localization and translational efficiency. The ability of a UTR to perform these functions depends on the sequence of the UTR and can differ between mRNAs. The stability of mRNAs may be controlled by the 5' UTR and/or 3' UTR due to varying affinity for RNA degrading enzymes called ribonucleases and for ancillary proteins that can promote or inhibit RNA degradation.

Translational efficiency, including sometimes the complete inhibition of translation, can be controlled by UTRs. Proteins that bind to either the 3' or 5' UTR may affect translation by influencing the ribosome's ability to bind to the mRNA. MicroRNAs bound to the 3' UTR also may affect translational efficiency or mRNA stability. Cytoplasmic localization of mRNA is thought to be a function of the 3' UTR. Proteins that are needed in a particular region of the cell can actually be translated there; in such a case, the 3' UTR may contain sequences that allow the transcript to be localized to this region for translation. Some of the elements contained in untranslated

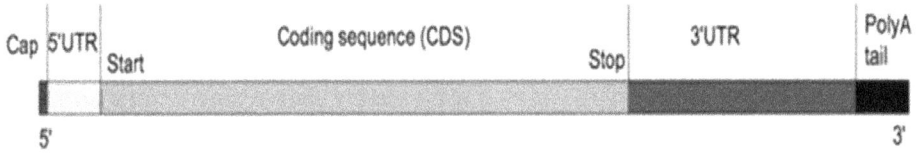

Figure 3.15: The structure of mature eukaryotic mRNA. A fully processed mRNA includes a 5' cap, 5' UTR, coding region, 3' UTR and poly (A) tail.

regions form a characteristic secondary structure when transcribed into RNA. These structural mRNA elements are involved in regulating the mRNA. Some, such as the SECIS element, are targets for proteins to bind. One class of mRNA element, the riboswitches, directly binds small molecules, changing their fold to modify levels of transcription or translation. In these cases, the mRNA regulates itself.

Poly (A) tail: The 3' poly (A) tail is a long sequence of adenine nucleotides (often several hundred) at the 3' end of the pre-mRNA. This tail promotes export from the nucleus and translation and protects the mRNA from degradation.

Monocistronic versus Polycistronic mRNA: An mRNA molecule is said to be monocistronic when it contains the genetic information to translate only a single protein. This is the case for most of the eukaryotic mRNAs. On the other hand, polycistronic mRNA carries the information of several genes, which are translated into several proteins. These proteins usually have a related function and are grouped and regulated together in an operon. Most of the mRNA found in bacteria and archea are polycistronic. Dicistronic is the term used to describe a mRNA that encodes only two proteins.

Circularization of mRNA

In eukaryotes it is thought that mRNA molecules form circular structures due to an interaction between the cap binding complex and poly (A)-binding protein. Circularization is thought to promote recycling of ribosomes on the same message leading to efficient translation.

Degradation

Different mRNAs within the same cell have distinct lifetimes (stabilities). In bacterial cells, individual mRNAs can survive from seconds to more than an hour; in mammalian cells, mRNA lifetimes range from several minutes to days. The greater the stability of an mRNA, the more protein may be produced from that mRNA. The limited lifetime of mRNA enables a cell to alter protein synthesis rapidly in response to its changing needs. There are many mechanisms which lead to the destruction of a message.

Prokaryotic mRNA Degradation: In prokaryotes the lifetime of mRNA is generally much shorter than in eukaryotes. The regulation of mRNA degredation in prokaryotes is much simpler than in eukaryotes. Prokaryotes have numerous RNases which degrade messages rapidly regardless of the sequence of the mRNA. Alternatively, small RNA molecules (sRNA) of tens to hundreds of nucleotides long can recognize specific mRNAs and stimulate their degredation. Complementary sequences in the sRNA bind to the mRNA creating a double-stranded RNA molecule which is a substrate for certain classes of RNAses. It was recently shown that bacteria also have a sort of 5' cap consisting of a triphosphate on the 5' end. Removal of two of the phosphates leaves a 5' monophosphate causing the message to be destroyed by the exonuclease RNAse E.

Eukaryotic mRNA Turnover: Inside eukaryotic cells there is a balance between the processes of translation and mRNA decay. Messages which are being actively translated are bound by polysomes, the eukaryotic initiation factors eIF-4E and eIF-4G and poly (A)-binding protein. The eIF-4E and eIF-4G block the decapping enzyme (DCP2) and poly(A)-binding protein blocks the exosome complex, protecting the message. In nutrient-starvation conditions or during viral infection translation may be compromised and decay is stimulated. The balance between translation and decay is reflected in the size and abundance of the cytoplasmic structures known as P-bodies. During rounds of translation the poly-A tail of the mRNA is shortened by exonucleases. This is thought to disrupt the circular structure of the message and destabilize the cap binding complex. The message is then subject to degradation by either the exosome complex or the decapping complex. In this way inactive messages are destroyed quickly and active messages remain intact leading to selection of those messages which the cell needs at the present time. The mechanism by which translation stops and the message and is handed-off to decay complexes is not understood in detail.

AU-rich Element Decay: The presence of AU-rich elements in some mammalian mRNAs tends to destabilize those transcripts through the action of cellular proteins that bind these sequences. Rapid mRNA degradation via AU-rich elements is a critical mechanism for preventing the overproduction of potent cytokines such as tumor necrosis factor (TNF) and granulocyte-macrophage colony stimulating factor (GM-CSF). AU-rich elements also regulate oncogenic transcription factors like c-Jun and c-Fos. Binding of proteins which recognize AU-rich elements is thought to promote decay by both the exosome complex and decapping complex.

Nonsense Mediated Decay: Eukaryotic messages are subject to surveillance by nonsense mediated decay (NMD) which checks for the presence of premature stop codons (nonsense codons) in the message. These can arise via alternative splicing, V (D) J recombination in the adaptive immune system, mutations in DNA, transcription errors, leaky scanning by the ribosome causing a frame shift and other causes. Detection of a premature stop codon results in decay by the decapping complex from the 5' end, the exosome complex from the 3' end or endonucleolytic cleavage.

Small interfering RNA (siRNA): In metazoans, small double-stranded RNA that is processed by Dicer is incorporated into a complex known as the RNA-induced silencing complex or RISC. This complex contains an endonuclease that cleaves the message leading to destruction of both fragments by exonucleases. The siRNA is commonly used in laboratories to block the function of genes in cell culture. It is thought to be part of the innate immune system as a defense against double-stranded RNA viruses.

Micro RNA (miRNA)

Micro RNA (miRNA) is small RNAs that are almost perfectly complementary to a sequence in a messenger RNA. Binding of the miRNA to the mRNA can lead to repression of translation of the message or removal of the 5' cap by the decapping complex. In genetics, microRNAs (miRNA) are single-stranded RNA molecules of 21-23 nucleotides in length, which regulate gene expression. The miRNAs are encoded by genes from whose DNA they are transcribed but miRNAs are not translated into protein (non-coding RNA); instead each primary transcript (a pri-miRNA) is processed into a short stem-loop structure called a pre-miRNA and finally into a functional miRNA. Mature miRNA molecules are partially complementary to one or more messenger RNA (mRNA) molecules and their main function is to down regulate gene expression. They were first described in 1993 by Lee and colleagues in the Victor Ambros lab, yet the term microRNA was only introduced in 2001 in a set of three articles in Science.

TRANSFER RNA (tRNA)

Transfer RNA (tRNA) is small RNA usually about 74-95 nucleotides that transfer a specific active amino acid to a growing polypeptide chain at the ribosomal site of protein synthesis during translation. It has a 3' terminal site for amino acid attachment. This covalent linkage is catalyzed by an aminoacyl tRNA synthetase. It also contains a three base region called the anticodon that can base pair to the corresponding three base codon regions on mRNA. Each type of tRNA molecule can be attached to only one type of amino acid, but because the genetic code contains multiple codons that specify the same amino acid, tRNA molecules bearing different anticodons may also carry the same amino acid. The existence of tRNA was first hypothesized by Francis Crick, based on the assumption that there exists an adapter molecule capable of mediating the translation of the RNA alphabet into the protein alphabet. Significant research on structure was conducted in the early 1960s by Alex Rich and Don Caspar, two researchers in Boston, Jacques Fresco group in Princeton University and a United Kingdom group at King's College London. A later publication reported the primary structure in 1965 by Robert W. Holley. The secondary and tertiary structures were derived from X-ray crystallography studies reported independently in 1974 by American and British research groups headed by Alexander Rich and Aaron Klug.

Structure of tRNA

The tRNA has primary structure, secondary structure usually visualized as the cloverleaf structure and tertiary structure. All tRNAs have a similar L-shaped 3D structure that allows them to fit into the P and A sites of the ribosome.

i. The acceptor stem is a 7-bp stem made by the base pairing of the 5'-terminal nucleotide with the 3'-terminal nucleotide (which contains the CCA 3'-terminal group used to attach the amino acid). The acceptor stem may contain non-Watson-Crick base pairs.

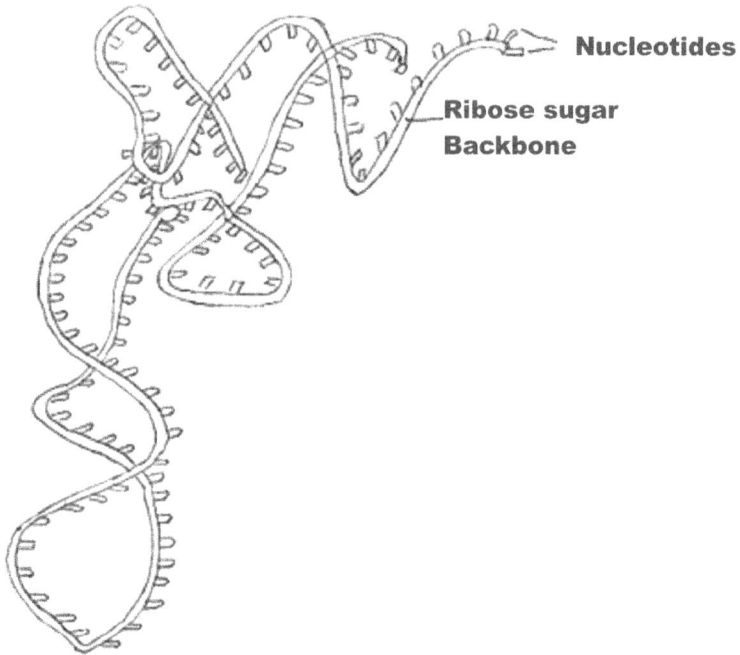

Figure 3.16: Structure of tRNA

ii. The CCA tail is a CCA sequence at the 3' end of the tRNA molecule. This sequence is important for the recognition of tRNA by enzymes critical in translation. In prokaryotes, the CCA sequence is transcribed. In eukaryotes, the CCA sequence is added during processing and therefore does not appear in the tRNA gene.

iii. The D arm is a 4 bp stem ending in a loop that often contains dihydrouridine.

iv. The anticodon arm is a 5-bp stem whose loop contains the anticodon. It also contains a Y that stands for a modified purine nucleotide.

v.   The T arm is a 5 bp stem containing the sequence TØC where Ø is a pseudouridine.

vi. Bases that have been modified, especially by methylation, occur in several positions outside the anticodon. The first anticodon base is sometimes modified to inosine (derived from adenine) or pseudouridine (derived from uracil).

Anticodon

An anticodon is a unit made up of three nucleotides that correspond to the three bases of the codon on the mRNA. Each tRNA contains a specific anticodon triplet sequence that cans base pair to one or more codons for an amino acid *e.g.* one codon for lysine is AAA; the anticodon of a lysine tRNA might be UUU. Some anticodons can pair with more than one codon due to a phenomenon known as wobble base pairing. Frequently, the first nucleotide of the anticodon is one of two not found on mRNA: inosine and pseudouridine, which can hydrogen bond to more than one base in the corresponding codon position. In the genetic code, it is common for a single amino acid to be specified by all four third position possibilities *e.g.* amino acid glycine is coded for by the codon sequences GGU, GGC, GGA and GGG. To provide a one-to-one correspondence between tRNA molecules and codons that specify amino acids, 61 tRNA molecules would be required per cell. However, many cells contain fewer than 61 types of tRNAs because the wobble base is capable of binding to several, though not necessarily all, of the codons that specify a particular amino acid.

Aminoacylation

Aminoacylation is the process of adding an aminoacyl group to a compound. It produces tRNA molecules with their CCA 3' ends covalently linked to an amino acid. Each tRNA is aminoacylated (charged) with a specific amino acid by an aminoacyl tRNA synthetase. There is normally a single aminoacyl tRNA synthetase for each amino acid, despite the fact that there can be more than one tRNA and more than one anticodon, for an amino acid. Recognition of the appropriate tRNA by the synthetases is not mediated solely by the anticodon and the acceptor stem often plays a prominent role.

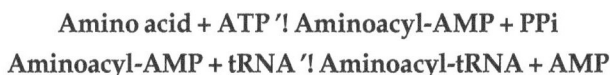

Amino acid + ATP '! Aminoacyl-AMP + PPi

Aminoacyl-AMP + tRNA '! Aminoacyl-tRNA + AMP

Binding to Ribosome

The ribosome has three binding sites for tRNA molecules; A, P and E sites. During translation the A site binds an incoming aminoacyl-tRNA as directed by the codon currently occupying this site. This codon specifies the next amino acid to be added to the growing peptide chain. The A site only works after the first aminoacyl-tRNA has attached to the P site. The P-site codon is occupied by peptidyl-tRNA that is a tRNA with multiple amino acids attached as a long chain. The P site is actually the first to bind to aminoacyl tRNA. This tRNA in the P site carries the chain of amino acids that has already been synthesized. The E site is occupied by the empty tRNA as it is about to exit the ribosome.

tRNA Genes

Organisms vary in the number of tRNA genes in their genome. The nematode worm *C. elegans* has 29647 genes in its nuclear genome, of which 620 code for tRNA. The budding yeast *Saccharomyces cerevisiae* has 275 tRNA genes in its genome. In the human genome, which according to current estimates has about 27161 genes in total, there are about 4421 non-coding RNA genes, which include tRNA genes. There are 22 mitochondrial tRNA genes; 497 nuclear genes encoding cytoplasmic tRNA molecules and there are 324 tRNA-derived putative pseudogenes. Cytoplasmic tRNA genes can be grouped into 49 families according to their anticodon features. These genes are found on all chromosomes, except 22 and Y chromosome. High clustering on 6p is observed (140 tRNA genes), as well on 1 chromosome. The tRNA molecules are transcribed in eukaryotic cells by RNA polymerase III, unlike messenger RNA which is transcribed by RNA polymerase II. Pre-tRNAs contain introns whereas in eukaryotes and archaea they are removed by tRNA splicing endonuclease.

Formation and Processing

The genes encoding miRNAs are much longer than the processed mature miRNA molecule; miRNAs are first transcribed as primary transcripts or pri-miRNA with a cap and poly-A tail and processed to short, 70-nucleotide stem-loop structures known as pre-miRNA in the cell nucleus. This processing is performed in animals by a protein complex known as the Microprocessor complex, consisting of the nuclease Drosha and the double-stranded RNA binding protein Pasha. These pre-miRNAs are then processed to mature miRNAs in the cytoplasm by interaction with the endonuclease Dicer, which also initiates the formation of the RNA-induced silencing complex (RISC). This complex is responsible for the gene silencing observed due to miRNA expression and RNA interference. The pathway in plants varies slightly due to their lack of Drosha homologs; instead, Dicer homologs alone affect several processing steps. The pathway is also different for miRNAs derived from intronic stem loops; these are processed by Dicer but not by Drosha. Either the sense strand or antisense strand of DNA can function as templates to give rise to miRNA.

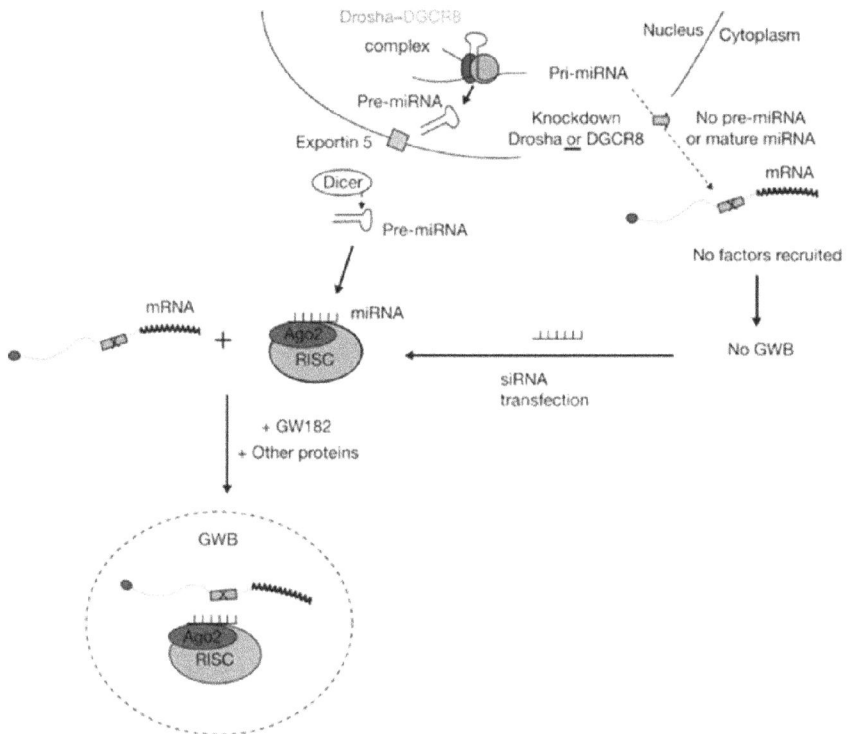

Figure 3.17: Formation of MicroRNA

Efficient processing of pri-miRNA by Drosha requires the presence of extended single stranded RNA on both 3'- and 5'-ends of hairpin molecule. These ssRNA motifs could be of different composition while their length is of high importance if processing is to take place at all. A bioinformatics analysis of human and fly pri-miRNAs revealed very similar structural regions called basal segments, lower stems, upper stems and terminal loops; based on these conserved structures, thermodynamic profiles of pri-miRNA have been determined. The Drosha complex cleaves the RNA molecule ~22 nucleotides away from the terminal loop. Most pre-miRNAs don't have a perfect double-stranded RNA (dsRNA) structure topped by a terminal loop. There are few possible explanations for such selectivity. One could be that dsRNAs longer than 21 base pairs activate interferon response and anti-viral machinery in the cell. Another plausible explanation could be that the thermodynamic profile of pre-miRNA determines which strand will be incorporated into Dicer complex. Indeed, clear similarities between pri-miRNAs encoded in respective (5'- or 3'-) strands have been demonstrated.

When Dicer cleaves the pre-miRNA stem-loop, two complementary short RNA molecules are formed, but only one is integrated into the RISC complex. This strand is known as the guide strand and is selected by the argonaute protein, the catalytically active RNase in the RISC complex, on the basis of the stability of the 5' end. The remaining strand, known as the anti-guide or passenger strand, is degraded as a RISC complex substrate. After integration into the active RISC complex, miRNAs base pair with their complementary mRNA molecules and inhibit translation or sometimes induce mRNA degradation by argonaute proteins, the catalytically active members of the RISC complex. It is as yet unclear how the activated RISC complex locates the mRNA targets in the cell, though it has been shown that the process is not coupled to ongoing protein translation from the mRNA.

Cellular Functions of miRNAs

The function of miRNAs appears to be in gene regulation. For that purpose, a miRNA is complementary to a part of one or more messenger RNAs (mRNAs). Animal miRNAs are usually complementary to a site in the 3' UTR whereas plant miRNAs are usually complementary to coding regions of mRNAs. The annealing of the miRNA to the mRNA then inhibits protein translation, but sometimes facilitates cleavage of the mRNA. This is thought to be the primary mode of action of plant miRNAs. In such cases, the formation of the double-stranded RNA through the binding of the miRNA triggers the degradation of the mRNA transcript through a process similar to RNA interference (RNAi), though in other cases it is believed that the miRNA complex blocks the protein translation machinery or otherwise prevents protein translation without causing the mRNA to be degraded. The miRNAs may also target methylation of genomic sites which correspond to targeted mRNAs. The miRNAs function in association with a complement of proteins collectively termed the miRNP. This effect was first described for the worm *C. elegans* in 1993 by Victor Ambros and coworkers. As of 2002, miRNAs have been confirmed in various plants and animals, including *C. elegans*, human and the plant *Arabidopsis thaliana*. Work at the University of Louisville has resulted in the production of microarrays containing all known miRNAs for human, mouse, rat, dog, *C. elegans* and *Drosophila* species, tools referred to as MMChips. Agilent has subsequently commercialized a human miRNA microarray.

Gene Activation

The dsRNA can also activate gene expression, a mechanism that has been termed small RNA-induced gene activation. ThedsRNA targeting gene promoters can induce potent transcriptional activation of associated genes. This was demonstrated in human cells using synthetic dsRNAs termed small activating RNA (saRNA), but has also been demonstrated for endogenous microRNA.

Detecting and Manipulating miRNA Signaling

The activity of a miRNA can be experimentally blocked using a locked nucleic acid oligo, a Morpholino oligo or a 2'-*O*-methyl RNA oligo. Steps in the maturation of miRNAs can be blocked by steric-blocking oligos. The target site of a miRNA on an mRNA can be blocked by a steric blocking oligo.

miRNA and Disease

Just as miRNA is involved in the normal functioning of eukaryotic cells, so has dysregulation of miRNA been associated with disease. Disease association in turn has led to increased funding opportunities for academic research and financial incentives for development and commercialization of miRNA based diagnostics and therapeutics. After early commercialization aimed at academic research support was established, the initial research focus based on products and services requested was on cancer and neuroscience research. During 2007, interests indicated by product and services requested broadened to include cardiac research, virology, cell biology in general and plant biology.

i) **miRNA and Cancer:** A study of mice altered to produce excess c-myc, a protein implicated in several cancers shows that miRNA has an effect on the development of cancer. Mice that were engineered to produce a surplus of types of miRNA found in lymphoma cells developed the disease within 50 days and died two weeks later. In contrast, mice without the surplus miRNA lived over 100 days. Another study found that two types of miRNA inhibit the E2F1 protein, which regulates cell proliferation. The miRNA appears to bind to messenger RNA before it can be translated to proteins that switch genes on and off. By measuring activity among 217 genes encoding miRNA, patterns of gene activity that can distinguish types of cancers can be discerned. The miRNA signatures may enable classification of cancer. This will allow doctors to determine the original tissue type which spawned a cancer and to be able to target a treatment course based on the original tissue type. The miRNA profiling has already been able to determine whether patients with chronic lymphocytic leukemia had slow growing or aggressive forms of the cancer. In 2008, the companies Asuragen and Exiqon were working to commercialize this potential for miRNAs to act as cancer biomarkers.

ii) **miRNA and Heart Disease:** The global role of miRNA function in the heart has been addressed by conditionally inhibiting miRNA maturation in the murine heart and has revealed that miRNAs play an essential role during its development. The miRNA expression profiling studies demonstrate that expression levels of specific miRNAs change in diseased human hearts, pointing to their involvement in cardiomyopathies. Furthermore, studies on specific miRNAs in animal models have identified distinct roles for miRNAs both during heart development and under pathological conditions, including the regulation of key factors important for cardiogenesis, the hypertrophic growth response and cardiac conductance. In 2008, academic work on the relationship between miRNA and heart disease had advanced sufficiently to lead to the establishment of a company, miRagen, with a primary focus on cardiovascular health and disease.

Similarities and Differences between DNA and RNA

They differ in composition *i.e.* the sugar in RNA is ribose, not the deoxyribose in DNA. The base uracil is present in RNA instead of thymine. They also differ in size and structure, RNA molecules are smaller (shorter) than DNA molecules, RNA is single stranded, not double-stranded like DNA. Another difference between RNA and DNA is in function. DNA has only one function *i.e.* storing genetic information in its sequence of nucleotide bases (Table 3.3).

Table 3.3: Similarities and Differences between DNA and RNA

S.No.	Characteristic	DNA	RNA
1.	Deoxyribonucleic acid	√	—
2.	Ribonucleic acid	—	√
3.	Ribose sugar present	—	√
4.	Deoxyribose sugar present	√	—
5.	It's sugar is linked to a phosphate group at one end and a nitrogenous base at the other end	√	√
6.	Polymer of nucleotides	√	√
7.	Nitrogenous bases:	—	—
	Adenine (A) present	√	√
	Thymine (T) present	√	
	Uracil (U) present	—	√
	Cytosine (C) present	√	√
	Guanine (G) present	√	√
8.	Two (2) double chains held in a double helix by hydrogen bonds	√	—
9.	Single stranded		√
10.	Contains a chemical code or message which must be transcribed.	√	—

Summary

1. DNA and RNA are two types of nucleic acids found in most of the organisms.

2. Nucleic acids are long polymers of nucleotides, while DNA stores genetic information.

3. RNA mostly helps in transfer and expression of information.

4. A gene is a unit of information that directs the activity of the cell or organism during its life time.

5. Genes are situated in chromosome. Every gene occupies a fixed position in the chromosome. They are arranged in a single linear order in a chromosome.

6. The most conclusive evidence in support of DNA as the genetic material came from transformation of bacteria. This was done by F. Griffith in 1928.

7. The quantity of DNA found in a diploid cell is approximately the twice that in a haploid germ cell.

8. The DNA from cells of widely differing species is less alike in composition than the DNA from closely related species.

9. Among the chemical and physical agents known to alter the chemical structure of DNA without killing the organism are those which cause mutation.

10. The wave lengths of UV light that cause a high incidence of mutation closely correspond to the wavelength absorbed by DNA.

11. On replication each DNA molecule gives rise to two DNA molecules, identical to each other as well as the parent molecule. The replication is semi-conservative, it is proposed by Watson and Crick.

12. In 1902, A. Garrod reported that some heredity human disease is caused by certain biochemical defects.

13. The disease is caused by the failure of an enzyme to catalyze a reaction in the metabolic pathway. Three human disease phenylketonuria, albinism and alkaptonuria are caused by failure within metabolic pathway.

14. All enzymes are protein molecules and proteins are complex molecule composed of one or more polypeptide chain.

15. The double stranded DNA gives rise to RNA, which functions as a messenger to programme the synthesis of a polypeptide. During transcription, a complementary m RNA strand is formed from a DNA strand.

16. In the translation process, the coded information coming originally from DNA, contained in mRNA and ribosome for the synthesis of protein molecule.

17. The genetic code is a sequence of nitrogenous bases along a sugar-phosphate strand of a DNA molecule.

18. AUG and GUG triplets are chain initiation codons. UAA, UAG and UGA triplets are chain termination codons.

19. Operon Modal proposed by Jacob and Monod (1961). An operon consists of an operator gene which controls the activity of a number of structural gene.

20. Eukaryotic cell employ a variety of mechanism to regulate gene expression.

21. The information on the eukaryotic gene for assembling a polypeptide is not continuous but split. RNA splicing discovered by Phillip Sharp in 1977.

22. The region of a split gene that becomes part of mRNA and codes for the different amino acids is called exons. The region of a gene that does not form part of mRNA and are removed during RNA processing during mRNA synthesis is known as introns.

23. The gene battery model proposed by Britten and Davidson in 1969. A set of structural genes controlled by one sensor site is known as battery.

24. One gene one enzyme hypothesis proposed by Beadle and Tatum (1940).

25. Seymom Benzer (1957) coined the term cistron, recon and muton.

26. According to unineme model, chromosome is one long coiled or folded DNA molecule which is associated with histone protein or nucleoprotein. Unineme model proposed by E.J.Du Praw (1965).

27. In nucleosome helix, successive turns come close together and form a structure is called solenoid.

28. Human genome project was a mega project that aimed to sequence every base in human genome. This project has yielded much new information. Many new area and avenues have opened up as a consequence of the project.

29. DNA Fingerprinting is a technique to find out the variations in individuals of a population at DNA level. It works on the principles of polymorphism in DNA sequences. It has immense application in the field of forensic science, genetic biodiversity and evolutionary biology.

Chapter 4
Cell Cycle and Cell Division

Introduction

With improvements in microscopy, biologists came to recognize two fundamentally different types of cellular organization; a simpler one characteristic of bacteria and a more complex one found in all other kinds of cells. The organization of organisms depends upon the ir type of cells and their division. The development of any kind of organisms starts from the cell and their cleavage. Multicellular organisms such as animal including human have distinctive type of cell division to make up a complete organism.

The study of cell cycle focuses on mechanisms that regulate the timing and frequency of DNA duplication and cell division. As a biological concept, the cell cycle is defined as the period between successive divisions of a cell. During this period, the contents of the cell must be accurately replicated. Microscopists had known about cell division for more than one hundred years, but not until the 1950s, through the pioneering work of Alma Howard and Stephen Pelc, did they become aware that DNA replication took place only at a specific phase of the cell cycle and that this phase was clearly separated from mitosis. Howard and Pelc's work in the broad bean, *Vicia faba*, revealed that cell goes through many discrete phases before and after cell division. From this understanding, scientists then identified the four characteristic phases of the cell cycle; mitosis (M), gap 1 (G1), DNA synthesis (S) and gap 2 (G2). The study of these phases, the proteins that regulate them and the complex biochemical interactions that stop or start DNA replication and cell division (cytokinesis) are the primary concerns of cell cycle biologists. The most significant progress in this research field came with the demonstration that specific protein complexes involving cyclins were critical for regulating the passage of cells through the cell cycle. These early observations came from biological studies of the cells of rapidly dividing fertilized frog eggs as well as mutant yeast cells that could not divide. The observations suggested that regulation of the cell cycle is conserved throughout eukaryotes, which has since proved to be the case. The mechanism of division in bacteria differs from that of eukaryotes, and the control of their cell cycle is also somewhat different, although again it is linked with DNA replication.

Although the cell cycle is a highly integrated process, distinct areas of interest within this field of study have emerged. For instance, many genes and proteins that influence the passage from one phase of the cell cycle to another have been identified. When their expression is altered by mutation or aberrant regulation, they are usually classed as oncogenes. Other proteins act to hold the cell at distinct points in the cycle (checkpoints) and are known as tumor suppressor genes. Apart from those with a clearly regulatory role, many proteins have important functions in other aspects of the cell cycle; one is replication of DNA and organelles, which is a fascinating process that includes its own repair mechanisms and self editing. Other fields focus primarily on the mechanical processes of cell cleavage into two daughter cells at the end of mitosis and on the condensation and decondensation of chromatin. Originally, cell cycle studies were the preserve of microscopy, but today many specific techniques in addition to those widely employed in cell and molecular biology are applied. Fluorescence activated cell sorting has allowed biologists to both identify cells at particular points of the cell cycle and isolate them. It is possible to monitor how cells that have been exposed to different agents can progress through the cycle.

Cell division is a very important process in all living organisms. During the division of a cell, DNA replication and cell growth also take place. All these processes *i.e.* cell division, DNA replication, and cell growth, hence, have to take place in a coordinated way to ensure correct division and formation of progeny cells containing intact genomes. The sequence of events by which a cell duplicates its genome, synthesises the other constituents of the cell and eventually divides into two daughter cells is termed cell cycle. Although, cell growth (in terms of cytoplasmic increase) is a continuous process, DNA synthesis occurs only during one specific stage in the cell cycle. Then replicated chromosomes (DNA) are distributed to daughter nuclei by a complex series of events during cell division. These events are themselves under genetic control.

Cell Cycle

The cell cycle or cell division cycle is the series of events that take place in a eukaryotic cell leading to its replication. These events can be divided in two broad periods; interphase during which the cell grows, accumulating nutrients needed for mitosis and duplicating its DNA and the mitotic (M) phase, during which the cell splits itself into two distinct cells called daughter cells. The cell division cycle is an essential process by which a single celled fertilized egg develops into a mature organism, as well as the process by which hair, skin, blood cells and some internal organs are renewed.

Phases of Cell Cycle

The cell cycle consists of four distinct phases G_1 phase, S phase, G_2 phase (interphase) and M phase. M phase is itself composed of two tightly coupled processes *i.e.* mitosis, in which the cell's chromosomes are divided between the two daughter cells and cytokinesis, in which the cell's cytoplasm divides forming distinct cells. Activation of each phase is dependent on the proper progression and completion of

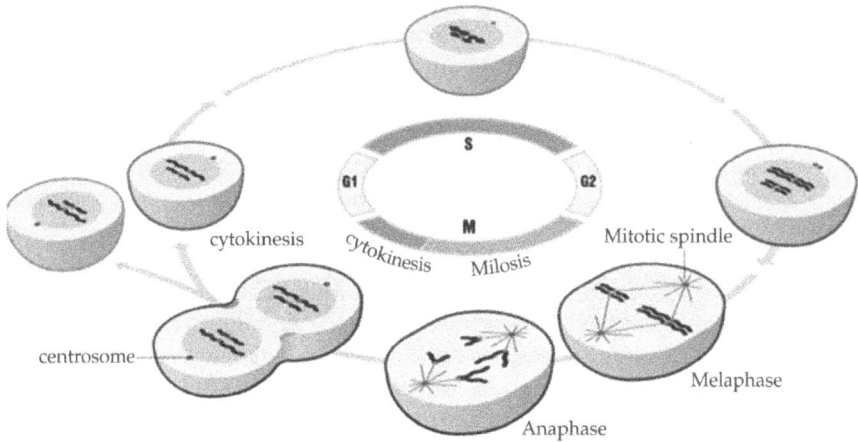

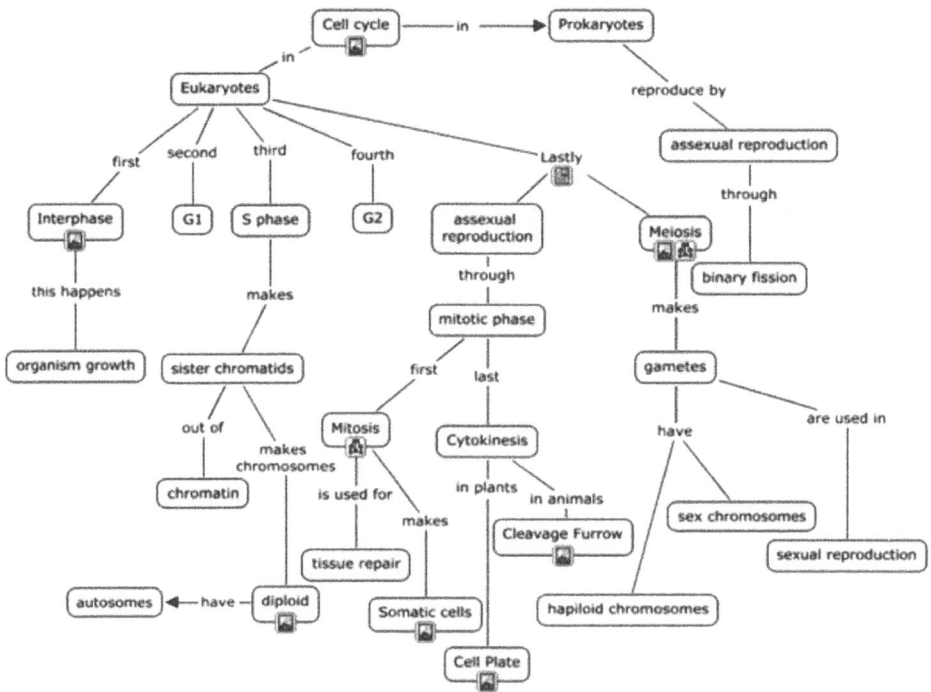

Figure 4.1: Schematic of Cell cycle

the previous one. Cells that have temporarily or reversibly stopped dividing are said to have entered a state of quiescence called G_0 phase.

M phase: The relatively brief M phase consists of nuclear division (mitosis) and cytoplasmic division (cytokinesis).

Interphase: After M phase, the daughter cells each begin interphase of a new cycle. Although the various stages of interphase are not usually morphologically distinguishable, each phase of cell cycle has a distinct set of specialized biochemical processes that prepare the cell for initiation of cell division.

G_1 phase: The first phase within interphase, from the end of the previous M phase till the beginning of DNA synthesis is called G_1 (G indicating gap or growth). During this phase the biosynthetic activities of the cell, which had been considerably slowed down during M phase, resume at a high rate. This phase is marked by synthesis of various enzymes that are required in S phase, mainly those needed for DNA replication. Duration of G_1 is highly variable, even among different cells of the same species.

S phase: The ensuing S phase starts when DNA synthesis commences; when it is complete, all of the chromosomes have been replicated, *i.e.*, each chromosome has two (sister) chromatids. Thus, during this phase, the amount of DNA in the cell has effectively doubled, though the ploidy of the cell remains the same. Rates of RNA transcription and protein synthesis are very low during this phase. An exception to this is histone production, most of which occurs during the S phase. The duration of S phase is relatively constant among cells of the same species.

G_2 phase: The cell then enters the G_2 phase, which lasts until the cell enters the next round of mitosis. Again, significant protein synthesis occurs during this phase, mainly involving the production of microtubules, which are required during the process of mitosis. Inhibition of protein synthesis during G_2 phase prevents the cell from undergoing mitosis.

G_0 phase: The term post mitotic is sometimes used to refer to both quiescent and senescent cells. Nonproliferative cells in multicellular eukaryotes generally enter the quiescent G_0 state from G_1 and may remain quiescent for long periods of time, possibly indefinitely as is often the case for neurons. This is very common for cells that are fully differentiated. Cellular senescence is a state that occurs in response to DNA damage or degradation that would make a cell's progeny nonviable; it is often a biochemical alternative to the self destruction of such a damaged cell by apoptosis. Some cell types in mature organisms, such as parenchymal cells of the liver and kidney, enter the G_0 phase semi-permanently and can only be induced to begin dividing again under very specific circumstances; other types, such as epithelial cells, continue to divide throughout an organism's life.

Cell Division

Cell division is a process by which a cell, called the parent cell, divides into two cells, called daughter cells. Cell division is usually a small segment of a larger cell cycle. In meiosis however, a cell is permanently transformed and cannot divide again. For simple unicellular organisms such as the Amoeba, one cell division reproduces an entire organism. On a larger scale, cell division can create progeny from multicellular organisms, such as plants that grow from cuttings. Cell division also enables sexually reproducing organisms to develop from the one celled zygote, which itself was produced by cell division from gametes. After growth, cell division allows for continual renewal and repair of the organism. The primary concern of cell division is the maintenance of the original cell's genome. Before division can occur, the genomic information which is stored in chromosomes must be replicated and the duplicated genome separated cleanly between cells. A great deal of cellular infrastructure is involved in keeping genomic information consistent between generations.

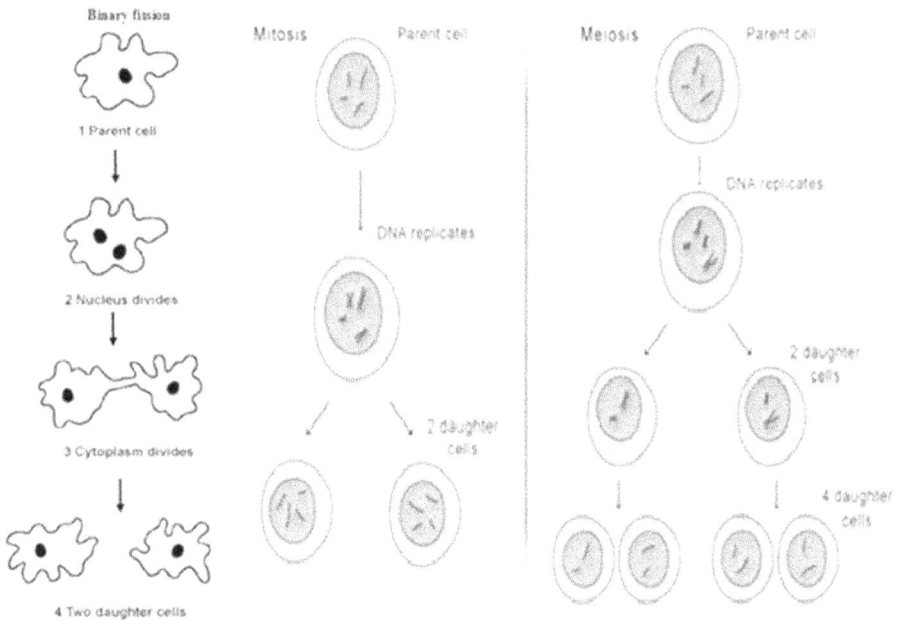

Figure 4.2: Differences in Binary fission, Mitosis and Meiosis

Types of Cell Division

Cells are classified into two categories: simple, non-nucleated prokaryotic cells and complex nucleated eukaryotic cells. Furthermore, the pattern of cell division that transforms eukaryotic stem cells into gametes (sperm in males or ova in females) is different from that of eukaryotic somatic (non-germ) cells.

Prokaryotic Cell Division

Prokaryotes are much simpler in their organization than are eukaryotes. There are a great many more organelles in eukaryotes, also more chromosomes. The usual method of prokaryote cell division is termed binary fission. The prokaryotic chromosome is a single DNA molecule that first replicates, then attaches each copy to a different part of the cell membrane. When the cell begins to pull apart, the replicate and original chromosomes are separated. Following cell splitting (cytokinesis), there are then two cells of identical genetic composition except for the rare chance of a spontaneous mutation. The prokaryote chromosome is much easier to manipulate than the eukaryotic one. One consequence of this asexual method of reproduction is that all organisms in a colony are genetic equals. When treating a bacterial disease, a drug that kills one bacterium will also kill all other members of that clone (colony) it comes in contact with.

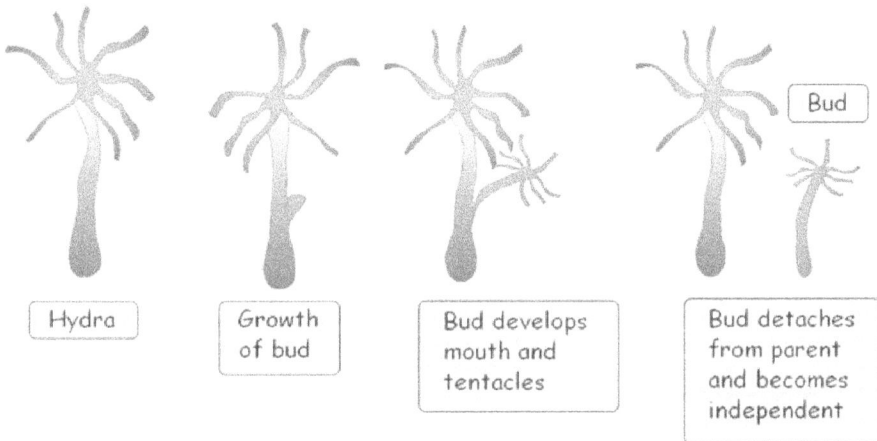

Figure 4.3: Budding in Hydra

Eukaryotic Cell Division

All cells arise by the division of an existing cell. The life of a cell from the time it is generated by the division of a progenitor cell to the time it in turn divides is called the cell division cycle or just the cell cycle for short. In humans the cells of some tissues, such as the skin, the lining of the gut and the bone marrow continue to divide throughout life. A human being is bigger than a mouse and smaller than an elephant. Allowing for some minor differences in basic design, this is because humans are made up of more cells than a mouse and less than an elephant. Due to their increased numbers of chromosomes organelles and complexity, eukaryote cell division is more complicated, although the same processes of replication, segregation and cytokinesis still occur. The three mechanisms are:

- **Mitosis**: The division of the nucleus, separating the duplicated genome into two sets identical to the parent's.

- **Cytokinesis**: The division of the cytoplasm, separating the organelles and other cellular components.

- **Meiosis**: The division of the nucleus in sex cells, making one cell into four sex cells identical to the parent sex cell.

Mitosis

Mitosis is the name given to basic cell division. Cells divide when hormones instruct them to; usually to replace dying cells or as part of the healing process. There are five stages to this division, the first of which is interphase. During interphase, the cell rests and the chromosomes make copies of themselves. After interphase comes prophase, the second stage of mitosis. During prophase, the chromosomes change shape and the walls of the nucleus begin to break down. The third phase is metaphase and it is when the chromosomes line up at their centers. During anaphase, the fourth stage, each forming cell is given its own identical set of chromosomes. The fifth stage, telophase, occurs when the two newly formed daughter cells pull away from each other and begin forming new nuclei. When these new nuclei are formed, the cells re-enter interphase and await their next division.

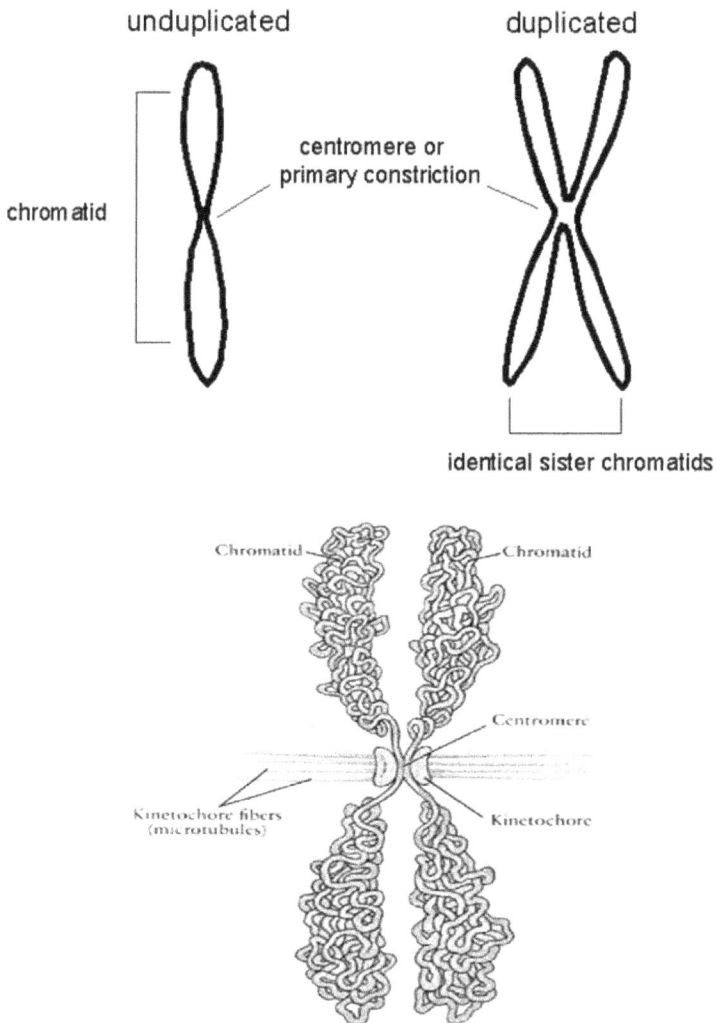

Figure 4.4: Chromatid

Stages of Mitosis

Mitosis is designed to produce two progeny cells each containing an identical set of the progenitor cell's chromosomes. Classically, mitosis is divided into five stages, each of which is characterized by changes in the appearance of the chromosomes and their organization with respect to a cellular structure, called the mitotic spindle and it is responsible for their segregation. One copy of our genome is encoded in 23 chromosomes and is made up of 3×10^9 base pairs. Human cells contain 46 chromosomes, 23 inherited from each parent. This state is called diploid in which each cell has two complete sets of chromosomes.

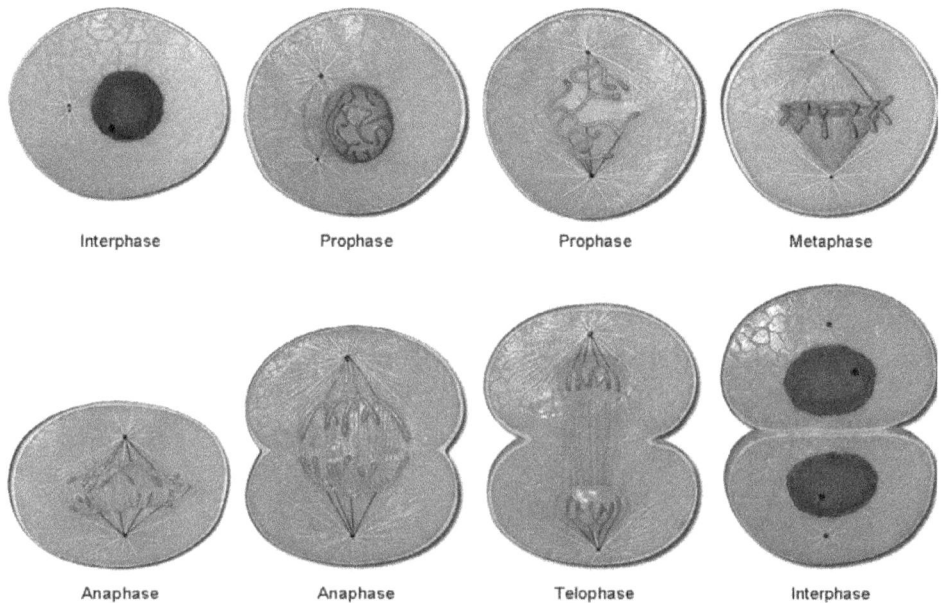

| Interphase | Prophase | Prophase | Metaphase |
| Anaphase | Anaphase | Telophase | Interphase |

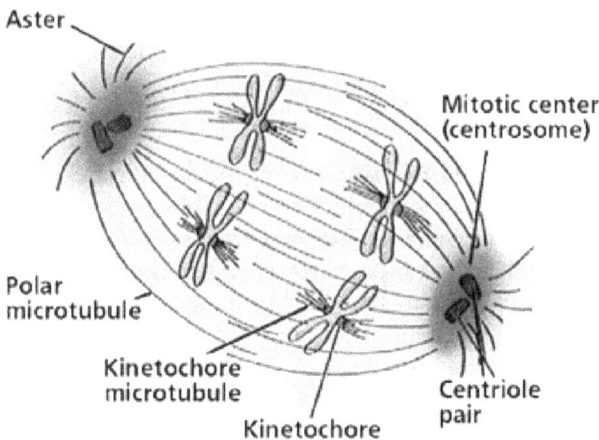

Figure 4.5: Satges of Mitosis

i.   Prophase : The first evidence of mitosis in most cells is the compaction of the threads of chromatin that existed through interphase into compact chromosomes that are visible in the light microscope. As the chromosomes compact, each can be seen to be paired structures composed of two chromatids. This is the visible effect of the DNA molecules having been replicated in interphase. Chromosome condensation reduces the chance of long DNA molecules becoming tangled and broken. Each chromosome has a constriction called the kinetochore, a structure that forms around a region rich in satellite DNA called the centromere. The kinetochore is the point of attachment of the chromosome to the spindle. At the same time as the chromosomes are condensing within the nucleus, the centrosomes, which lie on the cytoplasmic side of the nuclear envelope, begin to separate to establish the mitotic spindle.

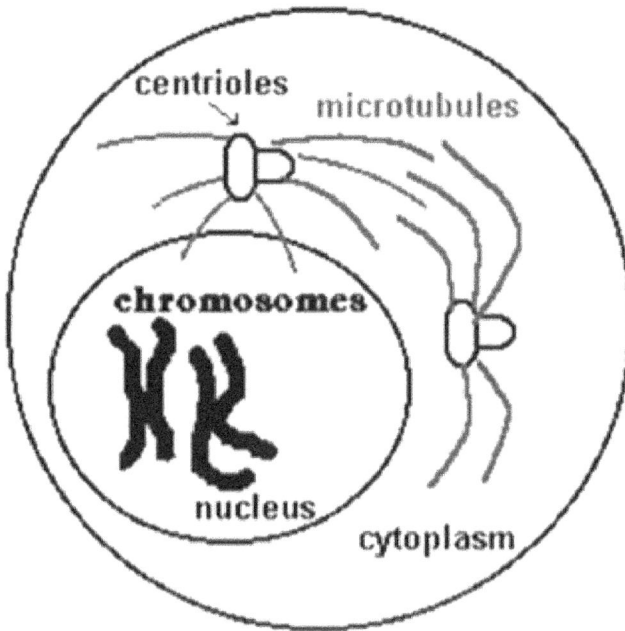

Figure 4.6: Prophase

ii.   Pro-metaphase : At the breakdown of the nuclear envelope, the chromosomes become free to interact with the forming spindle. Microtubule assembly from the centrosomes is random and dynamic. The growing ends of individual microtubules make chance contact with and are captured by the kinetochores. Because of the random nature of these events, the kinetochores of chromatid pairs are initially associated with different numbers of microtubules and the forces acting upon each chromosome are unbalanced. Initially the spindle is highly unstable and chromosomes make frequent excursions toward and away from the poles. Gradually, a balance of forces is established and the chromosomes become aligned at the equator, with the kinetochores of each member of a chromatid pair oriented toward opposite poles.

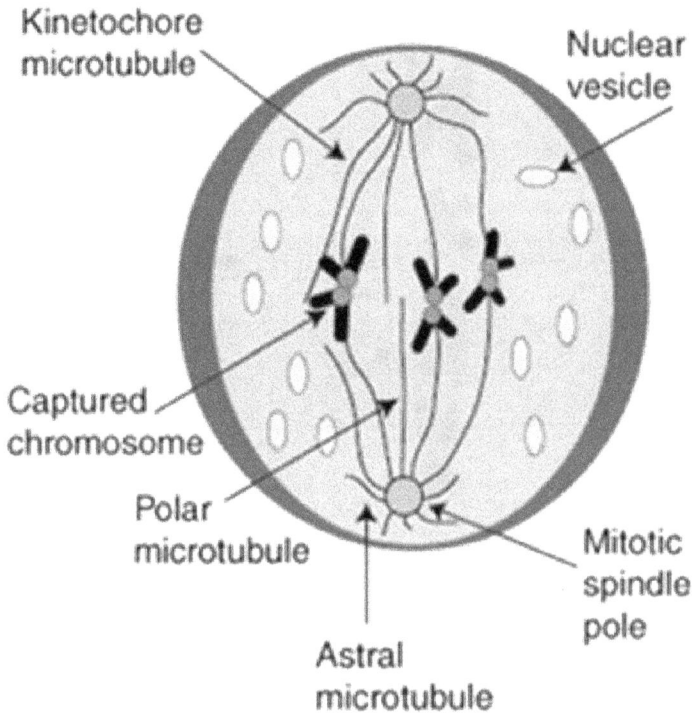

Figure 4.7: Pro-metaphase

iii. Metaphase : Metaphase is the most stable period of mitosis. The system can be regarded as being at steady state with the chromosomes lined up rather like athletes at the start of a race *e.g.* albeit half facing in one direction and half the other. The metaphase spindle consists of two major groups of microtubules: those connecting the chromatids to the poles and a second group extending from each pole toward the other. The second groups overlap at the spindle equator. If a single chromatid becomes detached from the spindle, it sends a signal that tells the other chromosomes not to start anaphase without it. The other chromosomes dutifully wait until the missing chromatid reattaches, whereupon all of the chromosomes enter anaphase together.

iv. Anaphase : The trigger for the separation of the paired chromatids and the start of their journey to the spindle poles is the degradation of the protein cohesin, which acts as the glue holding the pairs of chromatids together. In anaphase A the microtubules holding the chromosomes shorten, pulling the chromosomes to the spindle poles. The chromosomes move as a V with the kinetochores, at which the force for chromosome movement is applied, leading the way. In contrast, in anaphase B the microtubules that overlap at the spindle equator lengthen, extending the distance between the poles. Compared to other forms of cell motility, the movement of chromosomes at anaphase is extremely slow, less than 1 μm per minute.

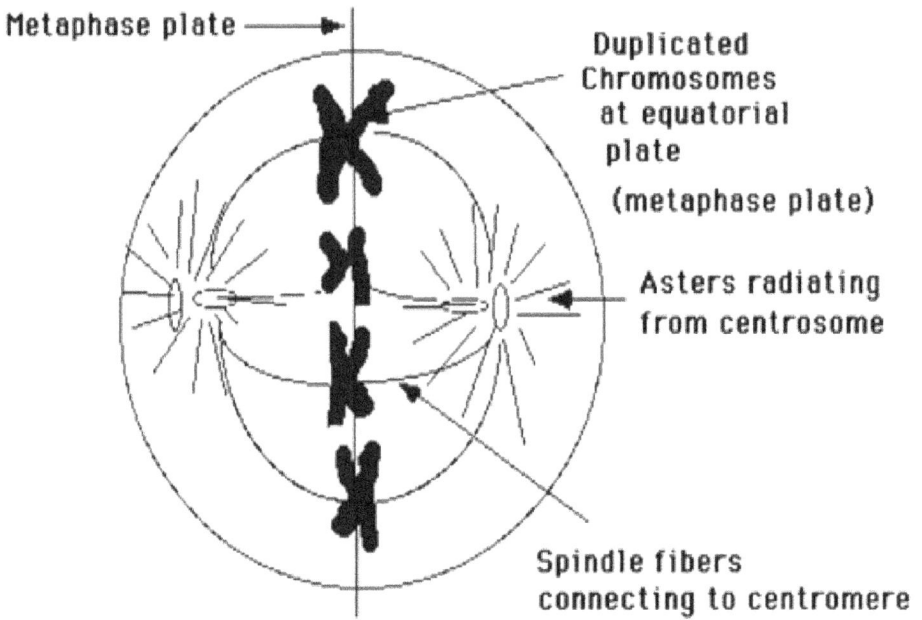

Figure 4.8: Metaphase

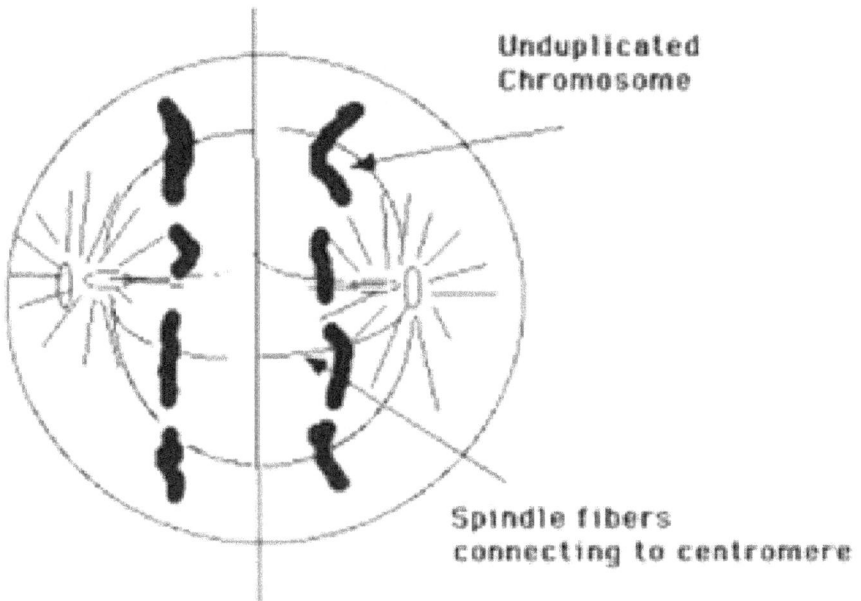

Figure 4.9: Anaphase

v. Telophase : This stage sees the reversal of many of the events of prophase; the chromosomes decondense, the spindle disassembles the nuclear envelope reforms, Golgi apparatus and endoplasmic reticulum reform and the nucleolus reappears. Each progeny nucleus now contains one complete copy of the genome from father and one copy from mother.

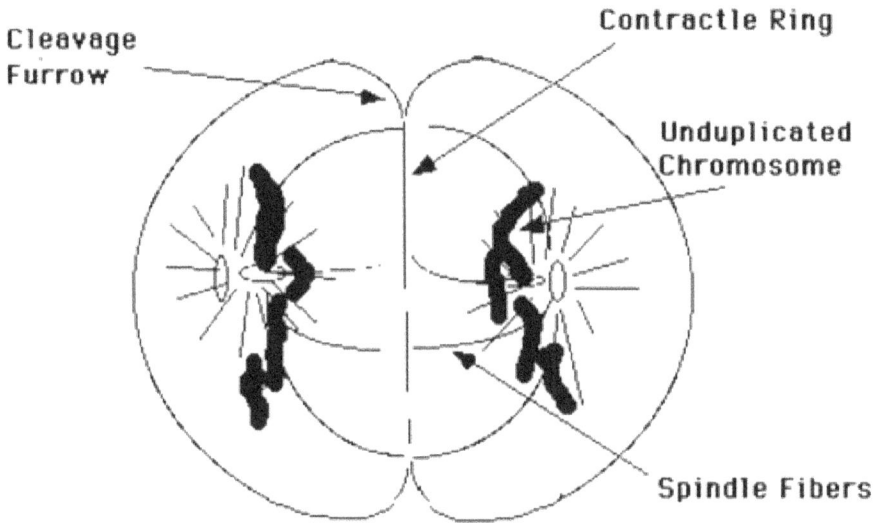

Figure 4.10: Telophase

vi. Cytokinesis : Cytokinesis is a separate process that begins after telophase. Cytokinesis is the process whereby the cytoplasm of a single cell is divided to spawn two daughter cells. Cytokinesis is technically not even a phase of mitosis, but rather a separate process, necessary for completing cell division. In animal cells, a cleavage furrow (pinch) containing a contractile ring develops where the metaphase plate used to be, pinching off the separated nuclei. In both animal and plant cells, cell division is also driven by vesicles derived from the Golgi apparatus, which move along microtubules to the middle of the cell. In plants this structure coalesces into a cell plate at the center of the phragmoplast and develops into a cell wall, separating the two nuclei. The phragmoplast is a microtubule structure typical for higher plants, whereas some green algae use a phycoplast microtubule array during cytokinesis. Each daughter cell has a complete copy of the genome of its parent cell. The end of cytokinesis marks the end of M-phase.

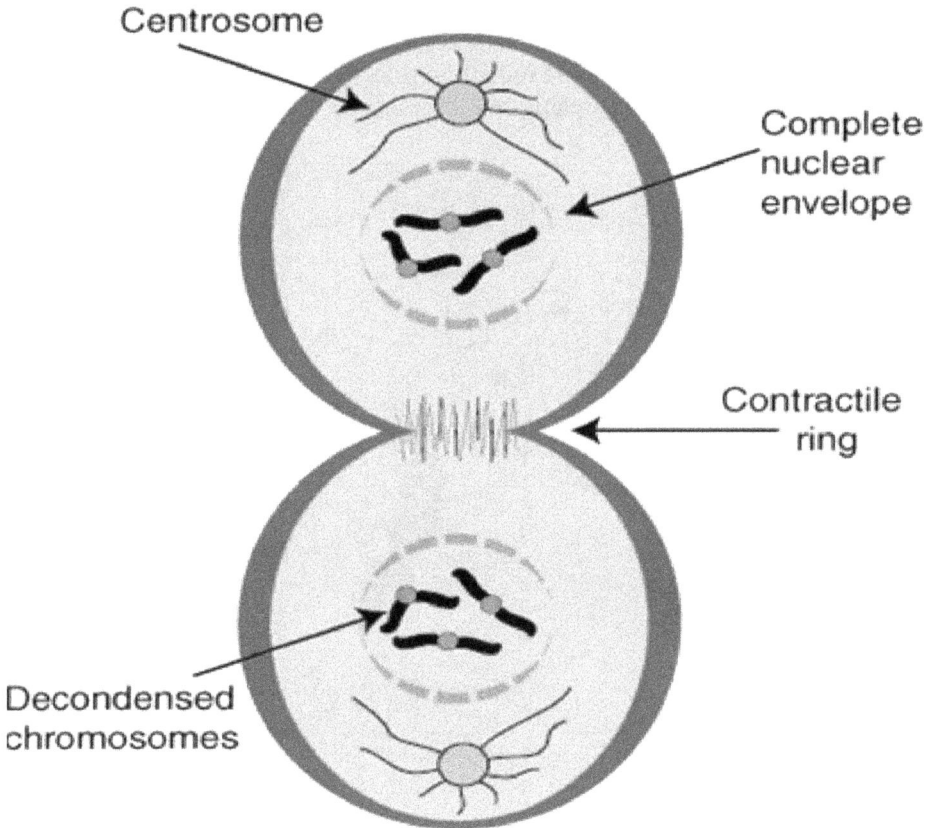

Figure 4.12:Cytokinesis

BOX 4.1

CYTOKINESIS IN ANIMAL, PLANT AND BACTERIA

Animal Cell Cytokinesis

During normal proliferative divisions, animal cell cytokinesis begins shortly after the onset of sister chromatid separation in the anaphase of mitosis. A contractile ring, comprised of non-muscle myosin II and actin filaments, assembles equatorially at the cell cortex (adjacent to the cell membrane). Myosin II uses the free energy released when ATP is hydrolysed to move along these actin filaments, constricting the cell membrane to form a cleavage furrow. Continued hydrolysis causes this cleavage furrow to ingress (move inwards), a stricking process that is clearly visible down a light microscope. Ingression continues until a so-called midbody structure composed of electron-dense, proteinaceous material is formed and the process of abscission then physically cleaves this midbody into two. Abscission depends on septin filaments beneath the cleavage furrow, which provide a structural basis to ensure completion of cytokinesis. After cytokinesis, non-kinetochore microtubules reorganize and disappear into a new cytoskeleton as the cell cycle returns to interphase.

Contractile ring positioning: The position at which the contractile ring assembles is dictated in part at least by the mitotic spindle. This seems to depend upon the GTPase RhoA, which influences several downstream effectors such as the protein kinases ROCK and citron to promote myosin activation and actin filament assembly at a particular region of the cell cortex.

Central spindle: Simultaneous with contractile ring assembly during anaphase, a microtubule based structure termed the central spindle or spindle midzone forms when non-kinetochore microtubule fibres are bundled between the spindle poles. A number of different species including *H. sapiens*, *D. melanogaster* and *C. elegans* require the central spindle in order to efficiently undergo cytokinesis, although the specific phenotype described when it is absent varies from one species to the next *e.g.* certain *Drosophila* cell types are incapable of forming a cleavage furrow without the central spindle, whereas in both *C. elegans* embryos and human tissue culture cells a cleavage furrow is observed to form and ingress, but then regress before cytokinesis is complete. Seemingly vital for the formation of the central spindle is a heterotetrameric protein complex called centralspindlin. Along with associated factors such as SPD-1 in *C. elegans*, centralspindlin plays a role in bundling microtubules to form the spindle midzone during anaphase. **Timing Cytokinesis:** Cytokinesis must be temporally controlled to ensure that it occurs only after sister chromatid separation during normal proliferative cell divisions. To achieve this, many components of the cytokinesis machinery are highly regulated to ensure that they are active only at a particular stage of the cell cycle.

Plant Cell Cytokinesis

Because plant cells have a cell wall, cytokinesis shows significant differences compared with the process in animals cells. Rather than forming a contractile ring, plant cells construct a cell plate in the middle of the cell. The Golgi apparatus releases vesicles containing cell wall materials. These vesicles fuse at the equatorial plane and form a cell plate. The cell plate begins as a fusion tube network, which then becomes a tubulo-vesicular network (TVN) as more components are added. The TVN develops into a tubular network, which then becomes a fenestrated sheet which adheres to the existing plasma membrane.

Bacterial Cell Cytokinesis

In bacterial cells, a tubulin-like protein called FtsZ was observed to be distributed equally in the cell, but seen to be forming a ring when cytokinesis takes place. The FtsZ ring becomes narrower by GTP hydrolysis. FtsZ employs other Fts proteins to the site, among other mureine transpeptidases. It is strongly suggested that the polar regions of a bacterium exclude FtsZ, thereby assuring that the contractile ring forms in the middle of the cell.

Endomitosis

Endomitosis is a variant of mitosis without nuclear or cellular division, resulting in cells with many copies of the same chromosome occupying a single nucleus. This process may also be referred to as endoreduplication and the cells as endoploid.

Consequences of errors

Although errors in mitosis are rare, the process may go wrong, especially during early cellular divisions in the zygote. Mitotic errors can be especially dangerous to the organism because future offspring from this parent cell will carry the same disorder. In non-disjunction, a chromosome may fail to separate during anaphase. One daughter cell will receive both sister chromosomes and the other will receive none. This results in the former cell having three chromosomes coding for the same thing (two sisters and a homologue), a condition known as trisomy and the latter cell having only one chromosome (the homologous chromosome), a condition known as monosomy. These cells are considered aneuploidic cells and these abnormal cells can cause cancer. Mitosis is a traumatic process. The cell goes through dramatic changes in ultrastructure, its organelles disintegrate and reform in a matter of hours and chromosomes are jostled constantly by probing microtubules. Occasionally, chromosomes may become damaged. An arm of the chromosome may be broken and the fragment lost, causing deletion. The fragment may incorrectly reattach to another, non-homologous chromosome, causing translocation. It may reattach to the original chromosome, but in reverse orientation, causing inversion. Or, it may be treated erroneously as a separate chromosome, causing chromosomal duplication. The effect of these genetic abnormalities depends on the specific nature of the error. It may range from no noticeable effect, cancer induction or organism death.

Meiosis

In biology, meiosis is the process by which one diploid eukaryotic cell divides to generate four haploid cells often called gametes. The word meiosis comes from Greek word *meioun*, meaning to make smaller, since it results in a reduction in chromosome number in the gamete cell. Among fungi, spores in which the haploid nuclei are at first disseminated are called meiospores or more specifically, ascospores in asci (Ascomycota) and basidospores on basidia (Basidiomycota). Meiosis was discovered and described for the first time in sea urchin eggs in 1876, by noted German biologist Oscar Hertwig (1849-1922). It was described again in 1883, at the level of chromosomes, by Belgian zoologist Edouard Van Beneden (1846-1910), in Ascaris worms' eggs. The significance of meiosis for reproduction and inheritance, however, was described only in 1890 by German biologist August Weismann (1834-1914), who noted that two cell divisions were necessary to transform one diploid cell into four haploid cells if the number of chromosomes had to be maintained. In 1911 the American geneticist Thomas Hunt Morgan (1866-1945) observed crossover in *Drosophila melanogaste*r meiosis and provided the first true genetic interpretation of meiosis.

Meiosis is essential for sexual reproduction and therefore occurs in all eukaryotes (including single celled organisms) that reproduce sexually. A few eukaryotes, notably the Bdelloid rotifers, have lost the ability to carry out meiosis and have acquired the ability to reproduce by parthenogenesis. Meiosis does not occur in archaea or bacteria, which reproduce via asexual processes such as mitosis or binary fission. During meiosis, the genome of a diploid germ cell, which is composed of long segments of DNA packaged into chromosomes, undergoes DNA replication followed by two rounds of division, resulting in haploid cells called gametes. Each gamete contains one complete set of chromosomes or half of the genetic content of the original cell. These resultant haploid cells can fuse with other haploid cells of the opposite sex or mating type during fertilization to create a new diploid cell or zygote. Thus, the division mechanism of meiosis is a reciprocal process to the joining of two genomes that occurs at fertilization. Because the chromosomes of each parent undergo genetic recombination during meiosis, each gamete and thus each zygote will have a unique genetic blueprint encoded in its DNA. In other words, meiosis and sexual reproduction produce genetic variation. Meiosis uses many of the same biochemical mechanisms employed during mitosis to accomplish the redistribution of chromosomes. There are several features unique to meiosis, most importantly the pairing and genetic recombination between homologous chromosomes.

Meiosis occurs in all eukaryotic life cycles involving sexual reproduction, comprising of the constant cyclical process of meiosis and fertilization. This takes place alongside normal mitotic cell division. In multicellular organisms, there is an intermediary step between the diploid and haploid transition where the organism grows. The organism will then produce the germ cells that continue in the life cycle. The rest of the cells, called somatic cells, function within the organism and will die with it. The organism phase of the life cycle can occur between the haploid to diploid transition and the diploid to haploid transition. Some species are diploid, grown from a diploid cell called the zygote. Others are haploid instead, spawned by the proliferation and differentiation of a single haploid cell called the gamete. Humans are diploid creatures. Human stem cells undergo meiosis to create haploid gametes, which are spermatozoa for males or ova for females. These gametes then fertilize in the Fallopian tubes of the female, producing a diploid zygote. The zygote undergoes progressive stages of mitosis and differentiation, turns into a blastocyst and then gets implanted in the uterus endometrium to create an embryo.

There are three types of life cycles that utilize sexual reproduction, differentiated by the location of the organism's stage. In the gametic life cycle, the living organism is diploid in nature. The organism's diploid germ-line stem cells undergo meiosis to create haploid gametes which fertilize to form the zygote. The diploid zygote undergoes repeated cellular division by mitosis to grow into the organism. Mitosis is a related process to meiosis that creates two cells that are genetically identical to the parent cell. The general principle is that mitosis creates somatic cells and meiosis creates germ cells. In the zygotic life cycle, the living organism is haploid. Two organisms of opposing gender contribute their haploid germ cells to form a diploid zygote. The zygote undergoes meiosis immediately creating four haploid cells. These cells undergo mitosis to create the organism. Many fungi and many protozoa are members of the zygotic life cycle. Finally, in the sporic life cycle, the living organism alternates between haploid and diploid states. Consequently, this cycle is also known as the alternation of generations. The diploid organism's germ-line cells undergo meiosis to produce gametes. The gametes proliferate by mitosis, growing into a haploid organism. The haploid organism's germ cells then combine with another haploid organism's cells creating the zygote. The zygote undergoes repeated mitosis and differentiation to become the diploid organism again. The sporic life cycle can be considered a fusion of the gametic and zygotic life cycles and indeed its diagram supports this conclusion.

Division Process

Because meiosis is a one-way process, it cannot be said to engage in a cell cycle as mitosis does. However, the preparatory steps that lead up to meiosis are identical in pattern and name to the interphase of the mitotic cell cycle. Interphase is divided into three phases:

*   **Growth 1 (G$_1$) phase:** Immediately follows cytogenesis. This is a very active period, where cell synthesizes its vast array of proteins, including the enzymes and structural proteins it will need for growth. In G1 stage each of the 46 human chromosomes consists of a single (very long) molecule of DNA.

*   **Synthesis (S) phase:** The genetic material is replicated: each of its chromosomes duplicates. The cell is still diploid, however, because it still contains the same number of centromeres. However, the identical sister chromatids are in the chromatin form because spiralisation and condensation into denser chromosomes have not taken place yet. It will take place in prophase I in meiosis.

*   **Growth 2 (G$_2$) phase:** The cell continues to grow making the cell larger.

    Interphase is immediately followed by meiosis I and meiosis II. Meiosis I consists of segregating the homologous chromosomes from each other, then dividing the diploid cell into two haploid cells each containing one of the segregates. Meiosis II consists of decoupling each chromosome's sister strands (chromatids), segregating the DNA into two sets of strands (each set containing one of each homolog) and dividing both haploid, duplicated cells to produce four haploid, unduplicated cells. Meiosis I and II are both divided into prophase, metaphase, anaphase and telophase subphases, similar in purpose to their analogous subphases in the mitotic cell cycle. Therefore, meiosis encompasses the interphase (G$_1$, S, G$_2$), meiosis I (prophase I, metaphase I, anaphase I, telophase I) and meiosis II (prophase II, metaphase II, anaphase II, telophase II).

Meiosis I

Prophase I

I.   Leptotene : The first stage of prophase I is the leptotene stage, also known as leptonema, from Greek words meaning thin threads. During this stage, individual chromosomes begin to condense into long strands within the nucleus. However the two sister chromatids are still so tightly bound that they are indistinguishable from one another.

II. Zygotene : The zygotene stage, also known as zygonema, from Greek words meaning paired threads, occurs as the chromosomes approximately line up with each other into homologous chromosomes. The combined homologous chromosomes are said to be bivalent. They may also be referred to as a tetrad, a reference to the four sister chromatids. The two chromatids become zipped together, forming the synaptonemal complex, in a process known as synapsis.

III. Pachytene : The pachytene stage, also known as pachynema, from Greek words meaning thick threads, contains the chromosomal crossover. Nonsister chromatids of homologous chromosomes randomly exchange segments of genetic information over regions of homology. Exchange takes place at sites where recombination nodules have formed. The exchange of information between the non-sister chromatids results in a recombination of information; each chromosome has the complete set of information it had before and there are no gaps formed as a result of the process unital cause the chromosomes cannot be distinguished in the diplotene stage.

IV. Diplotene : During the diplotene stage, also known as diplonema, from Greek words meaning two threads, the synaptonemal complex degrades and homologous chromosomes separate from one another a little. The chromosomes themselves uncoil a bit, allowing some transcription of DNA. However, the homologous chromosomes of each bivalent remain tightly bound at chiasmata, the regions where crossing over occurred.

V. Diakinesis : hromosomes condense further during the diakinesis stage, from Greek words meaning moving through. This is the first point in meiosis where the four parts of the tetrads are actually visible. Sites of crossing over entangle together, effectively overlapping, making chiasmata clearly visible. Other than this observation, the rest of the stage closely resembles prometaphase of mitosis; the nucleoli disappear, the nuclear membrane disintegrates into vesicles and the meiotic spindle begins to form.

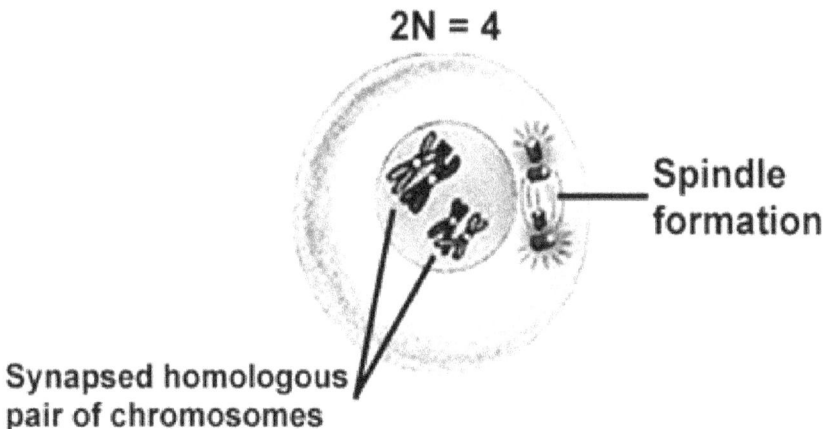

2N = 4

Spindle formation

Synapsed homologous pair of chromosomes

Figure 4.12: Prophase I

Synchronous Processes

During these stages, centrioles are migrating to the two poles of the cell. These centrioles, which were duplicated during interphase, function as microtubule coordinating centers. Centrioles sprout microtubules, essentially cellular ropes and poles, during crossing over. They invade the nuclear membrane after it disintegrates, attaching to the chromosomes at the kinetochore. The kinetochore functions as a motor, pulling the chromosome along the attached microtubule toward the originating centriole, like a train on a track. There are two kinetochores on each tetrad, one for each centrosome. Prophase I is the longest phase in meiosis. Microtubules that attach to the kinetochores are known as kinetochore microtubules. Other microtubules will interact with microtubules from the opposite centriole. These are called nonkinetochore microtubules.

Metaphase I

Homologous pairs move together along the phase plate: as kinetochore microtubules from both centrioles attach to their respective kinetochores, the homologous chromosomes align along an equatorial plane that bisects the spindle, due to continuous counterbalancing forces exerted on the bivalents by the microtubules emanating from the two kinetochores. The physical basis of the independent assortment of chromosomes is the random orientation of each bivalent along the metaphase plate.

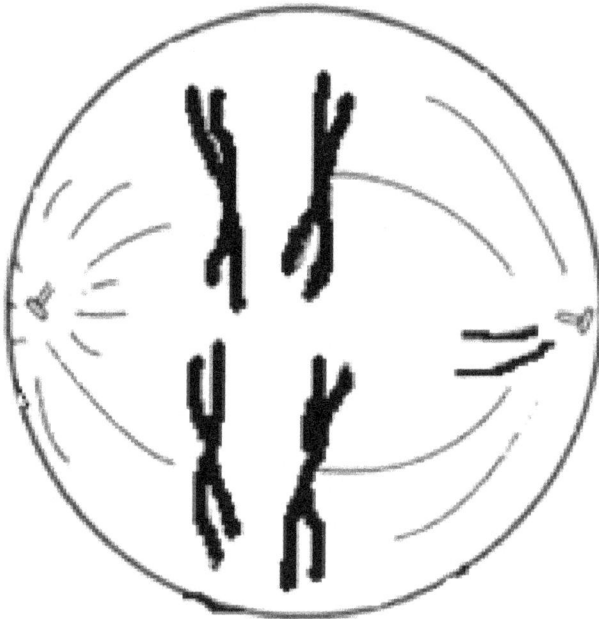

Figure 4.13: Metaphase-I

Anaphase I

Kinetochore microtubules shorten, severing the recombination nodules and pulling homologous chromosomes apart. Since each chromosome only has one kinetochore, whole chromosomes are pulled toward opposing poles, forming two diploid sets. Each chromosome still contains a pair of sister chromatids. Nonkinetochore microtubules lengthen, pushing the centrioles further apart. The cell elongates in preparation for division down the middle. In prophase I the DNA coils tightly and individual chromosomes become visible under the light microscope. Homologous chromosomes closely associated in synapsis and they exchange segments by crossing over.

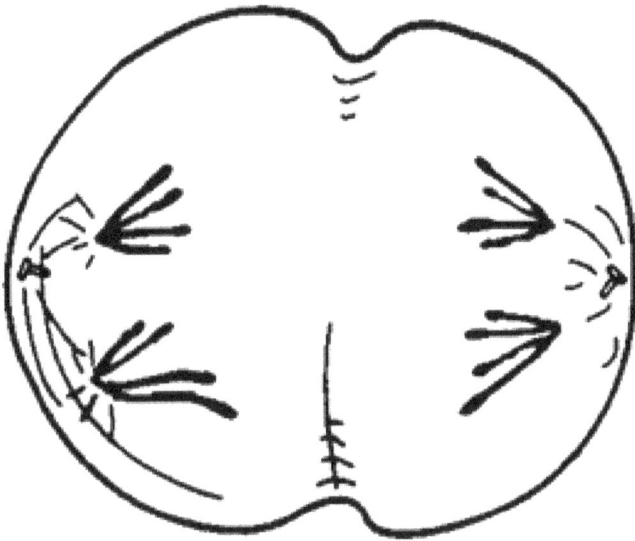

Figure 4.14: Anaphase-I

Telophase I

The first meiotic division effectively ends when the centromeres arrive at the poles. Each daughter cell now has half the number of chromosomes but each chromosome consists of a pair of chromatids. This effect produces a variety of responses from the neuro-synrchromatic enzyme, also known as NSE. The microtubules that make up the spindle network disappear and a new nuclear membrane surrounds each haploid set. The chromosomes uncoil back into chromatin. Cytokinesis, the pinching of the cell membrane in animal cells or the formation of the cell wall in plant cells, occurs, completing the creation of two daughter cells. Cells enter a period of rest known as interkinesis or interphase II. No DNA replication occurs during this stage. Many plants skip telophase I and interphase II, going immediately into prophase II.

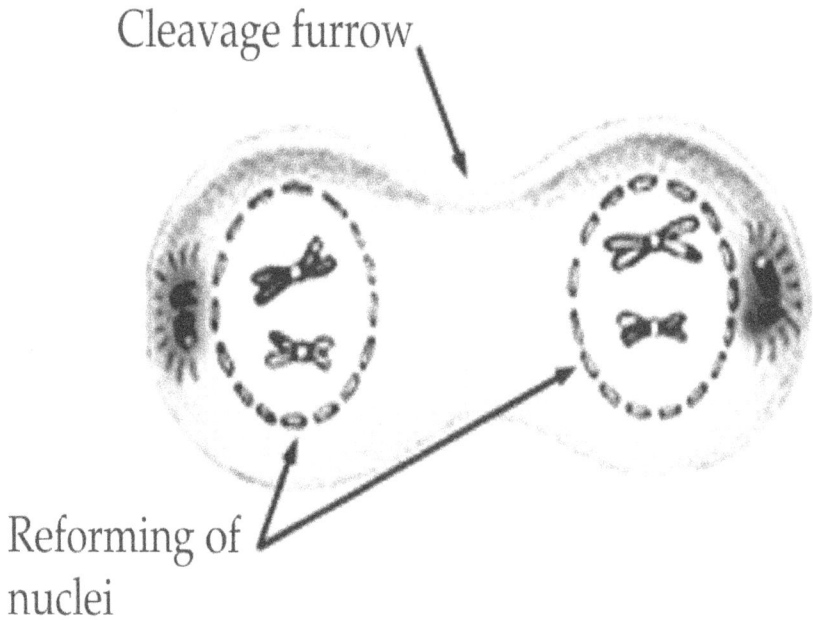

Cleavage furrow

Reforming of
nuclei

Figure 4.15: Telophase-1

Meiosis II

Prophase II takes inversely proportional time as compared to telophase I. In this prophase, the disappearance of the nucleoli is seen. The nuclear envelope and chromatids were observed. Centrioles move to the polar regions and are arranged by spindle fibres. The new equatorial plane is rotated by 90 degrees when compared to meiosis I, perpendicular to the previous plane. In metaphase II, the centromeres contain three kinetochores organizing fibers from the centrosomes on each side. This is followed by anaphase II, where the centromeres are cleaved, allowing the kinetochores to pull the sister chromatids apart. The sister chromatids by convention are now called sister chromosomes and they are pulled toward opposing poles. The process ends with telophase II, which is similar to telophase I, marked by uncoiling, lengthening and disappearance of the chromosomes occur as the disappearance of the microtubules. Nuclear envelopes reform; cleavage or cell wall formation eventually produces a total of four daughter cells, each with a haploid set of chromosomes. Meiosis is now complete.

Prophase II
($n = 2$)

Metaphase II

Anaphase II

Telophase II

Cytokinesis
($n = 2$)

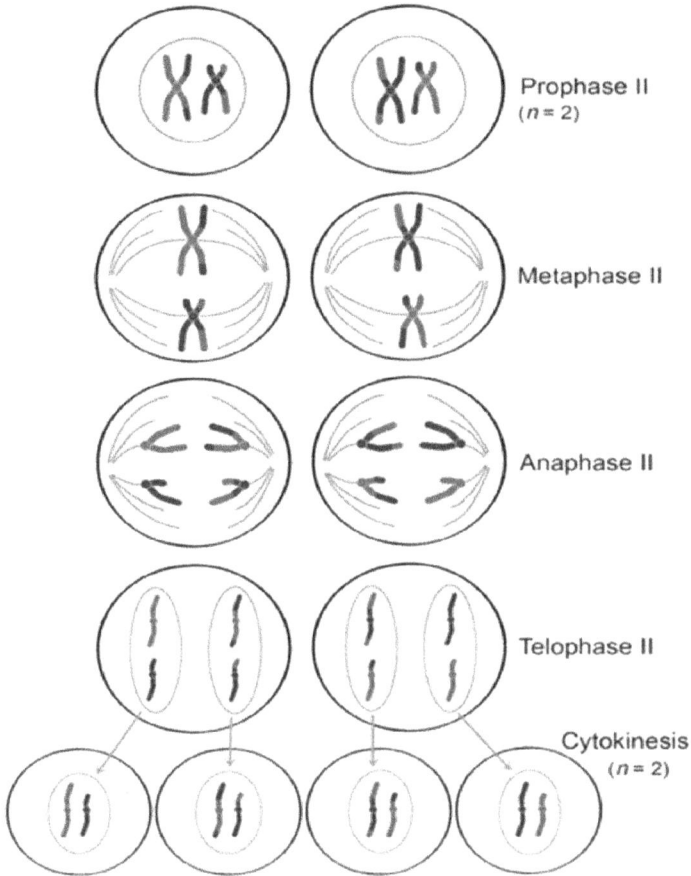

Figure 4.16: Meiosi II

Significance of Meiosis

Meiosis facilitates stable sexual reproduction. Without the halving of ploidy or chromosome count, fertilization would result in zygotes that have twice the number of chromosomes than the zygotes from the previous generation. Successive generations would have an exponential increase in chromosome count, resulting in an unwieldy genome that would cripple the reproductive fitness of the species. Polyploidy, the state of having three or more sets of chromosomes also results in developmental abnormalities or lethality. Polyploidy is poorly tolerated in animal species. Plants, however, regularly produce fertile, viable polyploids. Polyploidy has been implicated as an important mechanism in plant speciation. Meiosis produces genetic variety in gametes that propagate to offspring. Recombination and independent assortment allow for a greater diversity of genotypes in the population. As a system of creating diversity, meiosis allows a species to maintain stability under environmental changes.

Nondisjunction

The normal separation of chromosomes in Meiosis I or sister chromatids in meiosis II is termed disjunction. When the separation is not normal, it is called nondisjunction. This results in the production of gametes which have either more or less of the usual amount of genetic material and is a common mechanism for trisomy or monosomy. Nondisjunction can occur in the meiosis I or meiosis II, phases of cellular reproduction or during mitosis.

This is a cause of several medical conditions in humans, including:

*   Down's Syndrome - trisomy of chromosome 21

*   Patau Syndrome - trisomy of chromosome 13

*   Edward Syndrome - trisomy of chromosome 18

*   Klinefelter Syndrome - extra X chromosomes in males *i.e.* XXY, XXXY, XXXXY

*   Turner Syndrome - atypical X chromosome dosage in females *i.e.* XO, XXX, XXXX

*   XYY Syndrome - an extra Y chromosome in males

Meiosis in Humans

In females, meiosis occurs in precursor cells known as oogonia that divide twice into oocytes. These stem cells stop at the diplotene stage of meiosis I and lay dormant within a protective shell of somatic cells called the follicle. Follicles begin growth at a steady pace in a process known as folliculogenesis and a small number enter the menstrual cycle. Menstruated oocytes continue meiosis I and arrest at meiosis II until fertilization. The process of meiosis in females is called oogenesis and differs from the typical meiosis in that it features a long period of meiotic arrest known as the Dictyate stage and lacks the assistance of centrosomes. In males, meiosis occurs in precursor cells known as spermatogonia that divide twice to become sperm. These cells continuously divide without arrest in the seminiferous tubules of the testicles. Sperm is produced at a steady pace. The process of meiosis in males is called spermatogenesis.

Consequences of Meiosis

First, meiosis comprises two divisions; so each original cell produces four cells, there are exceptions to this generalization in many female animals. Second, chromosome number is reduced by half; so cells produced by meiosis are haploid. Third, cells produced by meiosis are genetically different from one another and from the parental cell. Genetic differences among cells result from two processes that are unique to meiosis. The first is crossing over, which takes place in prophase I. Crossing over refers to the exchange of genes between nonsister chromatids (chromatids from different homologous chromosomes). At one time, this process was thought to take place in pachytene and the synaptonemal complex was believed to be a requirement for crossing over. However, recent evidence from yeast suggests that the situation is more complex. Crossing over is initiated in zygotene, before the synaptonemal complex develops and is not completed until near the end of prophase I. After crossing over has taken place, the sister chromatids may no longer be identical. Crossing over is the basis for intrachromosomal recombination, creating new combinations of alleles on a chromatid. To see how crossing over produces genetic variation, consider two pairs of alleles, which abbreviated as Aa and Bb. Assume that one chromosome possesses the A and B alleles and its homolog possesses the a and b alleles. When DNA is replicated in the S stage, each chromosome duplicates and so the resulting sister chromatids are identical. In the process of crossing over, breaks occur in the DNA strands and the breaks are repaired in such a way that segments of nonsister chromatids are exchanged, the important thing here is that, after crossing over has taken place, the two sister chromatids are no longer identical chromatid has alleles A and B, whereas its sister chromatid has alleles a and B. Likewise, one chromatid of the other chromosome has alleles a and b and the other has alleles A and b. Each of the four chromatids now carries a unique combination of alleles: A B, a B, A b and a b. eventually, the two homologous chromosomes separate, each going into a different cell. In meiosis II, the two chromatids of each chromosome separate and thus each of the four cells resulting from meiosis carries a different combination of alleles. The second process of meiosis that contributes to genetic variation is the random distribution of chromosomes in anaphase I of meiosis following their random alignment during metaphase I. To illustrate this process, consider a cell with three pairs of chromosomes I, II and III. One chromosome of each pair is maternal in origin (Im, IIm and IIIm); the other is paternal in origin (Ip, IIp and IIIp).

The chromosome pairs line up in the center of the cell in metaphase I and in anaphase I, the chromosomes of each homologous pair separate. How each pair of homologs aligns and separates is random and independent of how other pairs of chromosomes align and separate. By chance, all the maternal chromosomes might migrate to one side, with all the paternal chromosomes migrating to the other. After division, one cell would contain chromosomes Im, IIm and IIIm and the other, Ip, IIp and IIIp. Alternatively, the Im, IIm and IIIp chromosomes might move to one side and the Ip, IIp and IIIm chromosomes to the other. The different migrations would produce different combinations of chromosomes in the resulting cells. There are four ways in which a diploid cell with three pairs of chromosomes can divide, producing a total of eight different combinations of chromosomes in the gametes. In general, the number of possible combinations is 2n, where n equals the number of homologous pairs. As the number of chromosome pairs increases, the number of combinations quickly becomes very large. In humans, who have 23 pairs of chromosomes, there are 8,388,608 different combinations of chromosomes possible from the random separation of homologous chromosomes. Through the random distribution of chromosomes in anaphase I, alleles located on different chromosomes are sorted into different combinations. Crossing over shuffles alleles on the same homologous chromosomes into new combinations, whereas the random distribution of maternal and paternal chromosomes shuffles alleles on different chromosomes into new combinations. Together, these two processes are capable of producing tremendous amounts of genetic variation among the cells resulting from meiosis.

Meiosis in Animal

The production of gametes in a male animal (spermatogenesis) takes place in the testes. There, diploid primordial germ cells divide mitotically to produce diploid cells called spermatogonia. Each spermatogonium can undergo repeated rounds of mitosis, giving rise to numerous additional spermatogonia. Alternatively, a spermatogonium can initiate meiosis and enter into prophase I. Now called a primary spermatocyte, the cell is still diploid because the homologous chromosomes have not yet separated. Each primary spermatocyte completes meiosis I, giving rise to two haploid secondary spermatocytes that then undergo meiosis II, with each producing two haploid spermatids. Therefore, each primary spermatocyte produces a total of four haploid spermatids, which mature and develop into sperm. The production of gametes in the female (oogenesis) begins much like spermatogenesis. Diploid primordial germ cells within the ovary divide mitotically to produce oogonia. Like spermatogonia, oogonia can undergo repeated rounds of mitosis or they can enter into meiosis. Once in prophase I, these still-diploid cells are called primary oocytes. Each primary oocyte completes meiosis I and divides. Here the process of oogenesis begins to differ from that of spermatogenesis. In oogenesis, cytokinesis is unequal: most of the cytoplasm is allocated to one of the two haploid cells, the secondary oocyte. The smaller cell, which contains half of the chromosomes but only a small part of the cytoplasm, is called the first polar body; it may or may not divide further. The secondary oocyte completes meiosis II and again cytokinesis is unequal most of the cytoplasm passes into one of the cells. The larger cell, which acquires most of the cytoplasm, is the ovum, the mature female gamete. The smaller cell is the second polar body. Only the ovum is capable of being fertilized and the polar bodies usually disintegrate. Oogenesis, then, produces a single mature gamete from each primary oocyte.

Crossing Over and Linkage

Prophase I end such a long time because the chromosomes deliberately tie themselves in knots and then untangle using topoisomerase II. The paternal and maternal chromosomes are composed of two chromatids and lined up side by side. The chromosome that originated from the father in light green and the maternal one in dark green during prophase 1 the chromosomes are cut and resealed at points called chiasmata (singular chiasma) so that lengths of paternal chromosome are transferred to a maternal one and vice versa. The rest of meiosis I proceeds, followed by meiosis II and the end result is that some gametes contain chromosomes that are neither completely paternal nor completely maternal but are a recombination of the two. The biological advantage of sexual reproduction is that it allows organisms to possess a random selection of the genes from their ancestors. Those individuals with a complement of genes that makes them better suited to their environment tend to do better, allowing evolution by natural selection of the individuals posessing the better genes. Without crossing over this could not happen: Those genes that are located on the same chromosome would remain linked down the generations, greatly reducing the number of gene permutations possible at each generation. Crossing over allows a child to inherit his grandmother's green eyes without also inheriting her defective sodium channel gene, although both genes are on chromosome 19. Even with crossing over, genes on the same chromosome are inherited together more than they would be if they were on different chromosoomes. The closer the genes, the less likely it is that a chisma will form between them and therefore the greater the probability that they will be inherited together. This phenomenon is used to help identify the genes responsible for specific diseases such as cystic fibrosis.

Chromosomal crossover or crossing over is the process by which two chromosomes pair up and exchange sections of their DNA. This often occurs during prophase 1 of meiosis in a process called synapsis. Synapsis begins before the synaptonemal complex develops and is not completed until near the end of prophase I. Crossover usually occurs when matching regions on matching chromosomes break and then reconnect to the other chromosome. The result of this process is an exchange of genes, called genetic recombination. Chromosomal crossovers also occur in asexual organisms and in somatic cells, since they are important in some forms of DNA repair.

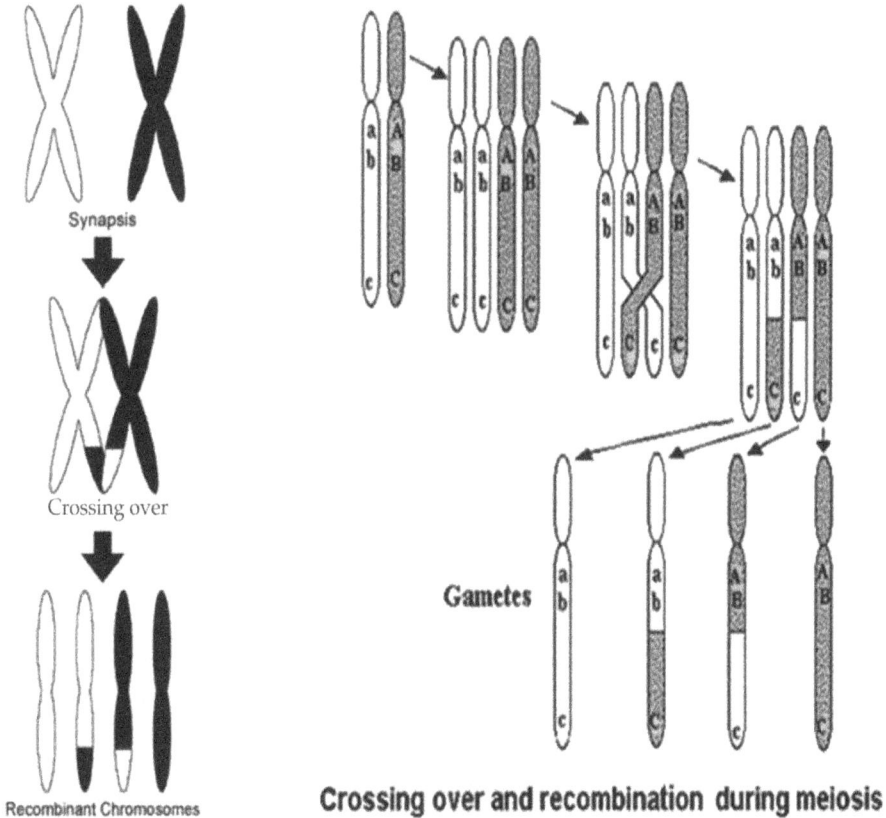

Crossing over and recombination during meiosis

Figure 4.17 : Recombination involves Breakage and Rejoining of parental Chromosomes

Crossing over was described by Thomas Hunt Morgan. He relied on the discovery of Belgian Professor Frans Alfons Janssens of University of Leuven who described the phenomenon in 1909 and called it chiasmatypie. The term chiasma is linked if not identical to chromosomal crossover. Morgan immediately saw the great importance of Janssens cytological interpretation of chiasmata to the experimental results of his research on the heredity of *Drosophila*. The physical basis of crossing over was first demonstrated by Harriet Creighton and Barbara McClintock in 1931. Meiotic recombination initiates with double-stranded breaks that are introduced into the DNA by the Spo11 protein. One or more exonucleases then digest the 5' ends generated by the double-stranded breaks to produce 3' single-stranded DNA tails. The meiosis specific recombinase Dmc1 and the general recombinase Rad51 coat the single stranded DNA to form nucleoprotein filaments. The recombinases catalyze invasion of the opposite chromatid by the single-stranded DNA from one end of the break. Next, 3' end of the invading DNA primes DNA synthesis, causing displacement of the complementary strand, which subsequently anneals to the single stranded DNA generated from other end of initial double stranded break. The structure that results is a cross, strand exchange, also known as a Holliday junction. The contact between two chromatids that will soon undergo crossing over is known as a chiasma. The Holliday junction is a tetrahedral structure which can be pulled by other recombinases, moving it along the four stranded structure.

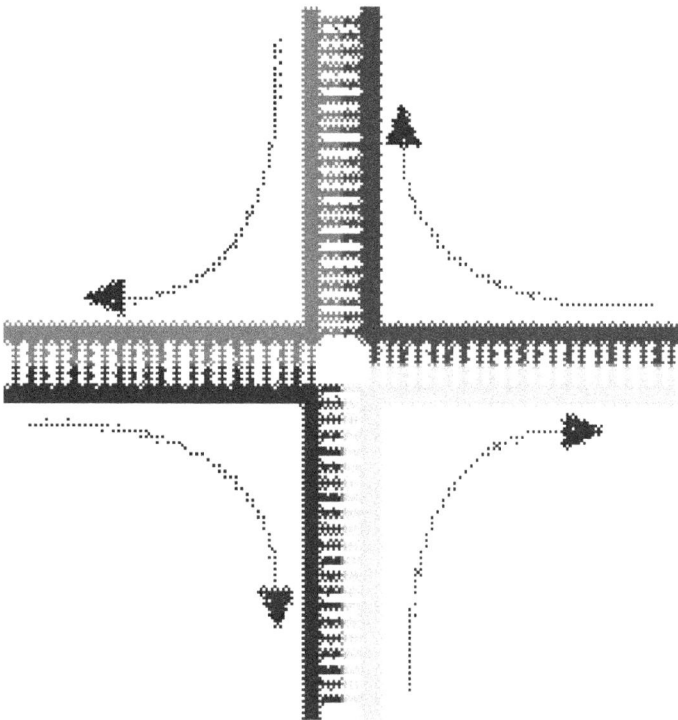

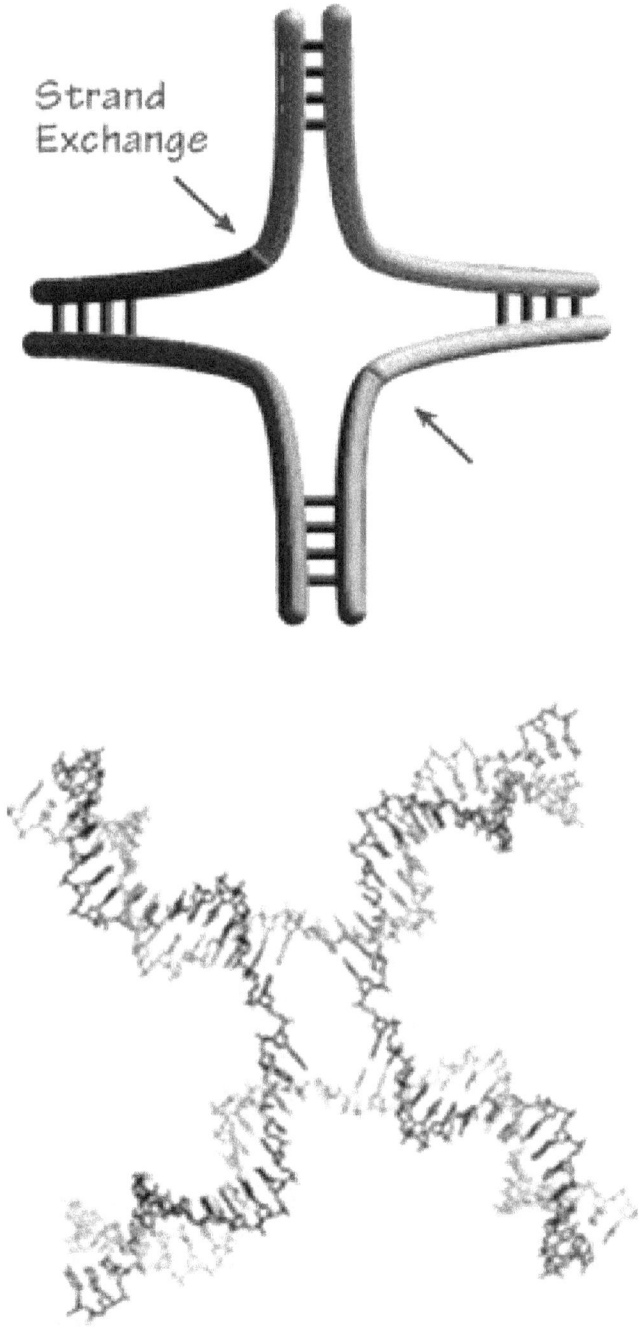

Strand
Exchange

Figure 4.18: Holliday Junction

Consequences

In most eukaryotes, a cell carries two copies of each gene, each referred to as an allele. Each parent passes on one allele to each offspring. An individual gamete inherits a complete haploid complement of alleles on chromosomes that are independently selected from each pair of chromatids lined up on the metaphase plate. Without recombination, all alleles for those genes linked together on the same chromosome would be inherited together. Meiotic recombination allows a more independent selection between the two alleles that occupy the positions of single genes, as recombination shuffles the allele content between homologous chromosomes. Recombination does not have any influence on the statistical probability that another offspring will have the same combination. This theory of independent assortment of alleles is fundamental to genetic inheritance. However, there is an exception that requires further discussion.

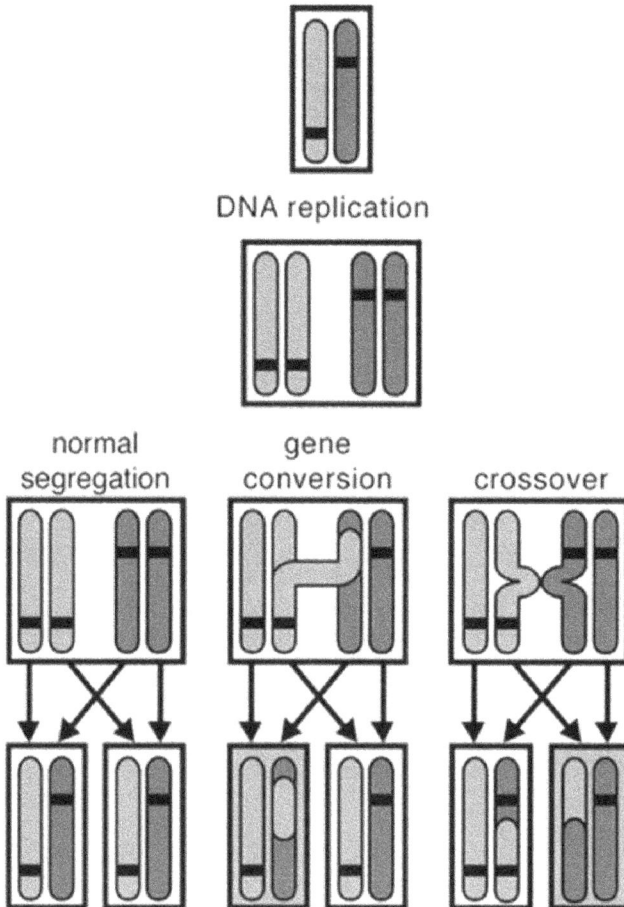

DNA replication

normal segregation   gene conversion   crossover

Figure 4.19: Difference between Gene conversion and Chromosomal Crossover

The frequency of recombination is actually not the same for all gene combinations. This leads to the notion of genetic distance, which is a measure of recombination frequency averaged over a (suitably large) sample of pedigrees. Loosely speaking, one may say that this is because recombination is greatly influenced by the proximity of one gene to another. If two genes are located close together on a chromosome, the likelihood that a recombination event will separate these two genes is less than if they were farther apart. Genetic linkage describes the tendency of genes to be inherited together as a result of their location on the same chromosome. Linkage disequilibrium describes a situation in which some combinations of genes or genetic markers occur more or less frequently in a population than would be expected from their distances apart. This concept is applied when searching for a gene that may cause a particular disease. This is done by comparing the occurrence of a specific DNA sequence with the appearance of a disease. When a high correlation between the two is found, it is likely that the appropriate gene sequence is really closer. Although crossovers typically occur between homologous regions of matching chromosomes, similarities in sequence can result in mismatched alignments. These processes are called unbalanced recombination. Unbalanced recombination is fairly rare compared to normal recombination, but severe problems can arise if a gamete containing unbalanced recombinants becomes part of a zygote. The result can be a local duplication of genes on one chromosome and a deletion of these on the other, a translocation of part of one chromosome onto a different one or an inversion.

Genetic Linkage

Genetic linkage occurs when particular genetic loci or alleles for genes are inherited jointly. Genetic loci on the same chromosome are physically connected and tend to stay together during meiosis and are thus genetically linked. This is called autosomal linkage. Alleles for genes on different chromosomes are usually not linked, due to independent assortment of chromosomes during meiosis. Because there is some crossing over of DNA when the chromosomes segregate, alleles on the same chromosome can be separated and go to different daughter cells. There is a greater probability of this happening if the alleles are far apart on the chromosome, as it is more likely that a cross-over will occur between them. The relative distance between two genes can be calculated using the offspring of an organism showing two linked genetic traits and finding the percentage of the offspring where the two traits do not run together. The higher the percentage of descendants that does not show both traits, the farther apart on the chromosome the two genes is. Among individuals of an experimental population or species, some phenotypes or traits occur randomly with respect to one another in a manner known as independent assortment. Today scientists understand that independent assortment occurs when the genes affecting the phenotypes are found on different chromosomes or separated by a great enough distance on the same chromosome that recombination occurs at least half of the time. An exception to independent assortment develops when genes appear near one another on the same chromosome. When genes occur on the same chromosome, they are usually inherited as a single unit. Genes inherited in this way are said to be linked and are referred to as linkage groups. In fruit flies, the genes affecting eye color and wing length are inherited together because they appear on the same chromosome.

But in many cases, even genes on the same chromosome that are inherited together produce offspring with unexpected allele combinations. This result from a process called crossing over. At the beginning of normal meiosis, a chromosome pair made up of a chromosome from the mother and a chromosome from the father, intertwines and exchange sections or fragments of chromosome. The pair then breaks apart to form two chromosomes with a new combination of genes that differs from the combination supplied by the parents. Through this process of recombining genes organisms can produce offspring with new combinations of maternal and paternal traits that may contribute to or enhance survival. Genetic linkage was first discovered by the British geneticists William Bateson and Reginald Punnett shortly after Mendel's laws were rediscovered.

Linkage Mapping

The observations by Thomas Hunt Morgan that the amount of crossing over between linked genes differs led to the idea that crossover frequency might indicate the distance separating genes on the chromosome. Morgan's student Alfred Sturtevant developed the first genetic map, also called a linkage map. Sturtevant proposed that the greater the distance between linked genes, the greater the chance that non-sister chromatids would cross over in the region between the genes. By working out the number of recombinants it is possible to obtain a measure for the distance between the genes. This distance is called a genetic map unit (m.u.) or a centimorgan and is defined as the distance between genes for which one product of meiosis in 100 is recombinant. A recombinant frequency (RF) of 1 % is equivalent to 1 m.u. A linkage map is created by finding the map distances between a numbers of traits that are present on the same chromosome, ideally avoiding having significant gaps between traits to avoid the inaccuracies that will occur due to the possibility of multiple recombination events.

Linkage mapping is critical for identifying the location of genes that cause genetic diseases. In an ideal population, genetic traits and markers will occur in all possible combinations with the frequencies of combinations determined by the frequencies of the individual genes *e.g.* if alleles *A* and *a* occur with frequency 90% and 10% and alleles *B* and *b* at a different genetic locus occur with frequencies 70% and 30%, the frequency of individuals having the combination *AB* would be 63%, the product of the frequencies of *A* and *B*, regardless of how close together the genes are. However, if a mutation in gene *B* that causes some disease happened recently in a particular subpopulation, it almost always occurs with a particular allele of gene *A* if the individual in which the mutation occurred had that variant of gene *A* and there have not been sufficient generations for recombination to happen between them (presumably due to tight linkage on the genetic map). In this case, called linkage disequilibrium, it is possible to search potential markers in the subpopulation and identify which marker the mutation is close to, thus determining the mutation's location on the map and identifying the gene at which the mutation occurred. Once the gene has been identified, it can be targeted to identify ways to mitigate the disease. Also, the location of a particular gene on a chromosome is called a gene locus.

Linkage Map

A linkage map is a genetic map of a species or experimental population that shows the position of its known genes and/or genetic markers relative to each other in terms of recombination frequency, rather than as specific physical distance along each chromosome. A genetic map is a map based on the frequencies of recombination between markers during crossover of homologous chromosomes. The greater the frequency of recombination (segregation) between two genetic markers, the farther apart they are assumed to be. Conversely, the lower the frequency of recombination between the markers, the smaller the physical distance between them. Historically, the markers originally used were detectable phenotypes (enzyme production, eye color) derived from coding DNA sequences; eventually, confirmed or assumed noncoding DNA sequences such as microsatellites or those generating restriction fragment length polymorphisms (RFLPs) have been used. Genetic maps help researchers to locate other markers, such as other genes by testing for genetic linkage of the already known markers. A genetic map is not a physical map or gene map.

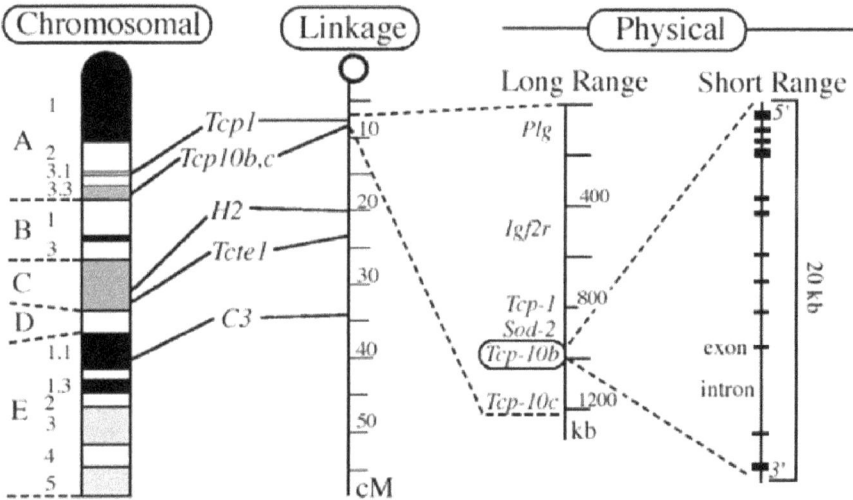

Figure 4.20: Chromosomal, Linkage and physical Map

LOD score

The LOD score (logarithm (base 10) of odds, also called logit by mathematicians) is a statistical test often used for linkage analysis in human populations and also in animal and plant populations. The test was developed by Newton E. Morton. Computerized LOD score analysis is a simple way to analyze complex family pedigrees in order to determine the linkage between Mendelian traits or between a trait and a marker or two markers. The method is described by Strachan and Read. Briefly, it works as follows:

i. Establish a pedigree.

ii. Make a number of estimates of recombination frequency.

iii. Calculate a LOD score for each estimate.

iv. The estimate with the highest LOD score will be considered the best estimate.

v. The LOD score is calculated as follows:

$$LOD = Z = \log 10 \frac{\text{probability of birth sequence with a given linkage value}}{\text{probability of birth sequence with no linkage}}$$

$$= \log 10 \frac{(1-\theta)^{NR} \times \theta^{R}}{0.5^{(NR+R)}}$$

NR denotes the number of non-recombinant offspring and R denotes the number of recombinant offspring. The reason 0.5 is used in the denominator is that any alleles that are completely unlinked *e.g.* alleles on separate chromosomes have a 50% chance of recombination, due to independent assortment. Theta is recombinant fraction which is equal to R / (NR + R). In practice, LOD scores are looked up in a table which lists LOD scores for various standard pedigrees and various values of recombination frequency. By convention, a LOD score greater than 3.0 is considered evidence for linkage. (A score of 3.0 means the likelihood of observing the given pedigree if the two loci are *not* linked is less than 1 in 1000). On the other hand, a LOD score less than -2.0 is considered evidence to exclude linkage. Although it is very unlikely that a LOD score of 3 would be obtained from a single pedigree, the mathematical properties of the test allow data from a number of pedigrees to be combined by summing the LOD scores.

Recombination Frequency

Recombination frequency (è) is the frequency that a chromosomal crossover will take place between two loci or genes during meiosis. Recombination frequency is a measure of genetic linkage and is used in the creation of a genetic linkage map. A centimorgan (cM) is a unit that describes a recombination frequency of 1%. During meiosis, chromosomes assort randomly into gametes, such that the segregation of alleles of one gene is independent of alleles of another gene. This is stated in Mendel's Second Law and is known as the law of independent assortment. The law of independent assortment always holds true for genes that are located on different chromosomes, but for genes that are on the same chromosome, it does not always hold true. As an example of independent assortment, consider the crossing of the pure-bred homozygote parental strain with genotype *AABB* with a different pure bred strain with genotype *aabb*. A and a and B and b represent the alleles of genes A and B. Crossing these homozygous parental strains will result in F_1 generation offspring with genotype AaBb. The F_1 offspring AaBb produces gametes that are AB, Ab, aB and ab with equal frequencies (25%) because the alleles of gene A assort independently of the alleles for gene B during meiosis. Note 2 of 4 gametes (50 %): Ab and aB, were not present in the parental generation. These gametes represent recombinant gametes. Recombinant gametes are those gametes that differ from both of the haploid gametes that made up the diploid cell. In this example, the recombination frequency is 50% since 2 of the 4 gametes were recombinant gametes. The recombination frequency will be 50% when two genes are located on different chromosomes or when they are widely separated on the same chromosome. This is a consequence of independent assortment.

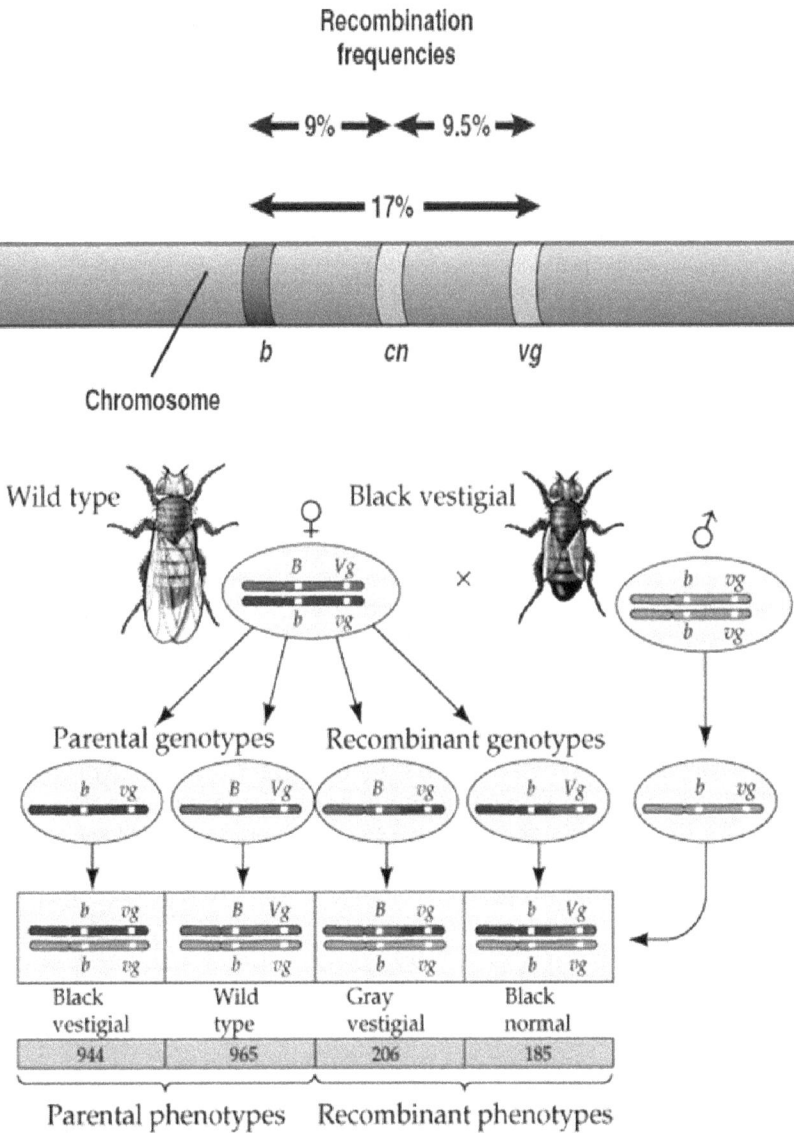

Figure 4.21: Recombination Frequency

When two genes are close together on the same chromosome, they do not assort independently and are said to be linked. Whereas genes located on different chromosomes assort independently and have a recombination frequency of 50%, linked genes have a recombination frequency that is less than 50%. As an example of linkage, consider the classic experiment by William Bateson and Reginald Punnett. They were interested in trait inheritance in the sweet pea and were studying two genes, the gene for flower color (*P*, purple and *p*, red) and the gene affecting the shape of pollen grains (*L*, long and *l*, round). They crossed the pure lines *PPLL* and *ppll* and then self crossed the resulting *PpLl* lines. According to Mendelian genetics, the expected phenotypes would occur in a 9:3:3:1 ratio of PL: Pl: pL: pl. To their surprise, they observed an increased frequency of PL and pl and a decreased frequency of Pl and pL.

Table 4.2: Bateson and Punnett Experiment

S.No.	Phenotype and Genotype	Observed	Expected from 9:3:3:1 Ratio
1.	Purple, long (*PpLl*)	284	216
2.	Purple, round (*Ppll*)	21	72
3.	Red, long (*ppLl*)	21	72
4.	Red, round (*ppll*)	55	24

Their experiment revealed linkage between the P and L alleles and the p and l alleles. The frequency of P occurring together with L and with p occurring together with l is greater than that of the recombinant Pl and pL. The recombination frequency cannot be computed directly from this experiment, but intuitively it is less than 50%. The progeny in this case received two dominant alleles linked on one chromosome referred to as coupling or cis arrangement. However, after crossover, some progeny could have received one parental chromosome with a dominant allele for one trait *e.g.* purple, linked to a recessive allele for a second trait *e.g.* round with the opposite being true for the other parental chromosome *e.g.* red and long. This is referred to as repulsion or a trans arrangement. The phenotype here would still be purple and long but a test cross of this individual with the recessive parent would produce progeny with much greater proportion of the two crossover phenotypes. While such a problem may not seem likely from this example, unfavorable repulsion linkages do appear when breeding for disease resistance in some crops. When two genes are located on the same chromosome, the chance of a crossover producing recombination between the genes is directly related to the distance between the two genes. Thus, the use of recombination frequencies has been used to develop linkage maps or genetic maps.

Summary

1. The process by which the cells arise is called cell division. The period from the end of one division of a cell to the end of the next division is called cell cycle.

2. The cell cycle is divisible into two phases: Interphase and Mitotic Phase. Interphase is the growth period between two successive divisions of a cell.

3. Interphase can be subdivided into three distinct period- G1 phase, S phase

and G2 Phase, on the basis of synthetic activities. During G1 phase the cell grows in size and there is active synthesis of RNA and proteins.

4. Mitotic cell division involves two process- Karyokinesis and Cytokinesis.

5. Mitosis has form four phases- Prophase, Metaphase, Anaphase and Telophase.

6. Mitosis helps in maintaining uniformity within a species. It restores the surface volume ratio of the cell. It results in the growth of the organism.

7. Meiosis is the process of nuclear division which takes place in reproductive cells. The daughter nuclei formed by this process contain only half number of chromosome of the parent cell. The term meiosis was coined by J.B. Farmer and J.E. Moore in 1905.

8. Meiosis is a complex process and comprises of two successive divisions, Meiosis I and Meiosis II.

9. Meiosis I is heterotype and is also called reduction division as the chromosome number halved.

10. Meiosis is called the reduction division since it reduces the chromosome number by half while making the gametes.

11. In sexual reproduction when the two gametes fuse the chromosome number is restored to the value in the parent.

12. Meiosis I has a long prophase, which is divided into five phases- leptotene, zygotene, pachytene, diplotene and diakinesis.

13. During metaphase I the bivalents arrange on the equatorial plate. This is followed by anaphase I in which homologous chromosomes move to the opposite poles with both their chromatids.

14. Meiosis II is similar to mitosis. During anaphase II the sister chromatids separate and at the end of meiosis four haploid cells are formed.

Chapter 5

Mendelian Genetics and Interaction of Genes

Principles of Genetics

It is common observation that seeds of mango trees grow into mango plants, dogs give birth to puppies and not into the young ones of any other animal. Humans give birth to human beings. The tendency of offspring to inherit parental characteristics is termed heredity and the science of heredity in Genetics. Genetics also seeks to answer questions like why two offspring of same parents look different, why some people dark and others are light skinned etc. In other words, why is there variation among individuals of the same kind? This lesson deals with heredity and variation. It also includes a section on hereditary disorders and gives an idea of the human genome too.

Heredity and Variation

Whenever an infant is born in a family, the relatives begin to wonder about the resemblance of the infant's eyes, facial features, complexion, colour of hair with those of the parents, siblings and grandparents. The source of such resemblances and differences are in the genes that are passed down from parents to children and so on generation after generation. New individual develop according to the genes inherited from their parents. The transmission of characters from one generation to the next that is from parents to offspring is known as heredity. It is further observed that siblings from same parents are unique and differ from each other except the identical twins. Such differences are termed variations. Variation means differences between parents and offspring or between offspring of same parents or between members of the same population. Variation in a population is very important. It has survival value for the population. This is because if the environment changes, some individuals (variants) may be able to adapt to new situations and save the population from dying out. Variation arises due to mutation or sudden change in the genes. Variation also arises because genes get shifted and exchanged during meiosis at formation of gametes, giving rise to new gene combinations. At fertilization, there is random mixing of parental chromosomes with different gene combinations. Such a source of variation which is most common is called recombination.

Mendel and his Experiments

Sir Gregor Johann Mendel (1822 to 1884) was Austrian monk who used garden pea (*Pisum sativum*) for his experiments and published his results in 1865. He started with 34 varieties of pea seeds in which he noticed 7 opposing characteristics among the plants. However his work was rediscovered in 1900, long after Mendel's death, by Tschermak, Correns and DeVries. But since Mendel was the first to suggest principles underlying inheritance he is regarded as the founder or father of genetics. Mendel designed his experiments such that a pure tall variety of pea plants could be crossed to a pure dwarf variety. The anthers from flowers of tall plants were removed and their stigmas dusted with pollen from flowers of dwarf plants. The reverse experiment was also carried out. In the following spring, seeds from the new plants were collected and sown. He found that all the plants of this generation called first filial generation or F_1 grew to be tall plants. He allowed them to self pollinate. Again he collected the seeds. The following year, after the seeds had been sown, he found that three quarters of these plants were tall and the rest dwarf. The change came in the next generation, in which, out of the 1,064 plants obtained, 787 were tall and 277 were dwarf. He repeated the experiment several times and found that the ratio of tall to dwarf plants was 3: 1.

Table 5.1: Characteristics of Dominant and Recessive traits

Dominant Traits	tall	colored seed coats	axial flowers	green pea pods	inflated pea pods	yellow peas	round peas
Recessive Traits	short	white seed coats	terminal flowers	yellow pea pods	constricted peas pods	green peas	wrinkled pea

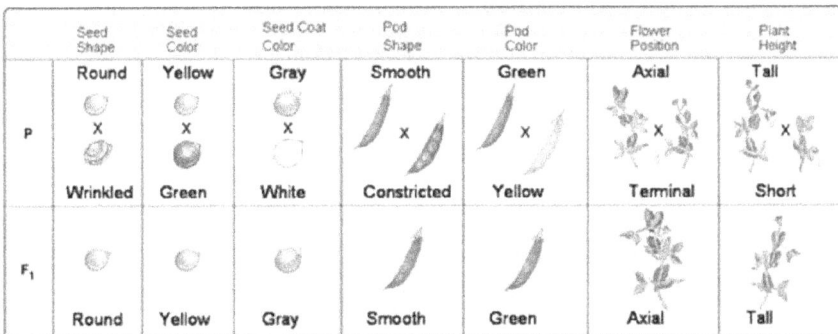

	Seed Shape	Seed Color	Seed Coat Color	Pod Shape	Pod Color	Flower Position	Plant Height
P	Round X Wrinkled	Yellow X Green	Gray X White	Smooth X Constricted	Green X Yellow	Axial X Terminal	Tall X Short
F_1	Round	Yellow	Gray	Smooth	Green	Axial	Tall

In this way he tried to cross pea plants with seven such contrasting characters. These were

i.   Red flowered and white flowered plants.

ii. Axillary flowered (flower arising in the axial of the leaf) and terminal flowered (flower arising at tip of stalk).

iii. Yellow seeded versus green seeded.

iv. Round seeded verses wrinkled seeded.

v.   Green pod versus yellow pod.

vi. Plants with inflated pods versus those with constricted pod.

vii. Pure tall plants versus pure dwarf plants.

Table 19: Comparison of Terms

S.No.	Mendel's Terminology	Current Terminology
1.	Unit factor	Gene
2.	Purebred/true breeding	Homozygous
3.	Hybrid	Heterozygous
4.	Two factors that control each trait	Allele

Plants with such contrasting characters exist in varieties that are self pollinating so that generation after generation they express only one type of feature. Crosses considering the inheritance of one feature only are called monohybrid crosses. Mendel also tried crosses involving two contrasting features, such as tall and red flowered with dwarf and white flowered plant such a cross is termed dihybrid cross. Basing on the results of his experiments, Mendel postulated the following laws of heredity.

Law of Dominance: Inheritance of many features *e.g.* eye colour, flower colour, seed shape etc. is controlled by one pair of genes. When the two genes are of the same kind *e.g.* brown colour of eyes, red colour of flower and the condition is termed homozygous. When a pair of chromosomes has the gene controlling the same feature (flower colour) in two different forms; red flower gene on one chromosome and white flower gene on its pair termed its homologue, the condition is termed heterozygous.

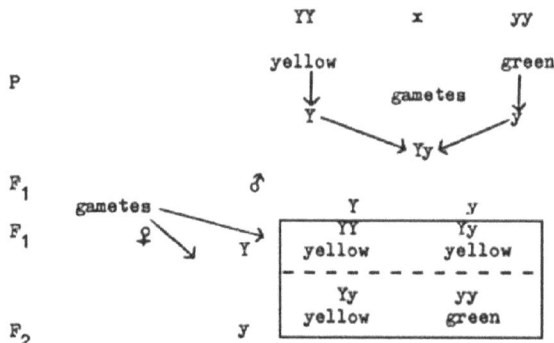

Law of Segregation or Purity of Gametes: At formation of gametes, the two chromosomes of each pair separate (segregate) into two different cell which form the gametes. This is a universal law and always during gamete formation in all sexually reproducing organisms, the two factors of a pair pass into different gametes. Each gamete receives one member of a pair of factors and the gametes are pure.

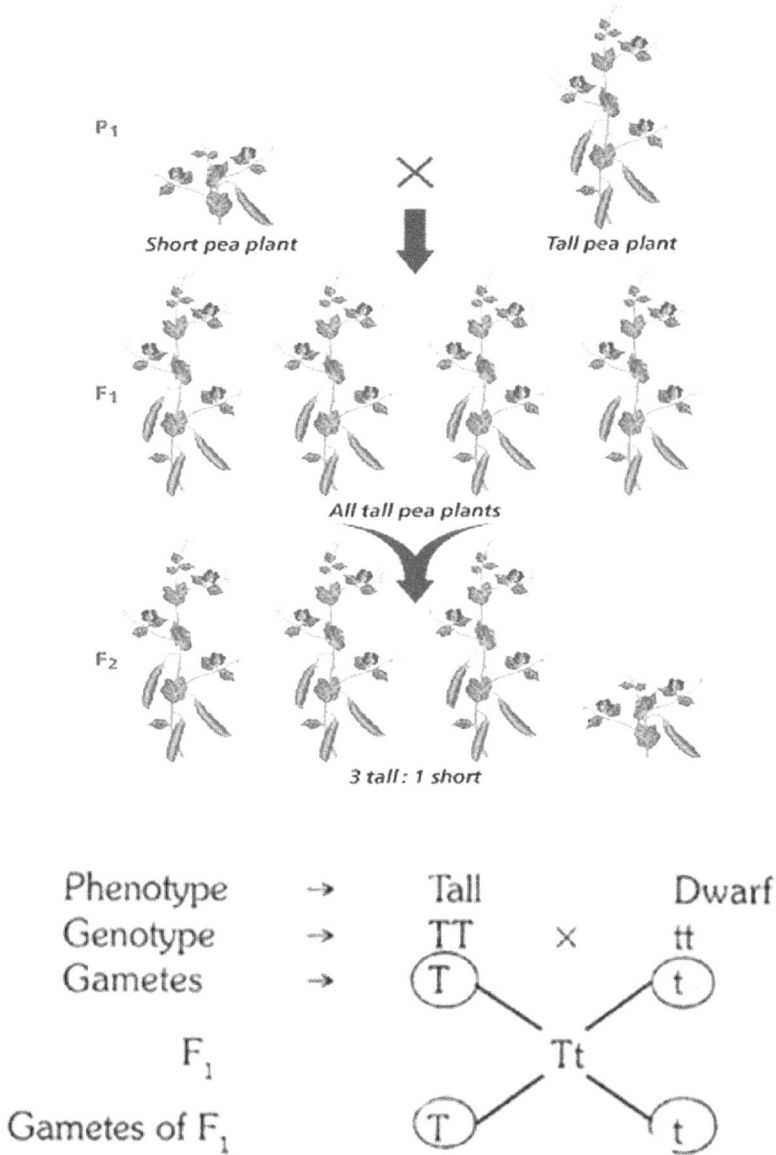

Figure 5.1: Segregation: An individual with the genotype Tt can make two types of gametes: T and t. Since this is a random process, the individual will make equal numbers of each gamete (Frequency of 1/2 for each gamete).

Law of Independent Assortment : The Law of Independent Assortment, also known as Inheritance Law, states that alleles of different genes assort independently of one another during gamete formation. While Mendel's experiments with mixing one trait always resulted in a 3:1 ratio between dominant and recessive phenotypes, his experiments with mixing two traits (dihybrid cross) showed 9:3:3:1 ratios. But 9:3:3:1 table shows that each of the two genes is independently inherited with a 3:1 ratio. Mendel concluded that different traits are inherited independently of each other, so that there is no relation between a cat's colour and tail length. This is actually only true for genes that are not linked to each other. Independent assortment occurs during meiosis I in eukaryotic organisms, specifically metaphase I of meiosis, to produce a gamete with a mixture of the organism's maternal and paternal chromosomes. Along with chromosomal crossover, this process aids in increasing genetic diversity by producing novel genetic combinations.

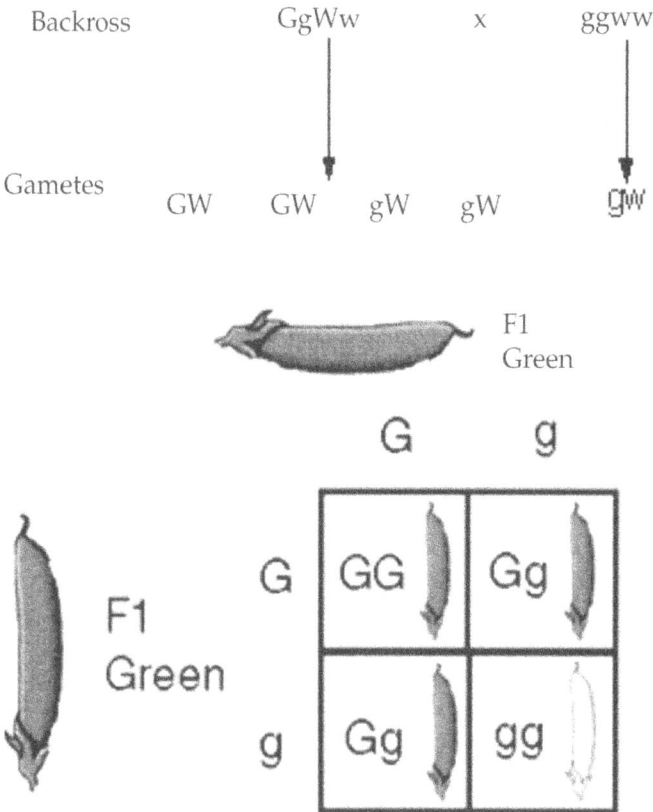

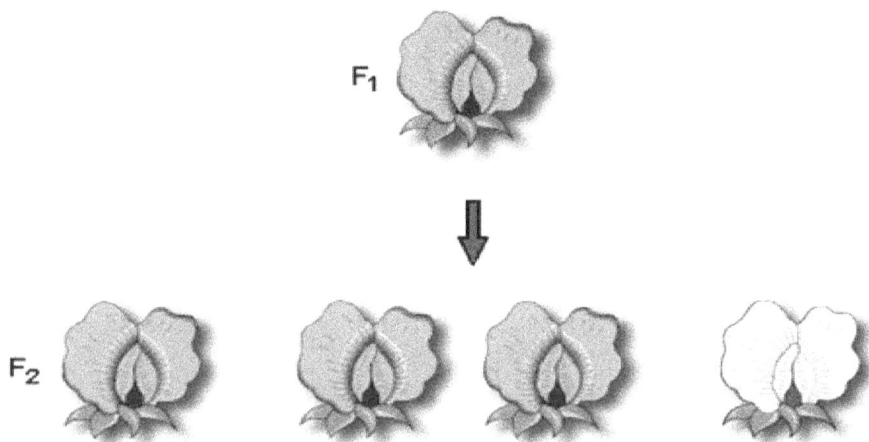

Figure 5.2: Independent Assortment

Of the 46 chromosomes in a normal diploid human cell, half are maternally derived (from mother's egg) and half are paternally derived (from father's sperm). This occurs as sexual reproduction involves the fusion of two haploid gametes (egg and sperm) to produce a new organism having the full complement of chromosomes. During gametogenesis; the production of new gametes by an adult- the normal complement of 46 chromosomes needs to be halved to 23 to ensure that the resulting haploid gamete can join with another gamete to produce a diploid organism. An error in the number of chromosomes, such as those caused by a diploid gamete joining with a haploid gamete, is termed aneuploidy. In independent assortment the chromosomes that end up in a newly formed gamete are randomly sorted from all possible combinations of maternal and paternal chromosomes. Because gametes end up with a random mix instead of a pre-defined set from either parent, gametes are therefore considered assorted independently. As such, the gamete can end up with any combination of paternal or maternal chromosomes. Any of the possible combinations of gametes formed from maternal and paternal chromosomes will occur with equal frequency. For human gametes, with 23 pairs of chromosomes, the number of possibilities is 2^{23} or 8,388,608 possible combinations. The gametes will normally end up with 23 chromosomes, but the origin of any particular one will be randomly selected from paternal or maternal chromosomes. This contributes to the genetic variability of progeny.

BOX 5.1

TERMINOLOGY FOR MENDELIAN GENETICS

Principle of Genes in Pairs: Genetic characters are controlled by unit factors (genes) that exist in pairs in individual organisms and are passed from parents to their offspring. When two organisms produce offspring, each parent gives the offspring one of the factors from each pair.

Principle of Dominance and Recessiveness: When two unlike factors responsible for a single character are present in a single individual, one factor can mask the expression of another factor; that is, one factor is dominant to the other, which is said to be recessive.

Principle of Segregation: During the formation of gametes, the paired factors separate (segregate) randomly so that each gamete receives one factor or the other.

Principle of Independent Assortment: During gamete formation, segregating pairs of factors assort independently of each other.

Factor: The unit responsible for the inheritance and expression of a particular character. Now factor replaced by the term gene.

Gene: It is a particular segment of a DNA molecule which determines the inheritance and expression of a particular character.

Alleles or Allelomorphs: Two or more alternative firms of a factor or a gene are called alleles. In pea plant, the gene for producing seed shape may occur in two alternative forms: round (R) and wrinkled (r). Genes for round and wrinkled seeds are alleles of each other. Similarly, there are three alleles for gene controlling blood group in man IA, IB, i (I = immunoglobulin gene). Alleles occupy same locus on homologous chromosomes.

Trait: is the expressed character *e.g.* colour of flower, shape of seed etc.

Dominant trait: Out of the two alternating forms (allelomorphs) of a trait, the one which expresses itself in a heterogygous organism in F^1 hybrid is called the dominant trait (dominant allele) and the phenomenon is called dominance. In an organism with Tt, T (tallness) expresses itself and t (dwarfness) cannot, so T is the dominant allele.

Recessive trait: Out of the two alternating alleles for a trait, the one which is suppressed (does not express) in the F^1 hybrid is called the recessive trait (recessive allele). Recessive allele expresses only in the homozygous state *e.g.* tt.

Genotype: The genetic constitution of an individual (which he/she inherits from the parents) is called the genotype *e.g.* the genotype of pure round seeded parent pea plant is RR.

Phenotype: The outward (morphological) appearance of an individual for any trait or traits is called the phenotype *e.g.* for seeds, round shape or wrinkled shape is the phenotype.

Homozygous: an individual possessing identical alleles for a trait is called homozygous or pure for that trait, *e.g.* plant with RR alleles is homozygous for the seed shape.

Heterozygous: An individual receiving dissimilar alleles for a trait is called (heterozygous or impure for that trait, *e.g.* a plant with Rr alleles is heterozygous for the seed shape.

Parent generations: The parents used for the first cross represent the parent or P_1 generation.

F_1 **generation:** The progeny produced from a cross between two parents (P_1) is called First filial or F_1 generation.

F_2 **generation:** The progeny resulting from self hybridization or inbreeding of F_1 individuals is called Second Filial or F_2 generation.

Monohybrid cross: The cross between two parents differing in a single pair of contrasting characters is called monohybrid cross and the F_1 offspring as the hybrid. The phenotypic ratio of 3 dominants: 1 recessive obtained in the F_2 generation from the monohybrid cross is called monohybrid phenotype ratio *e.g.* 3: 1 in Mendelian Inheritance.

Dihybrid cross: The cross between two parents in which two pairs of contrasting characters are studied simultaneously for the inheritance pattern is called dihybrid cross. The phenotypic ratio obtained in the F_2 generation from a dihybrid cross is called dihybrid ratio phenotypic *e.g.* 9: 3: 3: 1 in Mendelian crosses.

Hybridization: Crossing organisms belonging to different species for getting favourable qualities in the offspring.

Test cross: Crossing of the F_1 progeny with the homozygous recessive parent. If F_1 progeny is heterozygous then the test cross always yields the ratio of 1: 1.

Reciprocal cross: It is the cross in which the sex of the parents is reversed. That is if in the first cross father was dwarf and mother tall, then in the reciprocal cross, dwarf parent will be female and tall parent male.

Phenocopy

A phenocopy is an individual whose phenotype (generally referring to a single trait), under a particular environmental condition, is identical to the one of another individual whose phenotype is determined by the genotype. In other words the phenocopy environmental condition mimics the phenotype produced by a gene. An incorrect example of a phenocopy is a person with bleached brunette hair; the bleached hair is intended to mimic genetically determined blonde hair of actual blonde people. The false phenocopy can be easily distinguished by observing the roots of the hair or by shining an ultraviolet light on the bleached brunette hair. A correct example of a phenocopy is a person whose anti-psychotic medication causes them to manifest the same symptoms as the genetically determined Parkinsons disease. An example of a phenocopy is the Vanessa genus of butterflies who can change phenotype based on the local temperature. If introduced to Lapland they mimic butterflies localised to this area and if localised to Syria they mimic buterflies of this area. These phenotypes aren't inherited and are solely due to environment.

Pleiotropy

Pleiotropy occurs when a single gene influences multiple phenotypic traits. Consequently, a new mutation in the gene will have an effect on all traits simultaneously. This can become a problem when selection on one trait favours one specific mutant, while the selection on the other trait favours another mutant.

Pleiotropy describes the genetic effect of a single gene on multiple phenotypic traits. The underlying mechanism is that the gene codes for a product that is used by various cells or has a signaling function on various targets. A classic example of pleiotropy is the human disease PKU (phenylketonuria). This disease can cause mental retardation and reduced hair and skin pigmentation and can be caused by any of a large number of mutations in a single gene that codes for an enzyme (phenylalanine hydroxylase) that converts the amino acid phenylalanine to tyrosine, another amino acid. Depending on the mutation involved, this results in reduced or zero conversion of phenylalanine to tyrosine and phenylalanine concentrations increase to toxic levels, causing damage at several locations in body. PKU is totally benign if a diet free from phenylalanine is maintained.

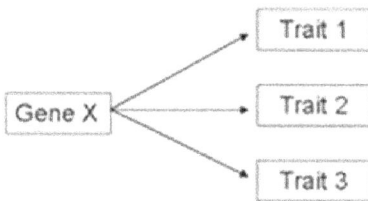

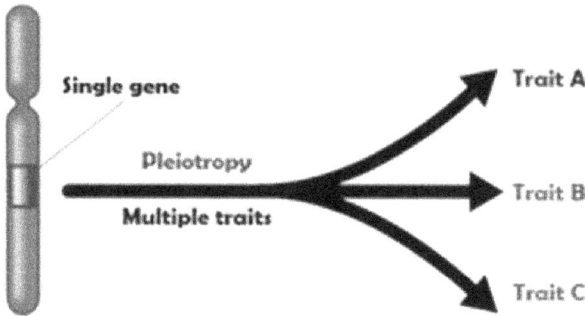

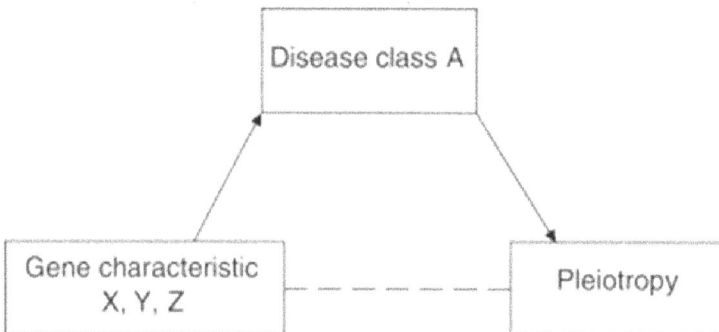

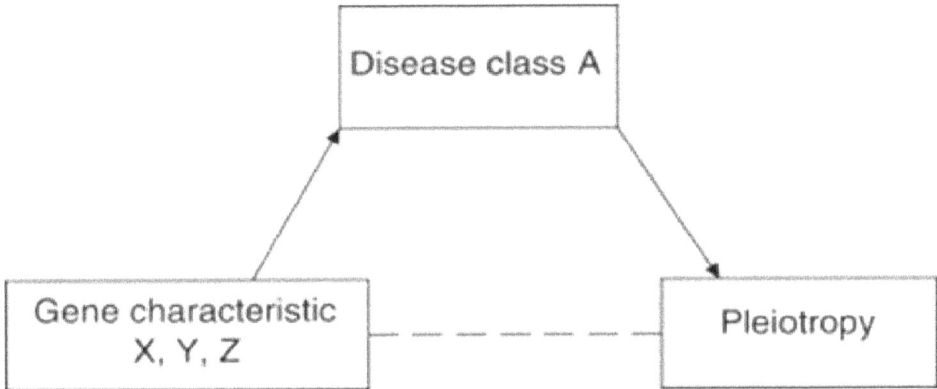

Figure 5.3: Pleiotopy

Sex linkage

Sex linkage is the phenotypic expression of an allele that is related to the chromosomal sex of the individual. This mode of inheritance is in contrast to the inheritance of traits on autosomal chromosomes, where both sexes have the same probability of expressing the trait. Since, in humans, there are many more genes on X than there are on Y, there are many more X-linked traits than there are Y-linked traits. In mammals, the female is the homogametic sex, having two X chromosomes (XX), while the male is heterogametic, having one X and one Y chromosome (XY). Genes that are present on the X or Y chromosome are called sex linked genes.

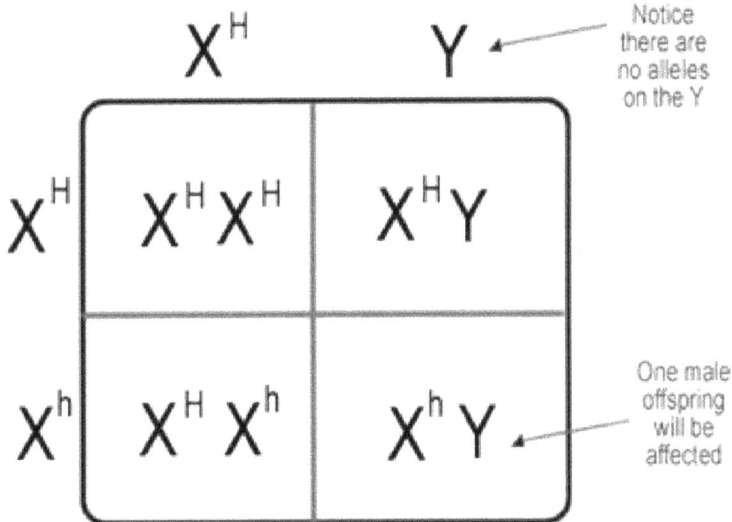

Punnett Squares

Punnett squares are helpful tools when determining the genotype of offspring and the probability of a certain genotype of the offspring of organisms. Cross a homozygous dominant pea plant (TT) short plant (tt).

	t	t
T	Tt	Tt
T	Tt	Tt

One dominant gene from the phenotypically (physical characteristic) tall plant (TT) is crossed with one recessive gene from the phenotypically short plant (tt) to produce plants with the genotype of Tt. It shows that 100% of the offspring of the cross between TT and tt will have a tall phenotype and Tt will be their genotype. If two Tt plants were to be crossed:

	T	t
T	TT	Tt
t	Tt	tt

Approximately, 25% of the offspring have the genotype of TT, 50% of the offspring have the genotype of Tt and 25% of the offspring have the genotype of tt. As a result:

a.75% of the offspring will have a tall phenotype.

b.25% of the offspring will have a short phenotype.

Let us change focus from the pea plant to animals. Pretend that for a certain type of rabbit, having black hair is a dominant trait over white hair. A rabbit with a heterozygous genotype is crossed with a rabbit with the same genotype. Use B for the dominant trait and b for the recessive trait.

	B	b
B	BB	Bb
b	Bb	bb

Ratio

The percent of each genotype and phenotype is in a ratio instead of listing out each of the different situations. The genotypic ratio is 1BB: 2Bb: 1bb. The correct notation for this is 1:2:1. The phenotypic ratio is 3B:1b or 3 black to 1 white. It is written as 3:1.

Incomplete Dominance

Incomplete dominance is the term given to the characteristic of certain organisms that have genes that do not dominate the other genes. In this situation, we obtain variations in physical appearance. A flower has genes for white petals (w) and red petals (r). When we mix white flowers with red flowers we get pink flowers. How is this possible? The w gene does not dominate over the r gene and vice versa.

	w	w
r	w r	w r
r	w r	w r

Both genes express themselves equally so we get a pink color in the petals. However, by crossing two pink flowers together there is a different outcome.

	w	r
w	ww	wr
r	wr	rr

There is a possibility of obtaining one white, two pink or one red flower. The phenotypic ratio is 1:2:1 and the genotypic ratio is 1:2:1.

Monohybrid Cross and Dihybrid Cross

A monohybrid cross is a cross dealing with only one characteristic such as height. This is oppposed to a dihybrid cross where two characteristics retaken into consideration *i.e.* height and color. In a dihybrid cross on a punnett square, the ratio and probability can be calculated and this gives the tall plant with a red bloom as opposed to a short plant with a white bloom. Punnett square used to show the outcome of crossing a tall plant with a white bloom with the genotype of TTrr and a tall plant with a red bloom with the genotype of TtRr. In this situation a red color trait dominates over a white color trait. The new generation obtains genes with the genotype of Tr from the 1st plant and obtains genes with the genotype of TR, tR, Tr or tr from the 2nd plant.

	Tr	Tr
TR	TTRr	TTRr
tR	TtRr	TrRr
Tr	TTrr	TTrr
tr	Ttrr	Ttrr

Dihybrid crosses can get trickier, though, when the next generation can receive a combination of TR, Tr, tR or tr from the first plant and the second plant.

	TR	Tr	tR	tr
TR	TTRR	TTRr	TtRR	TtRr
Tr	TTRr	TTrr	TtRr	Ttrr
tR	TtRR	TrRr	ttRR	ttRr
tr	TtRr	Ttrr	ttRr	ttrr

This chart gives us information that the odds of a plant in the next generation being tall with a red bloom are 9:7.

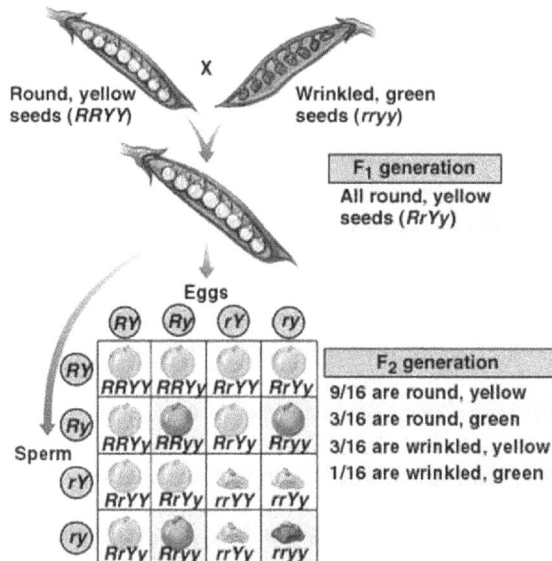

Back Cross

When F1 individuals are crossed with one of the two parents from which they have been derived, such cross is called back cross. In such cases, there are two possibilities:

A. When F^1 plant (Cc) is crossed to the Parent dominant phenotype *e.g.* homozygous for red colour (CC). In such z cross the plants will be 100% red.

B. When F^1 plant (Cc) is crossed to the parent with pure recessive (cc) white flowered plant, then in such a cross, 50% plants will be red and 50% plants will be white flowered.

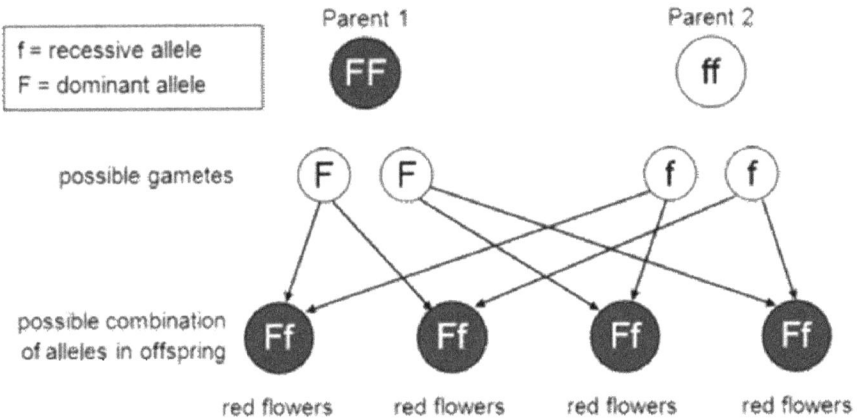

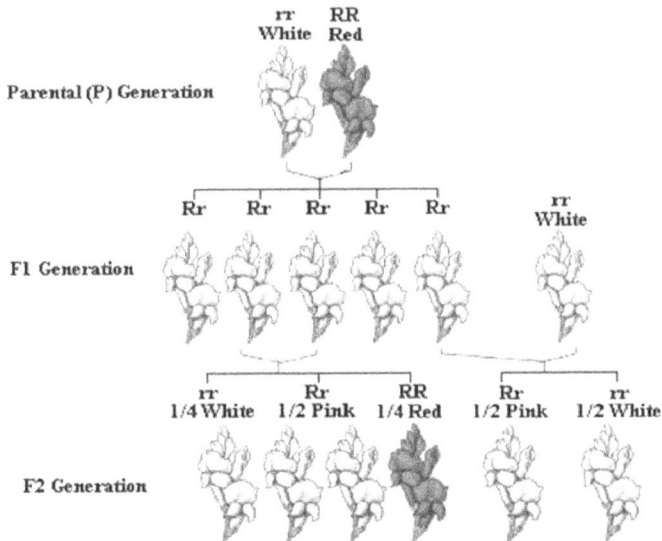

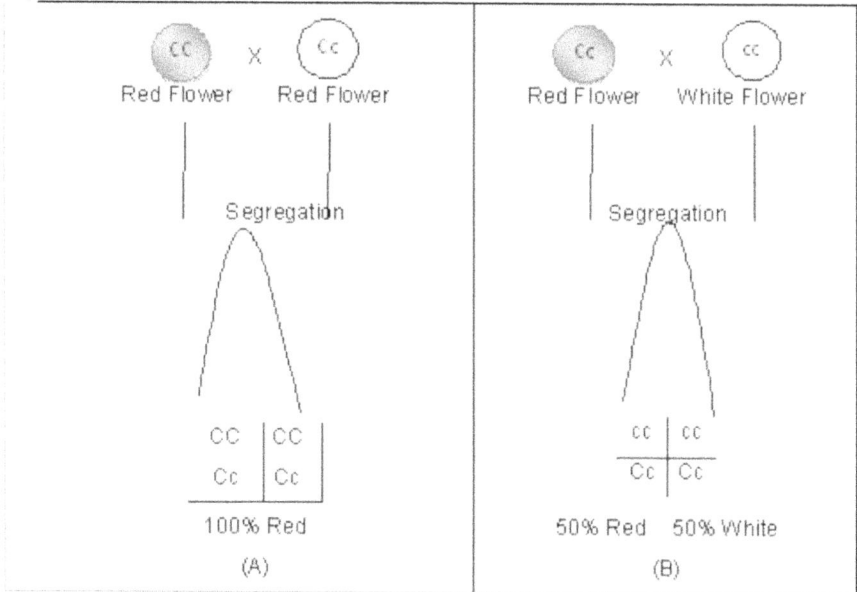

Figure 5.4: Back Cross

Test Cross

This cross is made in order to find out the genetic constitution of individual. In this cross the given individual is crossed with the homozygous recessive plant of the some trait. The phenotypes of the offspring produced by a test reveal the number of different gametes, formed by the parental genotype under test. These can be two possibilities of such a cross:

A. When impure dominant (Cc) is crossed with the pure recessive, then is this cross 50% plants will be red and 50% will be white.

B. When pure dominant (CC) is crossed with a pure recessive (cc), then is such a cross, 100% plants will be red flowered. Therefore, test cross revels whether the red flowered plants are homozygous or heterozygous.

i) A monohybrid test cross of a heterozygous dominant with pure recessive gives a 1:1 phenotypic ratio *i.e.* 50% each.

ii) A dihybrid test crosses of a heterozygous dominant with pure recessive gives a phenotypic ratio of 1:1:1:1 *i.e.* 25% each.

iii) Trihybrid test cross for heterozygous (Rr Yy Cc) with triple recessive (rr yy cc). The eight different phenotypes will be obtained 1:1:1:1:1:1:1:1, *i.e.* 12.5% each.

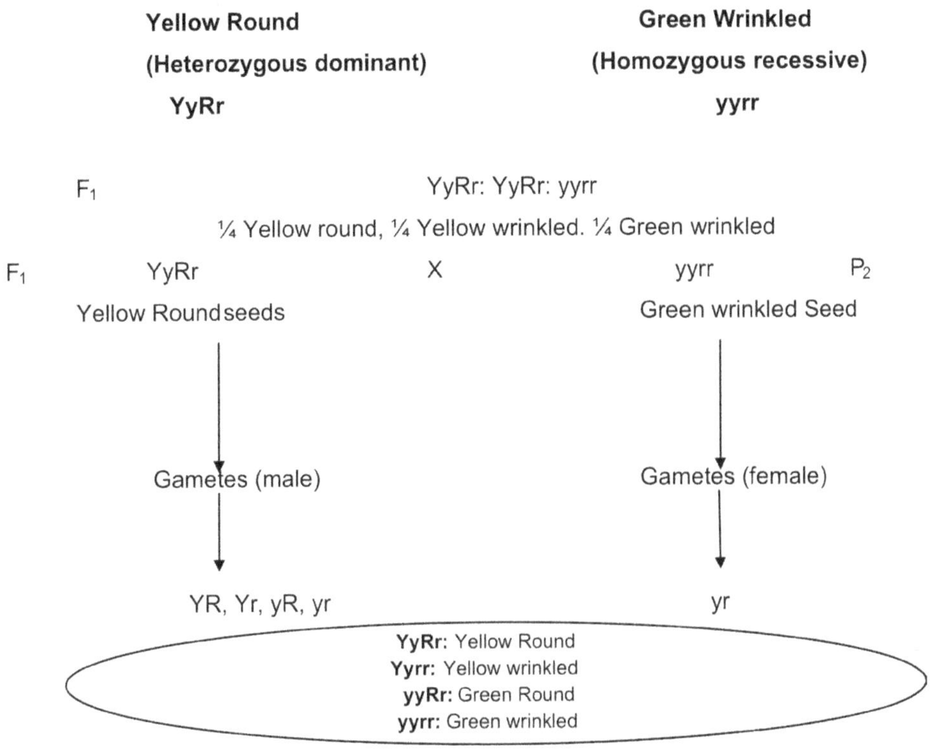

Yellow Round   Green Wrinkled

(Heterozygous dominant)   (Homozygous recessive)

YyRr   yyrr

F_1 YyRr: YyRr: yyrr

¼ Yellow round, ¼ Yellow wrinkled. ¼ Green wrinkled

F_1 YyRr   X   yyrr P_2

Yellow Round seeds   Green wrinkled Seed

Gametes (male)   Gametes (female)

YR, Yr, yR, yr   yr

YyRr: Yellow Round
Yyrr: Yellow wrinkled
yyRr: Green Round
yyrr: Green wrinkled

Figure 5.5 Test Cross

If test cross yields offsprings of which 50% show dominant character and 50% show recessive character, individual under test is heterozygous. If all offsprings show dominant trait individual being tested is homozygous dominant.

Non-Mendelian Inheritance

Non-Mendelian inheritance is a general term that refers to any pattern of inheritance in which traits do not segregate in accordance with Mendel's laws. These laws describe the inheritance of traits linked to single genes on chromosomes in the nucleus. In Mendelian inheritance, each parent contributes one of two possible alleles for a trait. If the genotypes of both parents in a genetic cross are known, Mendel's laws can be used to determine the distribution of phenotypes expected for the population of offspring. There are several situations in which the proportions of phenotypes observed in the progeny do not match the predicted values. Although inheritance of traits in fungi, viruses and bacteria are all non-Mendelian, the phrase non-Mendelian inheritance is usually only used to describe the exceptions which occur in eukaryotic reproduction.

Types of Non-Mendelian Inheritance

Extranuclear Inheritance : Extranuclear inheritance also known as cytoplasmic inheritance is a form of non-Mendelian inheritance first discovered by Carl Correns in 1908. While working with *Mirabilis jalapa* Correns observed that leaf color was dependent only on the genotype of the maternal parent. Based on this data, he determined that the trait was transmitted through a character present in the cytoplasm of the ovule. Later, Ruth Sager and others identified DNA present in chloroplasts as being responsible for the unusual inheritance pattern. Work on the poky strain of the mold Neurospora crassa begun by Mary and Hershel Mitchell ultimately led to the discovery of genetic material in mitochondria as well. According to the endosymbiont theory, mitochondria and chloroplasts were once free living organisms that were taken up by a eukaryotic cell. Over time, mitochondria and chloroplasts formed a symbiotic relationship with their eukaryotic hosts. Although the transfer of a number of genes from these organelles to the nucleus prevents them from living independently, each still possesses genetic material in the form of double stranded DNA. It is the transmission of this organellar DNA that is responsible for the phenomenon of extranuclear inheritance. Both chloroplasts and mitochondria are present in the cytoplasm of maternal gametes only. Thus, the phenotype of traits linked to genes found in either chloroplasts or mitochondria are determined exclusively by the maternal parent. In humans, mitochondrial diseases are a class of diseases, many of which affect the muscles and the eye.

Gene Conversion : Gene conversion can be one of major forms of non-Mendelian inheritance. Gene conversion is a reparation process in DNA recombination, by which a piece of DNA sequence information is transferred from one DNA helix which remains unchanged to another DNA helix, whose sequence is altered. This may occur as a mismatch repair between the strands of DNA which are derived from different parents. Thus the mismatch repair can convert one allele into the other. This phenomenon can be detected through the offspring non-Mendelian ratios and is frequently observed, *e.g.* in fungal crosses.

Infectious Heredity : Another form of non-Mendelian inheritance is known as infectious heredity. Infectious particles such as viruses may infect host cells and continue to reside in the cytoplasm of these cells. If the presence of these particles results in an altered phenotype, then this phenotype may be subsequently transmitted to progeny. Because this phenotype is dependent only on the presence of the invader in the host cell's cytoplasm, inheritance will be determined only by the infected status of the maternal parent. This will result in a uniparental transmission of the trait, just as in extranuclear inheritance. One of the most well studied examples of infectious heredity is the killer phenomenon exhibited in yeast. Two double-stranded RNA viruses, designated L and M, are responsible for this phenotype. The L virus codes for the capsid proteins of both viruses, as well as an RNA polymerase. Thus the M virus can only infect cells already harboring L virus particles. The M viral RNA encodes a toxin which is secreted from the host cell. It kills susceptible cells growing in close proximity to the host. The M viral RNA also renders the host cell immune to the lethal effects of the toxin. For a cell to be susceptible it must therefore be either uninfected or harbor only the L virus. The L and M viruses are not capable of exiting their host cell through conventional means. They can only transfer from cell to cell when their host undergoes mating. All progeny of a mating involving a doubly infected yeast cell will also be infected with L and M viruses. Therefore, the killer phenotype will be passed down to all progeny.

Heritable traits that result from infection with foreign particles have also been identified in Drosophila. Wild type flies normally full recover after being anesthetized with carbon dioxide. Certain lines of flies have been identified that die off after exposure to the compound. This carbon dioxide sensitivity is passed down from mothers to their progeny. This sensitivity is due to infection with Sigma virus, a rhabdovirus only capable of infecting Drosophila. Although this process is usually associated with viruses, *Wolbachia* bacterium is also capable of inserting its genome into that of its host.

Genomic Imprinting

Genomic imprinting represents yet another example of non-Mendelian inheritance. Just as in conventional inheritance, genes for a given trait are passed down to progeny from both parents. However, these genes are epigenetically marked before transmission, altering their levels of expression. These imprints are created before gamete formation and are erased during the creation of germ line cells. Therefore, a new pattern of imprinting can be made with each generation. Genes are imprinted differently depending on the parental origin of the chromosome that contains them. In mice, the insulin-like growth factor 2 gene undergoes imprinting. The protein encoded by this gene helps to regulate body size. Mice that possess two functional copies of this gene are larger than those with two mutant copies. The size of mice that are heterozygous at this locus depends on the parent from which the wild type allele came. If the functional allele originated from the mother, the offspring will exhibit dwarfism, whereas a paternal allele will generate a normal sized mouse. This is because the maternal Igf2 gene is imprinted. Imprinting results in the inactivation of the Igf2 gene on the chromosome passed down by the mother. Imprints are formed due to the differential methylation of paternal and maternal alleles. This results in differing expression between alleles from the two parents. Sites with significant methylation are associated with low levels of gene expression. Higher gene expression is found at unmethylated sites. In this mode of inheritance, phenotype is determined not only by the specific allele transmitted to the offspring, but also by the sex of the parent that transmitted it.

Mosaicism

Individuals who possess cells with genetic differences from the other cells in their body are termed mosaics. These differences can result from mutations that occur in different tissues and at different periods of development. If a mutation happens in the non-gamete forming tissues, it is characterized as somatic. Germline mutations occur in the egg or sperm cells and can be passed on to offspring. Mutations that occur early on in development will affect a greater number of cells and can result in an individual that can be identified as a mosaic strictly based on phenotype. Mosaicism also results from a phenomenon known as X-inactivation. All female mammals have two X chromosomes. To prevent lethal gene dosage problems, one of these chromosomes is inactivated following fertilization. This process occurs randomly for all of the cells in the organism's body. Because a given female's two X chromosomes will almost certainly differ in their specific pattern of alleles, this will result in differing cell phenotypes depending on which chromosome is silenced. Calico cats, which are almost all female, demonstrate one of the most commonly observed manifestations of this process.

Trinucleotide Repeat Disorders

Trinucleotide repeat disorders also follow a non-Mendelian pattern of inheritance. These diseases are all caused by the expansion of microsatellite tandem repeats consisting of a stretch of three nucleotides. In normal individuals, the number of repeated units is relatively low. With each successive generation, there is a chance that the number of repeats will expand. As this occurs, progeny can progress to permutation and ultimately affected status. Individuals with a number of repeats that falls in the permutation range have a good chance of having affected children. Those who progress to affected status will exhibit symptoms of their particular disease. Prominent trinucleotide repeat disorders include Fragile X syndrome and Huntington's disease. In the case of Fragile X syndrome it is thought that the symptoms result from the increased methylation and accompanying reduced expression of the fragile X mental retardation gene in individuals with a sufficient number of repeats.

Selective Breeding

Forever people have wanted the best plants or animals of a species. One method of obtaining the best species is called selective breeding. Selective breeding is the method of breeding certain organisms together that have desirable traits. Hopefully their offspring will inherit these desirable traits. For centuries it has been used to obtain desirable plants and animals. A recent selective breeding project on plants involved the work of Dr. Jerry Parsons, an Agricultural Specialist of Bexar County, Texas, United States. He began a project in 1984 to grow red bluebonnets. After searching, he found a rare patch of pink bluebonnets in Bexar County, Texas. When these bluebonnets reproduced, he called out the lighter pink ones and left the darker reddish ones. A few generations later he obtained maroon bluebonnets. Dr. Parsons was unable to breed red bluebonnets due to the blue nature of the plant. These maroon bluebonnets that he cultivated will be on the market after the 1999 crop matures. It took 15 years of selective breeding to get a maroon color trait to stand out in enough bluebonnets to sell on the market. Selective breeding is a slow and tedious process, but it works.

Multiple Alleles

Two or more alternative firms of a gene are called alleles. Some inherited traits involve more than two alleles of a single gene called multiple alleles. In humans, three alleles (A, B and O) determine blood type. A person can have only two of the alleles, but there are three different ones found in the human population. The A and B alleles are equally dominant. A child who inherits and A allele from one parent and a B allele from the other parent will have type AB blood. The O allele is recessive to both A and B alleles. A child who inherits an A allele from one parent and an O allele from the other parent will have a genotype of AO and a phenotype of Type A blood *e.g.* a man with type A blood marries a woman with type B blood. They have ten children together. All of the children have type AB blood. What do you suppose are the genotypes of each parent? The father must be either AA or AO. The mother must be BB or BO. If one parent had the recessive O gene, we would expect that some of the children would have type A or type B blood. If both parents had the recessive O gene, we would expect that some children would have type A, type B or type O blood. Since all ten children have type AB blood, it is likely that the father is AA and the mother is BB. Multiple allele inheritance shows many forms of a trait, but each individual has only two alleles for the trait. Polygenic inheritance shows a continuum of the forms of the trait, with each individual having many genes involved in the expression of the trait.

Blood Group and Rh Factor

A blood type, also called a blood group is a classification of blood based on the presence or absence of inherited antigenic substances on the surface of red blood cells (RBCs). These antigens may be proteins, carbohydrates, glycoproteins or glycolipids, depending on the blood group system and some of these antigens are also present on the surface of other types of cells of various tissues. Several of these red blood cell surface antigens that stem from one allele or very closely linked genes, collectively form a blood group system. Blood types are inherited and represent contributions from both parents. A total of 30 human blood group systems are now recognized by the International Society of Blood Transfusion (ISBT). Many pregnant women carry a fetus with a different blood type from their own and the mother can form antibodies against fetal RBCs. Sometimes these maternal antibodies are IgG, a small immunoglobulin, which can cross the placenta and cause hemolysis of fetal RBCs, which in turn can lead to hemolytic disease of the newborn, an illness of low fetal blood counts which ranges from mild to severe The two most significant blood group systems were discovered during early experiments with blood transfusion: the ABO group in 1901 and the Rhesus group in 1937. Development of the Coombs test in 1945, the advent of transfusion medicine and the understanding of hemolytic disease of the newborn led to discovery of more blood groups and now 30 human blood group systems are recognized by the International Society of Blood Transfusion (ISBT) and across the 30 blood groups, over 600 different blood group antigens have been found, but many of these are very rare or are mainly found in certain ethnic groups. Blood types have been used in forensic science and in paternity testing, but both of these uses are being replaced by genetic fingerprinting, which provides greater certitude.

BOX 5.2

RBC and WBC

Red blood cells are the most common type of blood cell and the vertebrate body's principal means of delivering oxygen to the body tissues via the blood. The cells are filled with hemoglobin, a biomolecule that can bind to oxygen. They take up oxygen in the lungs or gills and release it while squeezing through the body's capillaries. The blood's red color is due to the color of hemoglobin. In humans, red blood cells develop in the bone marrow, take the form of flexible biconcave disks, lack a cell nucleus, subcellular organelles and the ability to synthesize protein and live for about 120 days. Red blood cells are also known as RBCs, red blood corpuscles (an archaic term), haematids or erythrocytes (Greek erythros for red and kytos for hollow, with cyte translated as cell in modern usage). The capitalized term Red Blood Cells is the proper name in the US for erythrocytes in storage solution used in transfusion medicine. The first person to describe red blood cells was probably the young Dutch biologist Jan Swammerdam, who had used an early microscope in 1658 to study the blood of a frog. Unaware of this work, Anton van Leeuwenhoek provided another microscopic description in 1674. White blood cells (WBCs) or leukocytes are cells of the immune system defending the body against both infectious disease and foreign materials. Five different and diverse types of leukocytes exist, but they are all produced and derived from a multipotent cell in the bone marrow known as a hematopoietic stem cell. Leukocytes are found throughout the body, including the blood and lymphatic system. The number of leukocytes in the blood is often an indicator of disease. There are normally between 4×10^9 and 11×10^9 white blood cells in a litre of blood, making up approximately 1% of blood in a healthy adult. In conditions such as leukemia, the number of leukocytes is higher than normal and in leukopenia, this number is much lower. The physical properties of leukocytes, such as volume, conductivity and granularity, may change due to activation, the presence of immature cells or the presence of malignant leukocytes in leukemia.

The ABO blood group system comprises of four major groups A, B, AB and O and Rh positive or negative, depending on the presence or absence of corresponding antigen on red blood cells. Subgroup of A, B and D is known to exist and may show weaker haemagglutinaton reaction with Anti-A, Anti-B and Anti-D reagents. Approximately 39-41% of the causation population have the Antigen A, 9-11% have Antigen B, 4% have both A and B while remaining have neither A nor B antigen. The Rh system was discovered in 1940 by Landsteiner and Wiener. They injected rabbits and guinea pigs with the red cells from *Macacus rhesus* monkeys and the resulting antibody reacted with the red cells of 85% of New York blood donors. Those who reacted were said to have the Rhesus factor and were Rhesus positive, whilst those that did not react lacked the Rhesus factor and were Rhesus negative. The terms Rhesus positive or Rh positive and Rhesus negative or Rh negative are still used today, especially by clinical staff. In 1939, Levine and Stetson had described an antibody in a mother who had recently had a stillborn foetus. The antibody caused a haemolytic trans-fusion reaction when she was transfused with ABO-compatible blood from her husband. They suggested that the antibody had been produced in response to an antigen carried by the foetus, which had been inherited from the father. This antibody was subsequently shown to have the same reaction pattern as Landsteiner and Wiener's anti-Rh and so Rh haemolytic disease of the newborn was described for the first time.

By 1945, the original Rh factor had been renamed D and four more Rh antigens discovered. These were the antithetical antigens C and c and E and e. There are now

45 antigens in the Rh system but D, C, c, E and e are the most commonly identified and the most significant in blood transfu-sion. The Rh antigens are expressed on polypeptides. The Rh polypeptides span the red cell membrane exposing six extracellular loops on which are expressed the Rh antigens. These polypeptides are associated in the membrane with an Rh glycoprotein to form tetramers (two Rh polypeptides and two Rh glycoproteins), which form the Rh core complex. The Rh glyco-protein is essential for the formation of this Rh core complex. Mutations in the genes controlling the expression of the Rh polypeptides or the Rh glyco-proteins can result in the phenotype, in which no Rh antigens are expressed. Red cell defects seen in the phenotype include abnormal cation transport across the red cell membrane and red cell morphological abnormalities, in the form of stomatocytes, red blood cells that exhibit a slit or mouth-shaped pallor rather than a central pallor, which may cause a mild, compensated haemolytic anaemia. The function of the Rh polypeptide is not known for certain, but it seems likely that it is involved in cation transport across the red cell membrane. The Rh antigens are well developed before birth, being detectable in the 6 week old foetus. They are fully expressed on cord red blood cells. Rh antigens have not been demonstrated on leucocytes and platelets or found in saliva or amniotic fluid.

Table 5.3: ABO and Rh Blood Type Distribution by Nation (Population Averages)

Country	O+	A+	B+	AB+	O"	A"	B"	AB"
Australia	40%	31%	8%	2%	9%	7%	2%	1%
Austria	30%	33%	12%	6%	7%	8%	3%	1%
Belgium	38%	34%	8.5%	4.1%	7%	6%	1.5%	0.8%
Canada	39%	36%	7.6%	2.5%	7%	6%	1.4%	0.5%
Denmark	35%	37%	8%	4%	6%	7%	2%	1%
Estonia	30%	31%	20%	6%	4.5%	4.5%	3%	1%
Finland	27%	38%	15%	7%	4%	6%	2%	1%
France	36%	37%	9%	3%	6%	7%	1%	1%
Germany	35%	37%	9%	4%	6%	6%	2%	1%
Hong Kong, China	40%	26%	27%	7%	0.31%	0.19%	0.14%	0.05%
Iceland	47.6%	26.4%	9.3%	1.6%	8.4%	4.6%	1.7%	0.4%
Ireland	47%	26%	9%	2%	8%	5%	2%	1%M
Israel	32%	34%	17%	7%	3%	4%	2%	1%
New Zealand	38%	32%	9%	3%	9%	6%	2%	1%
Norway	34%	42.5%	6.8%	3.4%	6%	7.5%	1.2%	0.6%
Poland	31%	32%	15%	7%	6%	6%	2%	1%
Saudi Arabia	48%	24%	17%	4%	4%	2%	1%	0.23%
Spain	36%	34%	8%	2.5%	9%	8%	2%	0.5%
Sweden	32%	37%	10%	5%	6%	7%	2%	1%
Netherlands	39.5%	35%	6.7%	2.5%	7.5%	7%	1.3%	0.5%
Turkey	29.8%	37.8%	14.2%	7.2%	3.9%	4.7%	1.6%	0.8%

Contd.....

Table 5.3 Contd...

Country	O+	A+	B+	AB+	O"	A"	B"	AB"
UK	37%	35%	8%	3%	7%	7%	2%	1%
USA	37.4%	35.7%	8.5%	3.4%	6.6%	6.3%	1.5%	0.6%

Universal Donors and Universal Recipients

With regard to transfusions of whole blood or packed red blood cells, individuals with type O negative blood are called universal donors and those with type AB positive blood are called universal recipients; however, these terms are only generally true with respect to possible reactions of the recipient's anti-A and anti-B antibodies to transfused red blood cells and also possible sensitization to RhD antigens. Exceptions include individuals with hh antigen system who can only receive blood safely from other hh donors, because they form antibodies against the H substance. Blood donors with particularly strong anti-A, anti-B or any atypical blood group antibody are excluded from blood donation. The possible reactions of anti-A and anti-B antibodies present in the transfused blood to the recipients RBCs need not be considered, because a relatively small volume of plasma containing antibodies is transfused. Additionally, red blood cell surface antigens other than A, B and Rh D, might cause adverse reactions and sensitization, if they can bind to the corresponding antibodies to generate an immune response. Transfusions are further complicated because platelets and white blood cells (WBCs) have their own systems of surface antigens and sensitization to platelet or WBC antigens can occur as a result of transfusion. With regard to transfusions of plasma, this situation is reversed. Type O plasma can be given only to O recipients, while AB plasma (which does not contain anti-A or anti-B antibodies) can be given to patients of any ABO blood group.

Compatibility

In order to provide maximum benefit from each blood donation and to extend shelf life, blood banks fractionate some whole blood into several products. The most common of these products are packed RBCs, plasma, platelets, cryoprecipitate and fresh frozen plasma (FFP). FFP is quick frozen to retain the labile clotting factors V and VIII, which are usually administered to patients who have a potentially fatal clotting problem caused by a condition such as advanced liver disease, overdose of anticoagulant or disseminated intravascular coagulation (DIC). Units of packed red cells are made by removing as much of the plasma as possible from whole blood units. Clotting factors synthesized by modern recombinant methods are now in routine clinical use for hemophilia, as the risks of infection transmission that occur with pooled blood products are avoided.

Red Blood Cell Compatibility

- **Blood group AB** individuals have both A and B antigens on the surface of their RBCs and their blood serum do not contain any antibodies against either A or B antigen. Therefore, an individual with type AB blood can receive blood from any group (with AB being preferable), but can donate blood only to another type AB individual.

- **Blood group A** individuals have the A antigen on the surface of their RBCs and blood serum containing IgM antibodies against the B antigen. Therefore, a group A individual can receive blood only from individuals of groups A or O (with A being preferable) and can donate blood to individuals with type A or AB.

- **Blood group B** individuals have the B antigen on the surface of their RBCs and blood serum containing IgM antibodies against the A antigen. Therefore, a group B individual can receive blood only from individuals of groups B or O (with B being preferable) and can donate blood to individuals with type B or AB.

- **Blood group O** (or blood group zero in some countries) individuals do not have either A or B antigens on the surface of their RBCs, but their blood serum contains IgM anti-A antibodies and anti-B antibodies against the A and B blood group antigens. Therefore, a group O individual can receive blood only from a group O individual, but can donate blood to individuals of any ABO blood group (*i.e* A, B, O or AB). If anyone needs a blood transfusion in a dire emergency and if the time taken to process the recipient's blood would cause a detrimental delay, O Negative blood can be issued.

Inheritance and Nomenclature of Rh System

Two genetic systems were originally proposed to explain the relationships and inheritance of these five original Rh antigens. In the USA, Wiener proposed a system comprising a single locus producing factors he called agglutinogens, which could express multiple antigens. In the UK, Fisher and Race proposed a system of three closely linked loci for D/d, C/c and E/e, each gene coding for the production of a single antigen. Thus, the antigens C and c were thought to be the products of the co-dominant alleles *C* and *c*. Antigens E and e were thought to be the products of the co-dominant alleles E and e. The D antigen was the product of the D gene and the proposed allelic gene d was considered an amorph as no d antigen or anti-d antibody was ever discovered. Fisher also postulated that the order of the genes on a chromosome was DCE. It has become common practice to refer to them in this order.

The clinical significance of the Rh system has led to considerable investi-gation of the system. As new Rh antigens and phenotypes were discovered, it became apparent that neither Wiener's nor Fisher's system could explain every new finding. However, Fisher's system of three closely linked loci was the most complete and allowed the deduction of phenotypes of offspring from different mating types. Fisher's shorthand notation was also very conve-nient for communicating information regarding phenotypes and genotypes. It has now been shown by modern molecular biology techniques that neither of these earlier systems was completely correct and that in fact the Rh system is controlled by two closely linked loci. One carries the gene for the Rh D polypeptide and is known as the *RHD* locus. The other carries the genes for the CcEe polypeptide and is known as the *RHCE* locus. Despite current evidence concerning the genetics and biochemistry of the Rh system, Fisher's model and shorthand notation continue to be a convenient way to explain and communicate Rh phenotypes and genotypes.

Qualitative Differences in Rh Antigens

The Rh D antigen is now considered to contain at least 30 different epitopes, as revealed by tests using monoclonal antibodies. Rare individuals who lack certain epitopes are known as partial D and may be stimulated to produce antibodies to the missing epitopes by transfusion or pregnancy. The partial D type known as category DVI is the clinically most important partial D. Severe cases of haemolytic disease of the newborn have occurred in Rh D-positive babies born to category DVI mothers with anti-D antibody. Category DVI is the most common partial D occurring in 6–10% of weak D samples and 0.02–0.05% of all Caucasian samples. The majority of Rh D-positive individuals with allo-anti-D are category D. This partial D state may arise from the replacement of an exon segment from *RHD* by an equivalent segment from *RHCE,* creating a hybrid *RHD–CE–D* gene or as a result of point mutation within *RHD.* The replacement of several exon segments from *RHD* with the equivalent segments from *RHCE* can destroy the ability to produce D antigen altogether. Thus, the individual only expresses the C/c and E/e antigens and serologi-cally appears as Rh D negative although they do possess an *RHD* gene.

G antigen

The G antigen is usually only detected on red cells expressing D antigen or C antigen or both. Its expression appears to be dependent on amino acid sequences derived from exon 2 of the *RHD* gene. Anti-G has been impli-cated in haemolytic disease of the newborn. The presence of the G antigen explains the not uncommon observation that some non-transfused pregnant women apparently produce anti-C+D antibody even though the father of their foetus is found to be C negative. In such cases, the father has been shown to have passed an R2 chromosome (DcE) to the foetus. The G antigen would also be expressed by this gene arrangement. Thus, the mother has actually been immunized to produce anti-D and anti-G rather than anti-D and anti-C.

Compound Antigens

The C/c and E/e antigens are produced by the same gene, antibodies have been described which only react with compound antigens that are produced by the same gene. The antibody produced in response to the ce compound antigen is anti-ce (anti-f). This antibody will only react with cells expressing both c and e antigens derived from the same gene. This means that anti-ce will react with dce (r) or Dce (R_0) red cells but not with DCe/DcE (R_1R_2) cells where the c and e antigens have been produced by different genes. Other examples of compound antigens with corresponding antibodies are cE, CE and Ce.

Laboratory Aspects of Rh Blood Group Typing

Rh D Typing: When undertaking Rh D typing of patients and when selecting blood donors, consideration must be given to the qualitative and quantitative variations in the expression of the Rh D antigen. During D typing of patients, it is important to detect all but very weakest forms in order that the patient is not unnecessarily transfused with Rh D-negative blood, which would be wasteful of a scarce resource and also, when D typing babies of Rh D-negative women, it is important that the women receive anti-D prophylaxis, if the baby has a weak form of D. When D typing donors, it is essential to detect weak forms in order to avoid the chance of transfusing Rh D (weak)-positive donor blood to Rh D-negative patients. This could induce the production of anti-D antibody in the patient. The detection of partial D types is not necessary when typing patients. It is safer to treat them as Rh D negative for transfusion purposes. Patients with a partial D type may produce anti-D antibodies when exposed to normal Rh D-positive donor blood. The partial D expressed on a baby's cells is poorly immunogenic and it is therefore not necessary to offer anti-D prophylaxis to the Rh D-negative mothers of such infants. It is a different approach when D typing blood donors where it is necessary to detect partial D types in order to avoid mistakenly transfusing Rh D (partial)-positive to Rh D-negative patients, as this may result in the induction of anti-D antibody.

Phenotyping and Genotyping

It is necessary to make an assessment of the phenotype and genotype of an individual when selecting blood for transfusion to patients with Rh antibodies, assessing the likely effect on the foetus of a woman's Rh antibod-ies or when performing family studies. It is usually possible to derive the genotype from information about the phenotype in Rh D-negative individ-uals. However, it is usually impossible to tell whether Rh D-positive individ-uals are homozygous or heterozygous for D and therefore their genotype has to be assumed from the statistically most likely arrangement for their ethnic group. The presence of Rh antigens on red cells is most usually detected using the antisera anti-D, anti-C, anti-E, anti-c and anti-e. The phenotype of an individual may be established from the reactions of their red cells when added to these reagents.

Polygenic Traits

Polygenic traits are inherited characteristics where more than one gene is involved in determining the phenotype. Most of the traits you learned about earlier involved just two possibilities: attached or free earlobes can or cannot roll tongue, etc. Polygenic traits involve several possibilities. Hair color in humans is a polygenic trait. Eye color is, too. Height is also a polygenic trait, but nutrition during childhood also plays an important role in

	AB	**AB**
ab	AaBb	AaBb
ab	AaBb	AaBb

determining height. Even if the phenotype for height is six feet tall, without proper nutrition you won't reach that height. Kernel color in wheat is an interesting polygenic trait to study. There are two genes that work together to determine kernel color. Dark red kernel plants are AABB. White kernel plants are aabb. When you cross a dark red with a white, the combination looks like this:

The AaBb offspring have kernels that are an intermediate colour a medium pink.

Hemoglobin: Hemoglobin also spelled haemoglobin and abbreviated Hb or Hgb, is the iron-containing oxygen-transport metalloprotein in the red blood cells of vertebrates and the tissues of some invertebrates. In mammals, the protein makes up about 97% of the red blood cell's dry content and around 35% of the total content (including water). Hemoglobin transports oxygen from the lungs or gills to the rest of the body where it releases the oxygen for cell use. It also has a variety of other roles of gas transport and effect-modulation which vary from species to species and are quite diverse in some invertebrates. The oxygen-carrying protein hemoglobin was discovered by Hünefeld in 1840. In 1851, Otto Funke published a series of articles in which he described growing hemoglobin crystals by successively diluting red blood cells with a solvent such as pure water, alcohol or ether, followed by slow evaporation of the solvent from the resulting protein solution. Hemoglobin's reversible oxygenation was described a few years later by Felix Hoppe-Seyler. In 1959. Max Perutz determined the molecular structure of hemoglobin by X-ray crystallography. This work resulted in his sharing with John Kendrew the 1962 Nobel Prize in Chemistry. The role of hemoglobin in the blood was elucidated by physiologist Claude Bernard. The name hemoglobin is the concatenation of heme and globin, reflecting the fact that each subunit of hemoglobin is a globular protein with an embedded heme or haem group. Each heme group contains one iron atom that can bind one oxygen molecule through ion-induced dipole forces. The most common type of hemoglobin in mammals contains four such subunits.

Inter action of Genes

Mendel's great contribution to genetics was the idea that each character is controlled by a single gene or single factor, *e.g.* gene for tallness in pea can control only tallness and not others. But in reality there is no such thing as 1:1 ratio, between a character and a gene. It has been seen now that a gene produces not a single character but influences several characters of the individuals. The impact of a single gene on more than one characters or trait is called pleiotropy *e.g.* in human beings the gene for the disease phenylketonurea produces pleiotropic effects such as short stature, non-pigmented hairs and mental retardedation. Similarly quite often many genes, called compound gene are responsible for a single characters. The additive effect of two or more gene on single phenotypic characters is called as polygenic inheritance. Bateson called this phenomenon as factor hypothesis or factor interaction and lead to modification of basic Mendelian ratio *i.e.* 3:1 and 9:3:1 and so called modification F_2 factors. It has also been observed that a gene may sometimes interfere with the development and may cause the death of the individual. Similarly the dominant genes may interact and produces a new phenotype.

A. In Monohybrid Cross

i. Incomplete Dominance (1:2:1)

Correns (1903) while working on *Mirabilis jalapa* (Four O clock) found that when red flowered variety crossed with white flowered variety, the F_1 hybrid is pink and F_2 ratio is 1 red: 2 pink: 1 white. This shows that there is no complete dominance in the

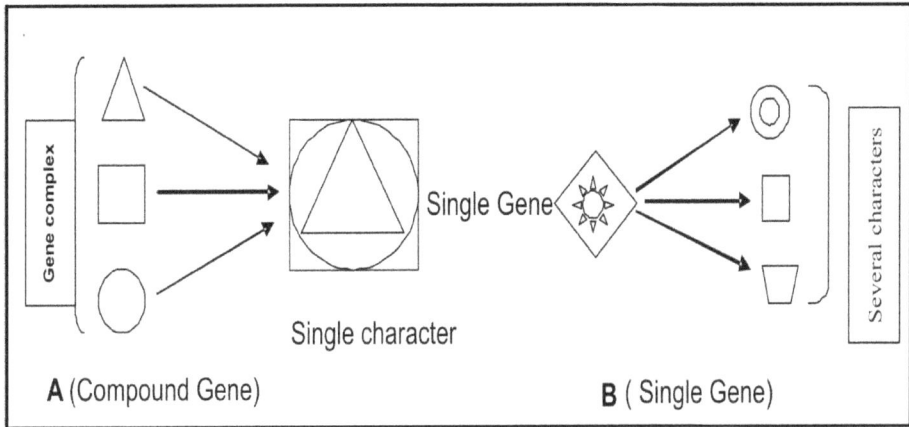

Figure 5.6: Effect of complex and single Gene

heterozygous plant which bears pink flowers. If the pair or alleles controlling flower colour be named Rr then red flowers develop on RR plants, white on rr plants, while heterozygous Rr plant develop pink flowers and not red ones which would have been the case, if there was complete dominance of R over r. This is also called blending inheritance as if the two colours have blended in the heterozygous. Other examples of incomplete dominance are *Antirrhinum* (Snapdragon), *Nicotiana tobaccum* (Tobacco) and *Oryza sativa* (Pady) etc.

ii. Lethel Gene (2:1)

It has been noticed that all genetic factors are not useful to the organisms. There are some factors which may even cause death of the progeny, *e.g.* Sanpdragon is characterized by variegated leaves. This golden variety on selfing gives two types of offspring, golden and green in the ratio 2:1 instead of 3:1. The green ones breed true and are recessive (gg) but the golden ones produce a mixed progeny on selfing being heterozygous. The dominant homozygous (GG) seedling are completely yellow, therefore, they will die because G in the homozygous conditiyon Shas lethal effect. Thus the ratio remains 2:1. Lethal genes were repeated by L. Cuenot (1905) in mouse body colour and by E. Baur (1907) in Snapdragon. Lethal gene has also reported in human beings. Sickle cell anemia and thallasemia are best known examples.

B. In Dihybrid Corss

iii. Simple Interaction (9:3:3:1)

Bateson and Punett gave classical example in fowl to show two genes influenciung the same character. There are four types of combs recongnised among fowls- pea, rose, walnut and single. These are caused by two allelomorphic pairs of

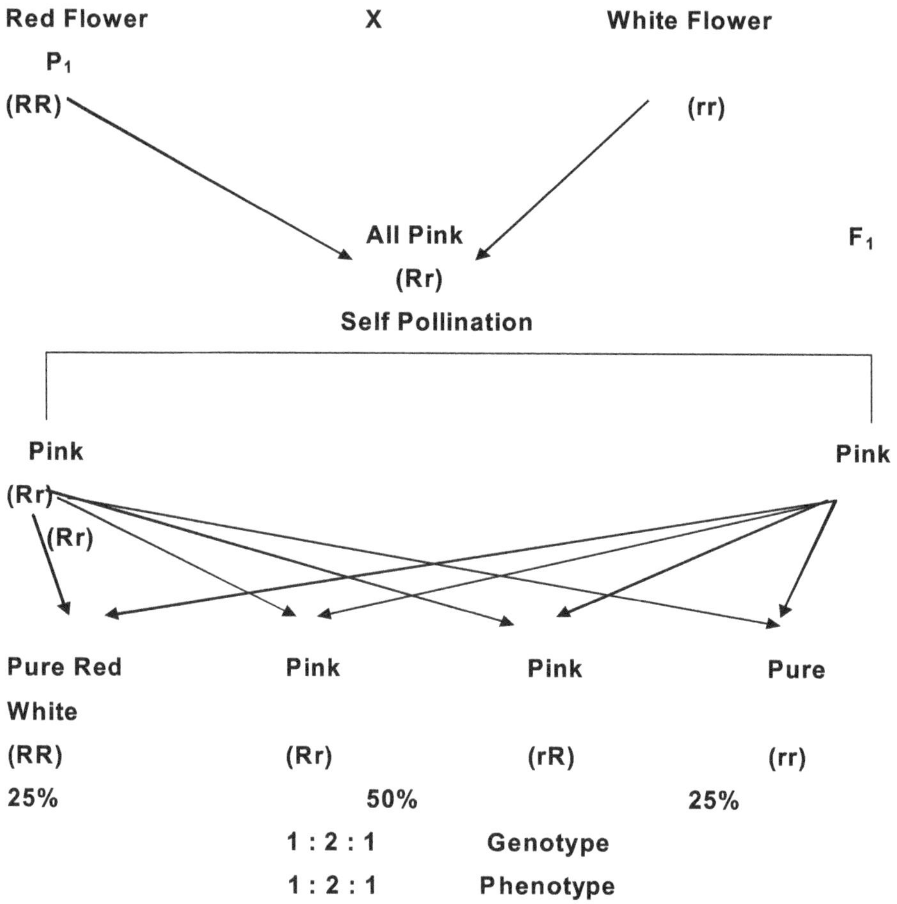

Red Flower   X   White Flower

   P₁

(RR)   (rr)

                All Pink   F₁

                 (Rr)

            Self Pollination

Pink   Pink

(Rr)   (Rr)

Pure Red   Pink   Pink   Pure

White

(RR)   (Rr)   (rR)   (rr)

25%   50%   25%

         1 : 2 : 1   Genotype

         1 : 2 : 1   Phenotype

Figure 5.7: Incomplete Dominance in *Miraqbilis jalapa*

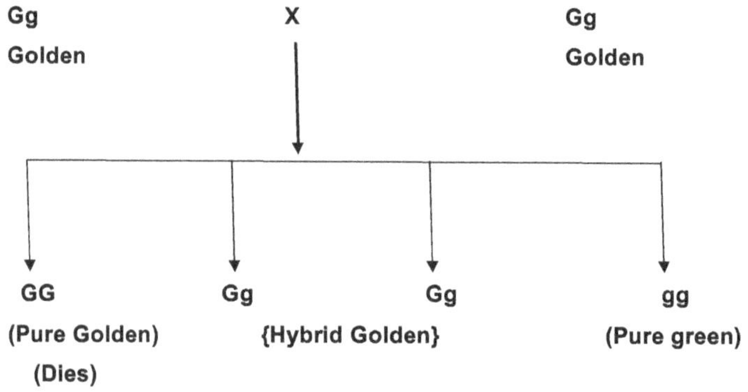

Gg   X   Gg

Golden   Golden

GG   Gg   Gg   gg

(Pure Golden)   {Hybrid Golden}   (Pure green)

  (Dies)

Figure 5.8: Lethal gene (GG) in *Antirrhinum*

genes symbolized by PPrr (Pea) ppRR (Rose). A cross between the two produces a new comb form in F^1 generation called walnut (RrPp). The F^1 generation on selfing produced F^2 generation as follows-9 walnut, 3 pea, 3 rose and 1 single. Thus when dominant gene P is present alone without other dominant gene R, the comb is pea type. When R is present alone, the comb is green or red or rose. But when both P and R are present there is an interaction and the comb becomes walnut. When no dominant gene present, comb is of double recessive *i.e.* single type.

iv. Complementary Factors (9:7)

Sometimes a trait is produced by the interaction of two or more genes situated on separate chromosomes which complement one another. In some varieties of sweet pea, the following interaction of two pairs of gene has been noted *i.e.* ccR-, C-rr and ccrr- white colour C-R red colour. It was observed by Bateson and Punnett in *Lathyrus odoratus*. Here gene C and R are complementary to each other and necessary for the production of colour in the flower. When they are together (C-R), red colour in petals develops.

Parents   CCrr   X   ccRR

                White   White

                                CcRr

                                Red

	Cr	Cr	cR	cr
CR	CCRR Red	CCRr Red	CcRR Red	CcRr Red
Cr	CCRr Red	CCrr White	CcRr Red	Ccrr White
cR	CcRR Red	CcRr Red	ccRR White	ccRr White
cr	CcRr Red	Ccrr White	ccRr White	ccrr White

Phenotype: 9 Red: 7 White

Figure 5.8: Complementary Factors

v. Supplementary Factors (9:3:4)

In this case one factor alone is sufficient to produce a visible results but the expression of character in question is changed by an additional factor which supplements the first factor, *e.g.* the red type anthocyanin colour of many flower is caused by two allele which may be termed as Aa and Bb in the Snapdragon flower.

A-B = Magenta flower

A-bb = Ivory flower

aaB and aabb = White flower

Thus in an ivory (AA bb) x white (aaBB) cross the F^1 (AaBb) is magenta and F^2 segregation ration is 9 Magnet (A-B-): 3 Ivory (A-bb) : 4 whte (aaB- and aabb).

This can be explained as follows:

Ivory flowers contain anthoxanthin and magenta flowers contain anthocyanin pigments. It is known that anthoxanthin and anthocyanin are synthesized out of the same raw materials; the former is synthesized in the first stage and the latter when some additional chemical reaction takes place. Thus it seems that pigments producing chemicals in the flower are brought to the anthoxanthin stage by gene A. When gene A is supplemented by the gene B, this reaction proceeds to a higher stage producing the anthocyanin pigment. Thus the magneta anthocyanin pigment may only be produced in two stages. The first stage is completed by A and the end product is Ivory (anthoxanthin). The second stage (anthocyanin) is brought about by B. Thus B is supplementary gene having no effect by itself.

vi. Inhibitory Factors (13:3)

In this type of modification, two pairs of factors are involved and one of the dominant factor suppresse or inhibits the expression of the other dominat factor. This may be explained by taking pigmentation in rice palnts. In the rice plants, the presence of gene P causes its leaves to be coloured deep purple. But if a gene I- is present then the purple colour is inhibited and the leaf becomes normally green. The I- gene is considered as inhibitory factors.

I-P-, I-pp, iipp = Green

Iipp = Purple

Thus in a green (IIpp) x purple (iiPP) cross the F_1 is green and F_2 generation comprises 13 green (I-P-, I-pp and iipp): 3 purple (iip-) as the presence of P- in the absence of 1I only cause the purple colour.

vii. Epistasis (12:3:1)

Epistasis means standing on. There are numerous cases where two different genes which are not alleles but effect the same trait of the organism, the expression of one cover up or hide the expression of the other. A gene that masks or prevents the expression of another is called epistatic to it and the gene that is hidden is known as hypostatic. Epistasis should not be confused with dominance. Epistasis is due to interaction of two separate genes while dominance is the interaction of two alleles of same pair. In summer squash (*Cucurbita pepo*), there are three common fruit colours, white, yellow and green. White is always found to be dominant and in cross between yellow and green, yellow will be dominant. Yellow colour is acts as a recessive in relation to white but as a dominant in relation to green. There is evidently a factor for white (W) which is epistatic to those for yellow and green as long as it is present, no colour is produced in the fruit. Where this factor for white is lacking (ww), the fruit colour is yellow, if the factor for Yellow Y is present and green if it is absent.

viii. Additive Factors (9:6:1)

The pericarp colour in wheat may be deep red and colourless, when deep red and colorless pericarp is crossed. The F_1 is deep red. In F_2, 9 deep red, 6 light red and 1 colourless types appears depending on the presence of the tow or single dominant gene. This phenomenon is called as polymerisms or additive.

ix. Pseudoalleles (Duplicate Factors- 15:1)

It was observed by G.H. Shull in Shepherd's purse (Capsella). When two or more genes localized on different chromosomes show the same phenotypic action, they are called duplicate genes or Pseudoalleles. For these reasons, the normal F^2 segregation ration (9:3:3:1) is not found and instead of the segregation ratio 15:1 is present *e.g.* endosperm colour in maize. In a pure yello (Y1Y1 Y2Y2) pure white (y1y1 y2y2) cross the F_1 will be yellow (Y1y1 Y2y2) and F_2 segregation will comprise 15 yellow: 1 white.

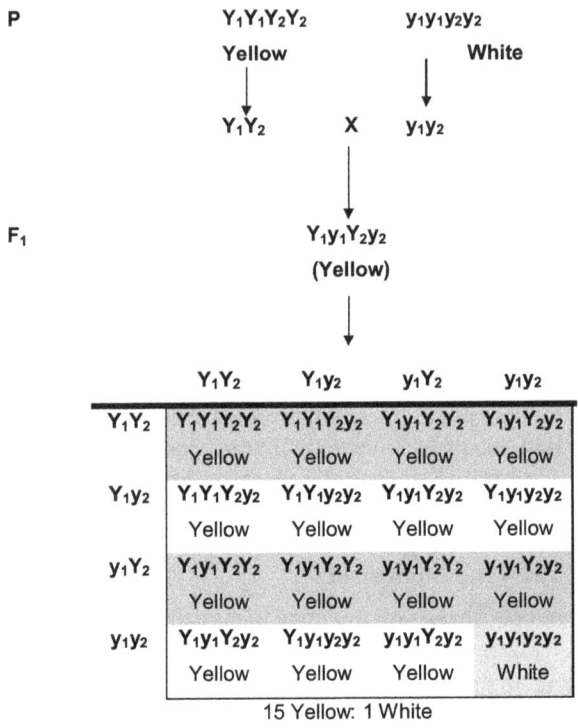

P $Y_1Y_1Y_2Y_2$ $y_1y_1y_2y_2$
                       Yellow   White

                       Y_1Y_2 X y_1y_2

F₁ $Y_1y_1Y_2y_2$
                               (Yellow)

	Y_1Y_2	Y_1y_2	y_1Y_2	y_1y_2
Y_1Y_2	$Y_1Y_1Y_2Y_2$ Yellow	$Y_1Y_1Y_2y_2$ Yellow	$Y_1y_1Y_2Y_2$ Yellow	$Y_1y_1Y_2y_2$ Yellow
Y_1y_2	$Y_1Y_1Y_2y_2$ Yellow	$Y_1Y_1y_2y_2$ Yellow	$Y_1y_1Y_2y_2$ Yellow	$Y_1y_1y_2y_2$ Yellow
y_1Y_2	$Y_1y_1Y_2Y_2$ Yellow	$Y_1y_1Y_2y_2$ Yellow	$y_1y_1Y_2Y_2$ Yellow	$y_1y_1Y_2y_2$ Yellow
y_1y_2	$Y_1y_1Y_2y_2$ Yellow	$Y_1y_1y_2y_2$ Yellow	$y_1y_1Y_2y_2$ Yellow	$y_1y_1y_2y_2$ White

15 Yellow: 1 White

Figure 5.10. Duplicate Factors

x. Multiple factors (Polygenic Inheritance)

Multiple factor inheritance implies that several pairs of alleles are interacting and that each has a similar and measurable effect on a characteristic, thus it is also called as Quantitative inheritance. Experimental evidence for polygenic inheritance was first obtained by a Swedish geneticist H. Nilsson Ehle in 1908. He found that the kernel colour in wheat is determined by three gene pairs. Davenport (1913) proposed that skin pigmentation is determined by at least two pairs of alleles and that each dominant gene is responsible for the synthesis of a fixed amount of melanin. The effect of all the gene is additive and the amount of melanin produced is always proportional to the number of dominant genes. Here 1:4:6:4:1 ratio is obtained on the basis of presence of 4, 3, 2, 1 and 0 dominant allele/s in the genotype respectively. Quite a few quantitative characters like plant height, yield of crop (size, shape and number of seeds and fruits per plant), intelligence in human beings, milk yield in animals, etc., have been found to be determined by many genes and their effects have been found to be combined.

xi. Modifies factor

Some factors modify the action of other factors or gene in some way or other. These are known as modifier genes. It is called suppressor, if it suppresses or called enhancer, if it enhances the visible effect of the other gene, *e.g.* in mice a gene W produces white spot on skin, however the degree of white spotting depends upon number of modifier gene. More the modifier genes, the greater the degree of spots is.

Pedigree Analysis

A pedigree is a diagram of family relationships that uses symbols to represent people and lines to represent genetic relationships. These diagrams make it easier to visualize relationships within families, particularly large extended families. Pedigrees are often used to determine the mode of inheritance (dominant/recessive) of genetic diseases. The analysis of segregation by generating controlled crosses and counting large numbers of progeny is not possible in human beings. But the mode of inheritance of a trait can sometimes be determined by examining pedigrees. A family tree that shows the phenotype of each individual is called pedigree. Important application of probability in genetics is its use in pedigree analysis.

Pedigree Problem: Because of the small number of progeny, pedigrees can often be ambiguous; more than one model may explain the observed pattern of inheritance. For this reason, we assume that the genetic abnormality is rare in the population. This means that, in a given family, very few (usually one) of the first generation individuals carry the abnormality and very few (usually none) individuals who marry into the family carry the abnormality.

Here is a sample human pedigree and one way to analyze it. Use A or a to represent the abnormality if it is dominant or recessive, respectively.

Parents connected by horizontal lines.

Vertical lines lead to their offspring.

Pedigree Symbols

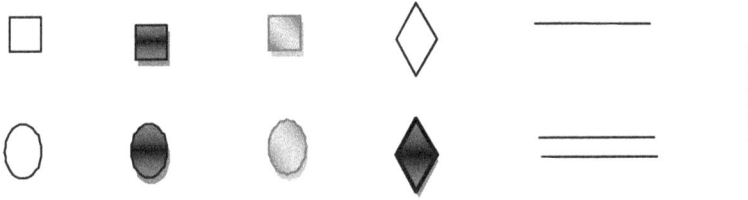

Meanings

1. *Circle:* female
2. *Square:* male
3. *Diamond:* sex unspecified
4. *Solid color:* affected individual
5. *Horizontal line connecting male and female:* a mating
6. *Two horizontal lines:* mating between relatives.
7. *Vertical line:* connects parents and offspring
8. *Symbol with slash:* deceased individuals

Figure 62: Symbols used Pedgree Analysis

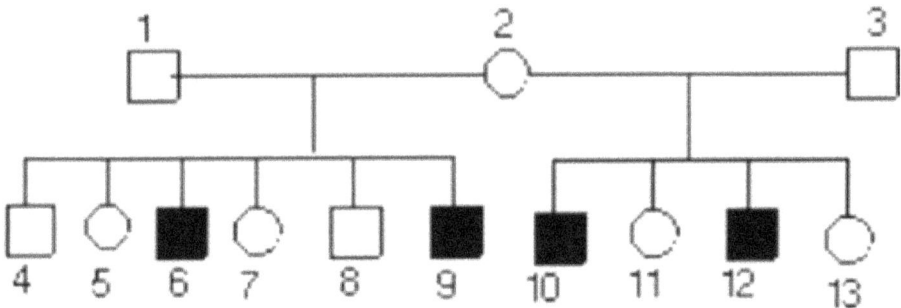

Prediction 1. If the abnormality were due to a dominant mutation in a gene on an autosome (autosomal dominant):

A - dominant abnormal allele

a - recessive normal allele

Then either 2 or both 1 and 3 would have to show the abnormality for it to be present in the children. This does not fit the data.

Prediction 2. If the abnormality were due to an autosomal recessive mutation:

a - recessive abnormal allele

A - dominant normal allele

In order for the second generation to have affected individuals (aa), both parents of each family must be carriers. That is: 1, 2 and 3 must be Aa. It is predicted that their children would have a 25% chance of being affected (aa). The observed frequencies are 33% and 50% in the two families which is not statistically significant for this small sample size. However, this model assumes that three non-blood relatives all carry the abnormal gene (1, 2 and 3). If we assume that the abnormality is rare, then the chance that three randomly selected individuals will have the abnormality is very small. Therefore, this model is a possible explanation of the data, but it is not the most likely.

Summary

1. Genetics is a branch of biology which deals the principles of inheritance and its practices. Genetics term coined by William Bateson in 1906.

2. The progeny resembling the parents in morphological and physiological features has attracted the attention of many biologists.

3. Mendel proposed the principles of inheritance, which are today referred as Mendel's Laws of Inheritance.

4. Heredity is the transmission of traits from one generation to the following generation.

5. G.J. Mendel performed a large number of experiments on common garden pea.

6. Mendel, the father of genetics, was born on 22 July, 1822 in Heizendrof in Austria. He procured seeds of 34 different varieties of peas from the local seedsman and grew them in the garden.

7. Mendel's first experiments were with the varieties of garden pea that differed in only one visible character.

8. The law of dominance states that out of a pair of allelomorphic characters, one is dominant and the other recessive.

9. The heredity units which are responsible for the appearance of characters in the off spring were said to be factors or determiners.

10. W. Johannsen (1909) gave the term gene.

11. The law of segregation states that when a pair of allelomorphs is brought together in the hybrid (F_1), they remain together in the hybrid without blending but separate complete and pure during gamete formation.

12. When two pairs of interdependent allele are brought together in the hybrid F_1, they show independent dominant effects. It is known as law of independent assortment.

13. Some characters are exceptions to Mendel's law of dominance and show incomplete dominance. It is found in *Mirabilis jalapa*.

14. In co-dominance, both allelic genes of a genetic trait are equally expressive.

15. Several genes present on different chromosome pairs interact in various ways and affect the production of single trait.

16. Chromosomes occur in pairs like the allele of a Mendelian factor. The homologous chromosomes separate during meiosis like the pair of similar or dissimilar alleles of a Mendelian factor separate at the time of gamete formation.

17. Different chromosomes orient and separate independently during meiosis like Mendelian factors. The tendency of two or more genes of the same chromosomes to remain together during the process of inheritance.

18. There are mainly two type of linkage, compete and incomplete linkage.

19. Complete linkage is exhibited when the genes for a particular character are present very close to one another. The best example of complete linkage is male Drosophila for grey body colour and long wings.

20. Incomplete linkage occurs when the genes for the different characters are separated at the time of chromosome pieces during meiosis.

21. Mutual exchange of blocks of homologous genes between a pair of homologous chromosomes is known as crossing over. Crossing over involves breaking and repairing of chromosomes in the synaptonemal complex.

22. The points where homologous are held together and exchange bits of chromatids are known as chiasmata.

23. As a result of crossing over, new gene combinations are produced when play an important role in micro-evolution.

24. The representation in figure of relative position of genes on the chromosome is known as chromosome map and the process of identifying is known as mapping.

25. Sex determination is concerned with the study of factors which are responsible for making an individual male, female or hermaphrodite.

26. According to the chromosomal theory f sex determination, two types of chromosomes (Autosomes and Sex chromosome) are present in each individual.

27. The male and female individuals differ in their sex chromosome constitution.

28. The balance theory of sex determination proposed by C.B. Bridge (1925).

29. In most unisexual organism, a pair of sex chromosomes is found besides a set of autosomes.

30. All genes situated on the sex chromosome show linkage. They are known as Sex linked trait. T.H. Morgan carried his experiments of inheritance on fruit fly.

31. Sex-linked character in human beings follows the same pattern as in Drosophila.

32. Colour blindness and hemophilia are two important examples of sex linked characters in human beings.

33. Sometimes the members of a chromosome pair fail to separate at the first meiotic division.

34. The non disjunction of sex chromosomes provides strong evidence in favour of the chromosomal theory of inheritance.

35. Mutations in a broad sense include all those heritable changes which alter the phenotype of an individual.

36. While working on evening primrose (*Oenothora lamarkiana*) Hugo-de Vries used the term mutation to describe phenotype changes which were heritable.

37. Mutations may occur spontaneously in nature or they may be artificially induced.

38. Mutations are of three type- gene mutation, chromosomal mutation and genomatic mutation.

39. A slight slip occurs in the replication of genes and this change in gene duplication is known as gene mutation.

40. The mutant gene and the original gene are situated at the same fixed point on a particular chromosome.

41. Since a gene is located at a fixed point on the chromosome, a gene mutation is called point mutation.

42. This type of mutation occurs at the molecular level usually at the time of DNA replication when new DNA strands are synthesized.

43. Gene mutation are also said to be copy-error mutations.

44. The structural changes in chromosomes which appear phenotypically are known as chromosomal mutations or aberrations.

45. These changes were first analyzed by H. J. Muller (1928) in Drosophila and by Barbara Mc Clintock in Maize.

46. The loss or absence of a section of a chromosome and may involve one or more gene is called Deficiency or Deletion.

47. The presence of a part of a chromosome in excess of the normal complement is known as duplication.

48. Individual carrying duplications shows various abnormalities in bodily characters and may be used to identify the carriers of the corresponding duplications.

49. Translocation involves the transfer of a part of a chromosome or set of genes to a non-homologous chromosome.

50. Due to independent segregation of chromosome translocation leads to the loss of genes in some of the cells and a reduction in the number of viable gametes or partial sterility.

51. Inversion involves a rotation of a part of a chromosome or a set of genes by 180° on its own axis.

52. Breakage and reunion are essential for inversion. The net result is neither a gain nor a loss in the genetic material but simply a rearrangement of the gene sequence.

53. Inversion may be paracentric or pericentric type.

54. In paracentric inversion centromere is located outside the inversion loop, whereas in pericentric inversion centromere is located inside the inversion loop.

55. Genomatic mutation involves variations in chromosome number of a whole genome.

56. These variations are mainly of two type- aneuploidy and euploidy.

57. Aneuploidy is the presence of a chromosome number which is different than the multiple of basic chromosome number.

58. This type of variation involves one or a few chromosomes but not the entire set. It is either due to loss of one or more chromosome or due to due to addition of one or more chromosomes to complete chromosome complement.

59. Aneuploidy mainly is of four types:- (i) Monosomics (ii) Nullisomics (iii) Trisomics (iv) Tetrasomics.

Chapter 6

Sex Determination and Sex Differentiation

Introduction

The concept of sex determination and differentiation has been baffling mankind since time immemorial. While Aristotle hypothesized in 335 BC that sex was determined by the heat generated during conception. In numerous cultures, women have been considered as the default state of men. However, in 17th century gradually it was discovered that the females produced eggs that transmitted parental traits. Later, in the 20th century Geddes and Thomson came forward with the hypothesis that constitution, age, nutrition and environment of parents decide the sex determination of the offspring. This environmental view of sex determination was again challenged by the discovery of sex chromosomes by McClung in 1902. Following this, more evidences gradually clinched to suggest the chromosomal concept of sex determination. Numerous experimental studies in vertebrates have established beyond doubt that sex is determined either by chromosomal factors, environmental influences or interplay of both depending on the species/groups.

Sex determination and sex differentiation are two separate but related phenomena. Sex differentiation is a programmed cascade of events in which the indifferent gonad develops as a testis or an ovary with the appropriate urogenital and secondary sex characters. Sex determination is the event that sets this cascade in motion. In placental mammals, there is good evidence that sex is determined by a gene on the Y chromosome (SRY) that initiates testis formation. In the absence of SRY an ovary develops. There are examples of placental mammals that develop as normal males with no detectable SRY. In reptiles, sex differentiation appears to be similar to mammals *i.e.* the same genes and hormones act in a similar manner but sex determination is clearly very differe nt. Ovarian differentiation in placental mammals can occur in the absence of estrogen or an estrogen receptor. Ovarian differentiation in reptiles requires the presence of estrogen. In the absence of estrogen a testis develops. In temperature sex determination, reptile embryos will develop as females when treated with estrogen, even if eggs are incubated at male inducing temperatures, it will develop as males when estrogen synthesis is blocked in eggs incubated at female-inducing temperatures. A number of other genes have also been shown to be important in mammalian sex determination. One of these genes Sox9, which is expressed in differentiating mouse testis, has recently been found to be expressed in embryonic reptile testis. Other genes that appear to be common to both mammals and reptiles in the sex determining cascade are SF-1, MIH and possibly DAX-1.

Genetic Sex

The first step in sex determination and differentiation is the establishment of genetic sex. When fertilization occurs between an oocyte (carrying an X chromosome) and a sperm (carrying either X or Y chromosome) the result is a zygote that is genetically female (46XX) or male (46XY). The formation of bipotential gonadal ridges, Müllerian and Wolffian duct structures common to both 46 XX and 46 XY embryos is evident by week 5 of gestation. Multiple transcription factors are involved in this phenomenon including LIM-1, EMX-2, PAX-2, WT-1, SF-1 and DAX-1 as well as the growth factors DMRT1, ATRX and insulin receptors. In mice, the development and maintenance of bipotential gonadal tissue requires expression of the genes M33, Emx2, Dhx9, Pod1 and Dmrt1 as well as Sf1 and Wt1.

Gonadal Sex

The differentiation of ovaries or testes from the bipotential gonadal ridge tissue is the next step in normal sex differentiation. In humans, differentiation of the testes and ovaries is initiated by 6 weeks and fully achieved by 13 to 14 weeks of fetal development. Testicular differentiation is controlled by a number of time and dosage sensitive genes that encode for transcription factors. These include genes WT-1, SOX-9 that are positive for the formation of testes and the sex determining region of the Y chromosome (SRY). Some factors *i.e.* DAX-1, SOX-3 and WNT-4 which inhibit testicular differentiation. Among 46 chromosomes, the XY chromosome affected by disorders of testicular differentiation and development, most of the identified mutations have been observed in SF-1, SOX-9 or SRY. Ovarian differentiation is less well understood and was previously believed to be the default state of gonadal differentiation. The ovarian development is an active process that occurs in the absence of SRY coupled with the expression of additional genes including FOXL-2, WNT-4 and possibly DAX-1.

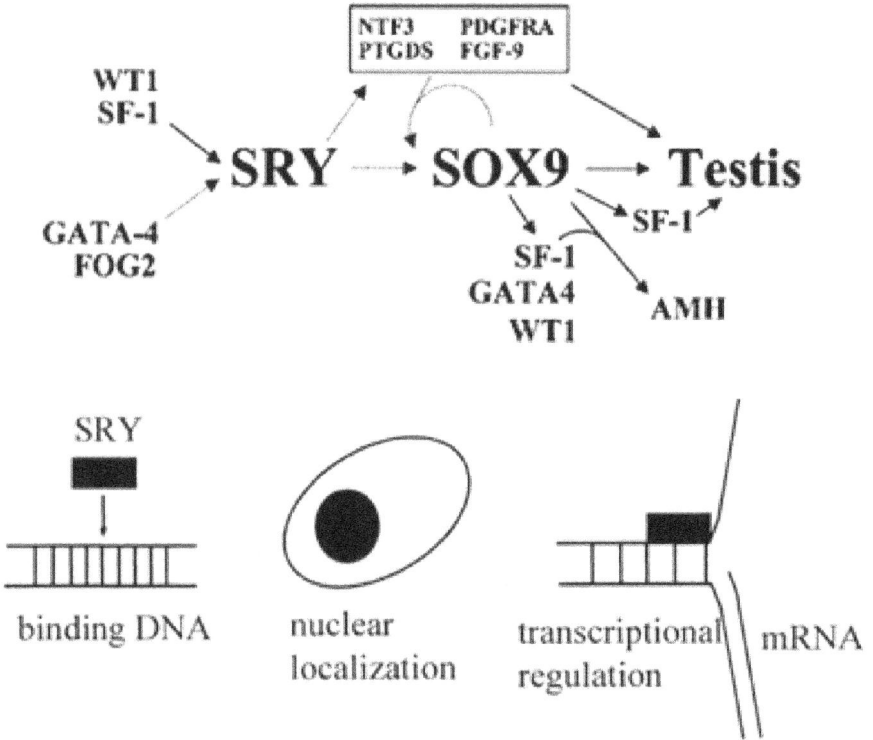

Figure 6.1 Molecular Action of SRY

Fetal Production of Gonadal Hormones

The fetal production of testicular androgens and Müllerian inhibiting substance (MIS) constitute the next step of sex differentiation and development. In males androgens are necessary to both masculinize the external genitalia and to support the maintenance of the Wolffian ducts, while MIS suppresses Mullerian duct development. The biosynthesis of testosterone by the Leydig cells requires the activity of a series of enzymes. Expression of androgenic effects by target tissues such as Wolffian duct structures requires the binding of testosterone to androgen receptors. In females, the foetal ovaries do not produce Müllerian inhibiting substance until after fetus is committed to developing along female lines; hence, development and maintenance of the Mullerian duct structures are permitted because the fetal ovaries do not secrete androgens. The Wolffian ducts become atrophic and the external genitalia continue to appear female in newborn girls.

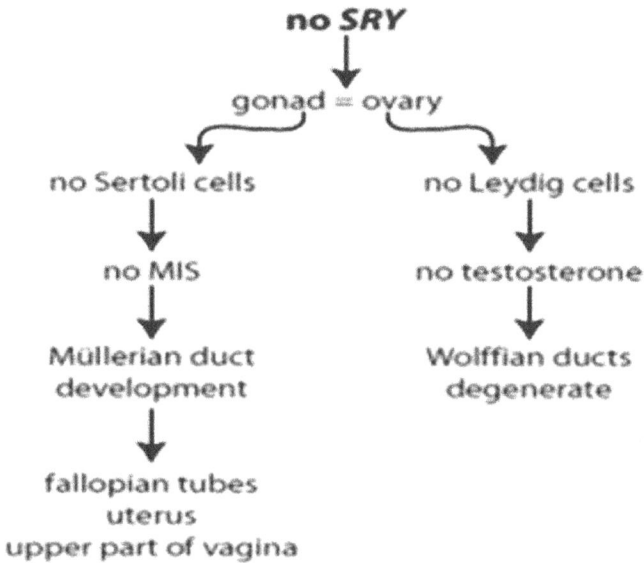

no SRY

↓

gonad = ovary

no Sertoli cells   no Leydig cells

↓   ↓

no MIS   no testosterone

↓   ↓

Müllerian duct   Wolffian ducts
development   degenerate

↓

fallopian tubes
uterus
upper part of vagina

Figure 6.2: Femele (XX)

BOX 6.1

CSD and ESD

CHROMOSOMAL SEX DETERMINATION (CSD)

Before the karyotyping of human chromosomes, it was considered that sex is determined by the number of X chromosomes present in an individual. It was observed that in drosophila, males had single X chromosome (XY or XO) and the presence of 2 or more X chromosomes (XX, XXX or XXY) always conferred female phenotype. It was thus considered that the Y chromosome was a null chromosome. However in 1966, a landmark observation was made by Jacobs and Ross. They described two sisters who had female external genitalia. It seemed that the testicular determining region of the Y chromosome normally resides in its short arm. This was confirmed by high resolution banding studies of an XX male which revealed that some material from the short arm of Y chromosome had been translocated to one of his X chromosomes. With advanced techniques it became apparent that sex determining gene on short arm of Y chromosome is responsible for the development of testis in mammals. Also testicular development is seen impaired in several clinical syndromes resulting from autosomal deletions or mutations. The autosomal genes such as SOX9, WNT4, SF1, DMRT1 etc. are shown to play a crucial role in the downstream events of sex differentiation initiated by SRY gene.

ENVIRONMENTAL SEX DETERMINATION (ESD)

In some cold blooded vertebrates *e.g.* fishes, reptiles etc. sex is determined not at the time of fertilization by sex chromosomes. It is determined by the environment in which the early embryonic development takes place. In various freshwater fishes as well as marine species from temperate or tropical habitats, it has been clearly shown that sex determination and consequent differentiation is influenced by the environmental factors like pH, salinity, social interaction and importantly, temperature. In most thermosensitive species *e.g.* Atherinids, Poecilids, Cichlids, Siluriform, high temperature increases male to female sex ratios and *vice-versa*. Exceptionally, in European sea bass, *Dicentrarchus labrax* and channel catfish, *Ictalurus punctatus* high temperature induces female sex differentiation. Density and pH also plays a sex determining role in fishes as evidenced in paradise fish *Macropodus opercularis,* where the number of females is directly proportional to the density and in all *Apistogramma* species (cichlids) the proportion of males is higher at an acidic pH (4.5) than at neutral pH (6.5). The complete sex reversal can also be accomplished by exposing gonochoristic fish to exogenous sex steroids during gonadal differentiation. In addition to gonochorism, several types of hermaphroditism are seen in fishes. Social interaction such as disappearance of a male or female from a mixed group causes sex inversion in these species like from male to female known as protoandrous *e.g.* sea anemone fish *(Amphiprion clarkii),* from female to male known as protogynous *e.g.* Red sea fish *(Anthias squamipinnis)* and a few can change sex either way or multiple times *e.g.* serial sex change in gobiid fish *(Trima okinawae).*

External Genitalia

In 46 chromosomes, the female-appearing external genitalia (XY fetuses) start to masculinize at 8-9 weeks of gestation when the potent androgen dihydrotestosterone (DHT) is present. DHT is required for fusion of the urethral and labioscrotal folds, lengthening of the genital tubercle and regression of the urogenital sinus. Steroid 5á-reductase-2 is the enzyme required to convert testosterone that is produced by the fetal Leydig cells to DHT. Steroid 5á-reductase-2 is located in androgen target cells of the developing external genitalia, but not in the testes. Complete masculinization of the external genitalia by DHT is accomplished by week 14 of gestation. In the absence of either testosterone secretion or 5á-reductase-2, the fetal external genitalia continue to develop along female lines. Specifically without DHT the labioscrotal and urethral folds form the labia majora and minora respectively. The genital tubercle develops into a clitoris and the urogenital sinus gives rise to the urethral opening and anterior portion of the vagina. The posterior portion of the vagina develops from the Mullerian ducts in the absence of Müllerian inhibiting substance (MIS).

Prenatal Diagnosis of Chromosomal Disorders

The standard measures for population health outcomes are based on maternal, infant and under five mortality rates. Health care of mother and unborn child is the most important part of population health. Therefore the care for mother and child health during pregnancy and delivery, assessment of all risks during pregnancy is of utmost importance of any health care system. It is known that prenatal mortality is caused in 20-25 per cent of cases by inherited anomalies of fetuses and many of these might be explained by genetic disorders. In general genetic disorder is a condition caused by abnormalities in genes or chromosomes. Chromosomes are complex bodies in cell nucleus as carriers of genes. While some diseases are due to genetic abnormalities acquired in a few cells during life, the term genetic disease most commonly refers to diseases present in all cells of the body and present since conception. Some genetic disorders are caused by chromosomal abnormalities due to errors in meiosis, the process which produces reproductive cells such as sperm and eggs. Examples include Down syndrome (extra chromosome 21), Turner Syndrome (45X0) and Klinefelter's syndrome (a male with 2X chromosomes). Other genetic changes may occur during the production of germ cells by the parent. One example is the triplet expansion repeat mutations which can cause fragile X syndrome or Huntington's disease. Defective genes may also be inherited intact from the parents. In this case the genetic disorder is known as a hereditary disease. This can happen unexpectedly when two healthy carriers of a defective recessive gene reproduce.

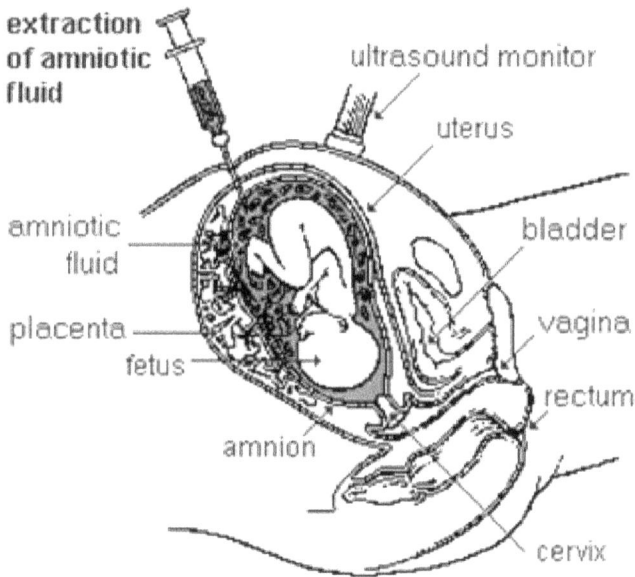

Figure 6.3: Prenatal diagnosis of Chromosomal Disorders

Chromosomal Abnormalities

Chromosomal abnormalities are disruptions in the normal chromosomal content of cell and are a major cause of genetic diseases in humans and some chromosomal abnormalities do not cause disease in carriers such as translocations or chromosomal inversions although they may lead to higher proportions of chromosomal disorder in child. Abnormal number of chromosomes or chromosome sets called aneuploidy may cause letal condition or give rise in genetic disorders. Furthermore the gain or loss of chromosome material may lead to genetic disorder (deletion, extra copy as trisomy). Chromosomal mutations produce changes in whole chromosomes (more than one gene) or in the number of chromosomes present. The risk for chromosomal abnormalities increases with increasing maternal age, mainly because non-dysfunctional events in meiosis are more likely and result in trisomies. To make it more complex the mosaicism must be added. A mosaic is a person with a combination of two cell lines with different karyotypes (normal and abnormal). When karyotyping is performed, multiple cells are analyzed to rule out this possibility. The mosaic condition is not as severe as the completely abnormal karyotype and the features may not be as marked and live births may be possible. Sometimes the mosaic is confined to the placenta or placental mosaicism.

A placenta with an abnormal karyotype may lead to stillbirth, even though the fetus has a normal karyotype. A placenta with a normal karyotype may allow longer survival for a fetus with a chromosomal abnormality. Rarely a translocation of part of one chromosome to another in the parent will be passed on to the child as a partial trisomy which may not be as severe as a complete trisomy. A host of other chromosomal abnormalities are possible. In general, fetal loss earlier in gestation and multiple fetal losses, more strongly suggests a possible chromosomal abnormality.

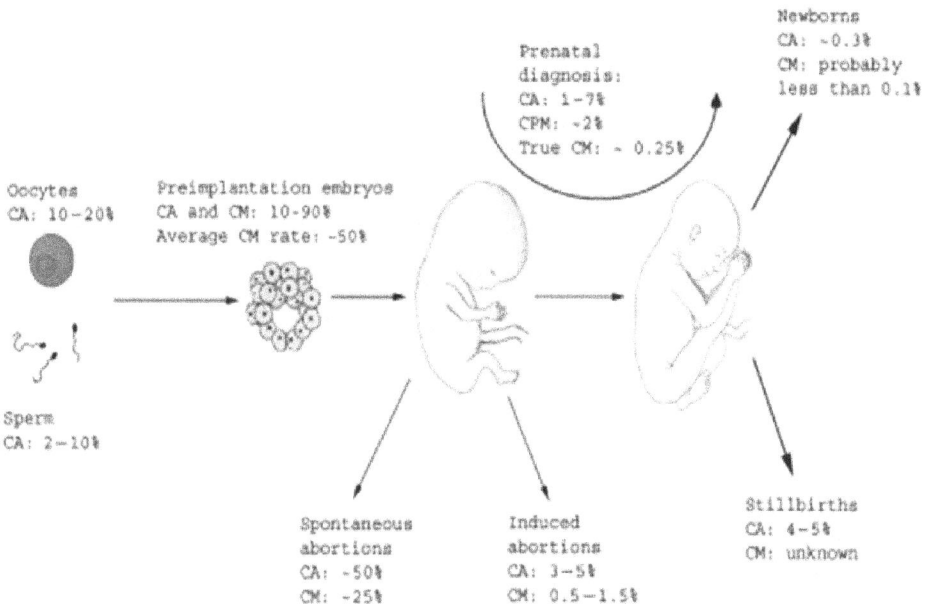

Figure 6.4: Chromosomal Abnormalities

BOX 6.2

CHROMOSOMAL DISORDERS

1. **Trisomy 21 (extra chromosome 21):** Down syndrome; incidence based upon maternal age, though translocation type is familial; features can include: epicanthal folds, simian crease, brachycephaly, cardiac defects.

2. **Trisomy 18 (47XY+18):** Features include micrognathia, overlapping fingers, horseshoe kidney, rocker bottom feet, cardiac defects, diapragmatic hernia and omphalocele.

3. **Trisomy 13 (Patau Syndrome/D-Syndrome):** Features include microcephaly, cleft lip and/or palate, polydactyly, cardiac defects, holoprosencephaly.

4. **Trisomy 16:** Seen in abortuses from first trimester. Never liveborn.

5. **Monosomy X:** Turner's syndrome (45X0); can survive to adulthood; features include short stature, cystic hygroma of neck (leading to webbing), infertility, coarctation.

6. **Klinefelter's syndrome** (XXY, a male with 2 X chromosomes); features include elongated lower body, gynecomastia, testicular atrophy (incidence: 1/500 males)

7. **Triploidy:** There is often a partial hydatidiform mole of placenta. Fetal features include 3-4 syndactyly, indented nasal bridge, small size.

8. **Idic 15 or isodicentric 15**: inverted duplication of chromosome 15 or tetrasomy 15 Jacobsen syndrome also called the terminal 11 q deletion disorder. This is a very rare disorder. Those affected have normal intelligence or mild mental retardation, with poor expressive language skills. Most have a bleeding disorder.

9. **XYY syndorme.** XYY boys are usually taller than their siblings. Like XXY boys and XXX girls, they are somewhat more likely to have learning difficulties.

   Triple XXX syndrome: XXX girls tend to be tall and thin. They have a higher incidence of dyslexia.

Prenatal Diagnosis

Prenatal diagnosis employs a variety of techniques to determine the health and condition of an unborn fetus. Without knowledge gained by prenatal diagnosis, there could be an untoward outcome for the fetus or the mother or both. Specifically, prenatal diagnosis is helpful for:

i. Managing the remaining weeks of the pregnancy

ii. Determining the outcome of the pregnancy

iii. Planning for possible complications with the birth process

    iv. Planning for problems that may occur in the newborn infant

    v.   Deciding whether to continue the pregnancy

    vi. Finding conditions that may affect future pregnancies

There are a variety of non-invasive and invasive techniques available for prenatal diagnosis. Each of them can be applied only during specific time periods during the pregnancy for greatest utility. Indications for prenatal diagnostic testing include age of mother, Down syndrome in previous pregnancy or family, structural aberrations in previous pregnancies or in family members, autosomal genopaties, X-linked genetic disorders, neuronal tube defects in previous pregnancies, mental retardation in family (linked to fragile X) present ultrasound suspicion, consanguinity, pathological finding in prenatal serum screening, other reasons like viral infection, radiation.

Samples for Prenatal Testing

Prenatal diagnosis of chromosomopathies as well as genetic disorders is based on invasive and non-invasive techniques are called chorionic villi sampling (CVS). In this procedure, a catheter is passed via the vagina through the cervix and into the uterus to the developing placenta under ultrasound guidance. Alternative approaches are transvaginal and transabdominal. The introduction of the catheter allows sampling of cells from the placental chorionic villi. These cells can then be analyzed by a variety of techniques. The most common test employed on cells obtained by CVS is chromosome analysis to determine the karyotype of the fetus. The cells can also be grown in culture for biochemical or molecular biologic analysis. CVS can be safely performed between 9.5 and 12.5 weeks gestation. CVS has the disadvantage of being an invasive procedure and it has a small but significant rate of morbidity for the fetus; this loss rate is about 0.5 to 1% higher than for women undergoing amniocentesis. Rarely CVS can be associated with limb defects in the fetus. The possibility of maternal Rh sensitization is present. There is also the possibility that maternal blood in the developing placenta will be sampled instead of fetal cells and confound chromosome analysis. The obtained material is used for fluorescent in situ hybridization (FISC), short tandem repeats (STR), DNA and some biochemical analyses. Amniocenthesis (transvaginal aspiration of amnionic fluid 15-20 weeks of pregnancy) is the most used method (risk below 0, 5 %) for sample for all kind of analyses.

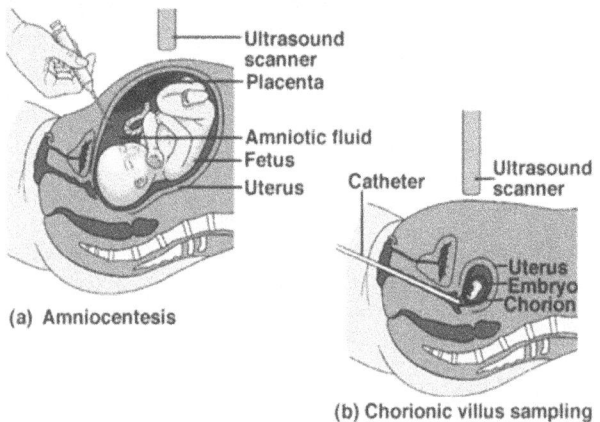

(a) Amniocentesis

(b) Chorionic villus sampling

Figure6.5: Sampling

Preconception–preimplantation diagnosis is possibility applied in connection with in vitro fertilization (IVF) to make diagnosis at the gamete stage or performing the biopsy of one or two blastomeres by aspiration with micropipette. Preimplantation diagnosis is offered as an alternative to conventional prenatal diagnosis in following cases: recessive or dominant hereditary disorders linked to chromosome X, monogenic disorders of authosomal inheritance (recessive or dominant) and the detection of translocations (couples who are carriers of chromosome abnormality of number or structure). Maternal blood sampling for fetal blood cells is a new non-invasive technique that makes use of the phenomenon of fetal blood cells gaining access to maternal circulation through the placental villi. Ordinarily, only a very small number of fetal cells enter the maternal circulation in this fashion not enough to produce a positive Kleihauer-Betke test for fetal-maternal hemorrhage. The fetal cells can be sorted out and analyzed by a variety of techniques to look for particular DNA sequences, but without the risks that these latter two invasive procedures inherently have. Fluorescence *in-situ* hybridization (FISH) is one technique that can be applied to identify particular chromosomes of the fetal cells recovered from maternal blood and diagnose aneuploid conditions such as the trisomies and monosomy X. The problem with this technique is that it is difficult to get many fetal blood cells. There may not be enough to reliably determine anomalies of the fetal karyotype or assay for other abnormalities.

Molecular Analysis

The technologies developed for the Human Genome Project, the recent surge of available DNA sequences resulting from it and the increasing pace of gene discoveries and characterization have all contributed to new technical platforms that have enhanced the spectrum of disorders that can be diagnosed prenatal. The importance of determining the disease-causing mutation or the informative ness of linked genetic markers before embarking upon a DNA-based prenatal diagnosis is, however, still emphasized. Different fluorescence in situ hybridization (FISH) technologies provide increased resolution for the elucidation of structural chromosome abnormalities that cannot be resolved by more conventional cytogenetic analyses, including micro deletion syndromes, cryptic or subtle duplications and translocations, complex rearrangements involving many chromosomes and marker chromosomes. Interphase FISH and the quantitative fluorescence polymerase chain reaction are efficient tools for the rapid prenatal diagnosis of selected aneuploidies, the latter being considered to be most cost-effective if analyses are performed on a large scale. There is some debate surrounding whether this approach should be employed as an adjunct to karyotyping or whether it should be used as a stand-alone test in selected groups of women. Interphase and metaphase FISH, either as a single probe analysis or using multiple chromosome probes, can give reliable results in different clinical situations. It should be noted that there may be variation in probe signals both between slides, depending on age, quality, etc. of metaphase spreads and within a slide. Where a deletion or a rearrangement is suspected, the signal on the normal chromosome is the best control of hybridisation efficiency and control probe also provides an internal control for the efficiency of the FISH procedure.

Depending on the sensitivity and specificity of the probe and on the number of cells scored, the possibility of mosaicism should be considered and comments made where appropriate. By using locus-specific probes at least 5 cells should be scored to confirm or exclude an abnormality. Three cells per probe should be scored to confirm a normal signal pattern in multiprobe where an abnormal pattern is detected. In prenatal interphase screening for aneuploidy signals should be countered in at least 30 cells for each probe set. A minimum 100 cells should be scored. When hybridisation is not optimal, the test should be repeated. When a deletion or another rearrangement is suspected, the results must be confirmed with at least one other probe. Results should preferably be followed up by karyotype analysis. This is essential when there are discrepancies between the expected laboratory findings and the clinical referral. Before introducing interphase FISH as a diagnostic technique, staff need appropriate training on the type of samples to be analysed. Laboratories should set standards for classification of observations and interpretation of results. The new method for fast identification of chromosomal abnormalities has been developed as high resolution array comparative genomic hybridization (aCGH) which provides genome wide analysis of chromosome copy number and structural change. The chip technology provides investigation of genetic causes associated with dysmorphic features, mental retardation, developmental delay, multiple congenital abnormalities. The commercial chip includes more tha 40 abnormalities including duplications and microdeletion regions. It is expected that evaluation of this technique will prove scientifically based evidence for named advantages.

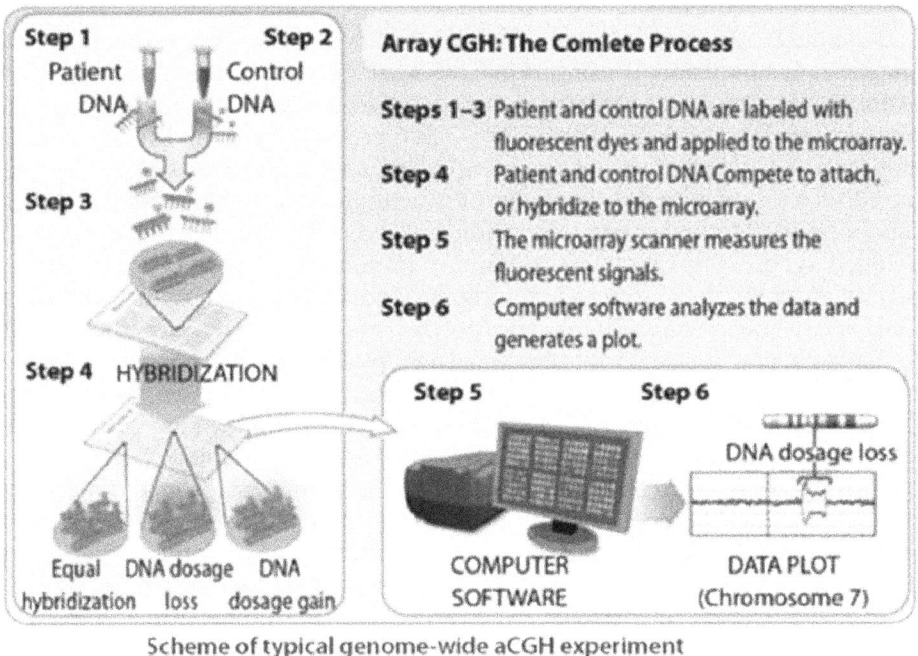

Scheme of typical genome-wide aCGH experiment

Figure 6.6: Scheme of typical genome-wide aCGH experiment

BOX 6.3

AMNIOCENTESIS

Amniocentesis in a technique by which hereditary disorders due to defects in genes can be detected. In this technique a small sample of amniotic fluid which surrounds the foetus is syringed out. This fluid has cells which break off from the skin of the foetus. When the baby is in the womb it is surrounded by amniotic fluid. This fluid contains cells that have the same genetic make-up as the baby. The small amount of this fluid is used to check the genes or chromosomes of the baby. This may not always be the most appropriate procedure for prenatal detection of genetic diseases. The first report of fetal karyotyping by Steele and Breg (1966) after amniocentesis in early pregnancy on prenatal diagnosis of genetic diseases has now become important. Prenatal chromosome analysis has become routine and the number of inborn errors of metabolism which can be detected in cultured amniotic fluid cells has steadily increased. Though theoretically over 40 metabolic disorders are now detectable in cultured amniotic fluid cells, only limited experience with each of these diseases has been gained. A few small series have been accumulated for GM2 gangliosidosis type 1 (Tay-Sachs' disease), glycogenosis type II (Pompe's disease) and the mucopolysaccharidoses. Conventional biochemical analysis requires relatively large cell numbers, which sometimes resulted in long waiting periods for the parents (4 to 8 weeks). The development of microchemical techniques enabled enzyme assays on small numbers of cultured amniotic fluid cells and a reduction in the time required for parental diagnosis. The alpha fetoprotein level in amniotic fluid is increased when the fetus has an open defect of the neural tube. When relatively new techniques like those of prenatal diagnosis are used full assessment of the scope and risks of the various procedures is possible only when sufficiently large series of diagnoses for different groups of genetic diseases can be analysed, including follow-up studies on children after amniocentesis. The present report describes 350 prenatal diagnoses performed in pregnancies at risk for a chromosomal aberration, X-linked disease, neural tube defect or 1 of 11 different metabolic diseases.

There is a small risk of miscarriage associated with amniocentesis. Some studies have suggested that if an amniocentesis is carried out before 14 weeks of pregnancy there is an increased risk of miscarriage. This is why the amniocentesis is usually performed between 15 and 16 weeks. Having an amniocentesis increases the risk of miscarriage by between 0.5% and 1% over the background risk for that stage of pregnancy about 0.5% for all women. Unfortunately, if a woman miscarries there is no way of knowing whether this was due to the amniocentesis or whether it would have happened anyway, even if she hadn't had the procedure. An amniocentesis is done by passing a fine needle through the woman's abdominal wall into the fluid around the baby. The needle is carefully observed on ultrasound scan all the time to ensure that it is correctly positioned in the fluid. Approximately 15–20ml (3–4 teaspoonfuls) of fluid is taken and sent to the laboratory. Occasionally, the amount of fluid retrieved at the first attempt is insufficient and the needle needs to be inserted again. Some women are blood group Rhesus negative. It is important that give these women an injection after the test to prevent complications related to this blood group. If someone is Rhesus positive then do not need an injection.

Sex Linkage

Sex linkage was first discovered by Thomas H. Morgan (Father of Modern genetics), (1910) in *Drosophila melanogaster*. Morgan observed a few white eyed mutant males in the population of red eyed individuals. When the white eyed male is crossed to a normal red eyed female, in the first generation all the males and females were red eyed. First generation red eyed female was crossed to a red eyed male, in the second generation all the females were red-eyed and 50% males were white eyed. These patterns of inheritance are called crisscross inheritance or skip generation inheritance, in which a character is inherited to the second generation through the carrier of first generation. The white eyed character from the male is inherited to the male of the 2nd generation through carrier female. In a reciprocal cross that involved a second cross of same traits but carried by sexes reversed, the results were different. A white eyed female was crossed to a red eyed male, in the first generation all the females were red eyed and males were white eyed. Morgan observed that the difference was due to the inheritance of a recessive gene located on X-chromosome. Males always get the sex linked recessive characters from females. The genes which are located on X-chromosome appear in two doses in female and one dose in males in both of *Drosophila* and humanbeings. A recessive gene gives its expression in the male due to a single recessive allele on X-chromosome. In females the same phenotypic expression is due to two recessive genes.

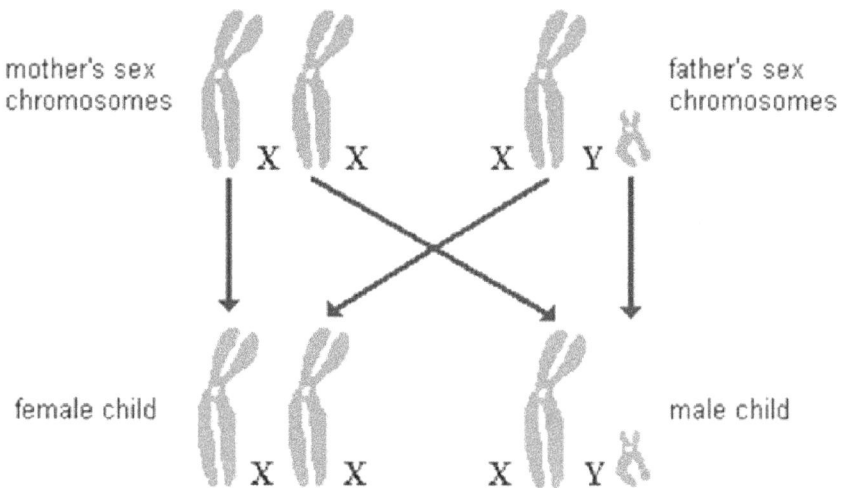

Figure 6.7 : Linkage

Genes on Sex Chromosomes

The genes located on the X chromosome, whose alleles are absent on the Y chromosome are called X-linked genes. These genes are hemizygous in males and holozygous (homozygous or heterozygous) in females. The genes located on Y chromosome, whose alleles are absent on the X chromosome are Y-linked genes or holandric genes (hemizygous). X linked and Y linked genes do not undergo pairing or crossing over during meiosis. The genes which are located on the homologous segments of the X and Y chromosomes are called XY linked genes and these regions are the pseudoautosomal regions. These regions undergo pairing and crossingover during meiosis. XY linked genes are incompletely sex linked genes, as they may undergo crossing over during meiosis like autosomes, but differ from autosomes in their inheritance in reciprocal crosses.

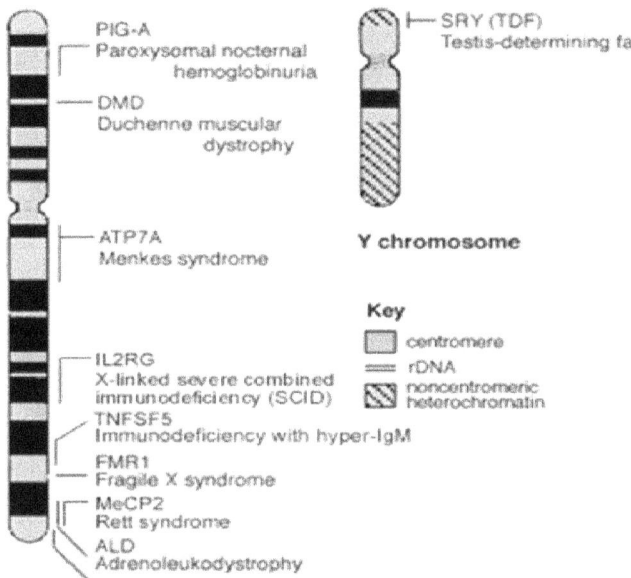

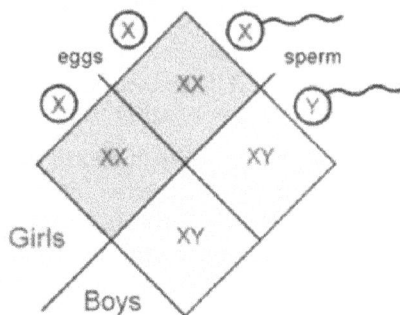

Figure 6.8: Sex Chromosome

Genetic and Hereditary Disorders

Genetic disorder is either hereditary disorders or a result of mutations. Some disorders may confer an advantage, at least in certain environments. There are a number of pathways to genetic defects, the simplest of which are summarized below.

- There are genetic disorders caused by the abnormal chromosome number as in Down syndrome (three instead of two number 21 chromosomes, therefore total of 47).

- Triplet expansion repeat mutations can cause fragile X syndrome or Huntington's disease by modification of gene expression or gain of function respectively.

- Defective genes are often inherited from the parents. In this case, the genetic disorder is known as a hereditary disease. This can happen unexpectedly when two healthy carriers of a defective recessive gene reproduce, but can also happen when the defective gene is dominant.

Types of Genetic Disorders

The genetic disorders which depend on the deletion, addition or aberration of chromosome are classified into four major groups:

a) Single gene disorders including Mendelian Disorders *i.e.* follow Mendelian order of inheritance *i.e.* Autosomal and X linked and Y linked and none Mendelian disorders *i.e.* do not follow Mendelian order of inheritance *e.g.* mitochondrial inheritance.

b) Multi factorial and polygenic disorders.

c) Disorders with variable modes of transmission.

d) Cytogenetic disorder including autosomal disorders and sex chromosome disorders.

BOX 6.4

GENETIC CHARACTERS DUE TO CHROMOSOMAL ABNORMALITIY

1. **Sex Linked Characters:** Sex linked is X Linked characters. Their inheritance is due to X linked genes. The X linked recessive characters follow crisscross pattern of inheritance or skip generation inheritance.

2. **XY Linked Characters:** The genes which are located in the homologous regions of X and Y chromosomes are the XY-linked genes. In *Drosophila*, XY-linked allele for bobbed bristles occurs on both the X chromosomes in females. These alleles are present on the X chromosome of male and short arm of Y chromosome. Bobbed condition in Drosophila is a recessive mutation (b). The normal allele is wild (b⁺). These genes are also called incompletely sex linked genes. Their inheritance is similar to that of autosomes, except in the results of reciprocal cross.

---

3. **Sex Limited Characters:** Sex limited genes are autosomal genes of both males and females, whose phenotypic expression is limited to one sex only. Secondary sexual characters in the human beings like development of beard in man, breast in woman are sex limited traits. Their expression is limited to one sex due to the internal hormonal environment.

4. **Sex Influenced Characters:** Sex influenced genes are the autosomal genes in both males and females, whose phenotypic expression is different in different sexes, dominant in one sex and recessive in the other *e.g.* Pattern baldness, one form of white forelock, a patch of white hair and the absence of upper lateral incisor teeth are some of the sex influenced traits in human beings.

Pattern baldness is a condition in which a fringe of hair is present low on the head in human beings. It is a genetically inherited condition. The gene as for baldness B is dominant in males and recessive in females. In heterozygous condition males are bald and females are nonbald. If a heterozygous nonbald woman marries a heterozygous bald man, in the offspring males are bald and nonbald in 3:1 ratio and females are nonbald and bald in 3:1 ratio.

Genotype	Phenotype	
BB	Bald	Bald
Bb	Non-bald	Bald
bb	Non-bald	Non-bald

PREVALENCE OF GENETIC CONDITIONS / BIRTH DEFECTS

1. **Down syndrome** (1/600 live births and increases with advanced maternal age)

2. **Pregnant and age 35 or above** (risk of chromosome aneuploidy)

3. **Cystic Fibrosis** (1/2500)

4. **Fragile X syndrome** (1/1,000 males and 1/800 female carriers of which 30% will be mentally retarded)

5. **Sickle cell disease** (1/500 of African American births)

6. **Hemophilia** - Factor VIII Deficiency (48/100,000 male births)

7. **Duchenne muscular dystrophy** (200/million male births)

8. **Hemochromatosis** (1/450 individuals)

9. **Breast cancer** (1/8 women of which 5-10% of will have a genetic predisposition)

Single Gene Disorders

Where genetic disorders are the result of a single mutated gene they can be passed on to subsequent generations. Genomic imprinting and uniparental disomy may affect inheritance patterns. The divisions between recessive and dominant are not hard and fast although the divisions between autosomal and X linked are related to the position of the gene *e.g.* achondroplasia is typically considered a dominant disorder, but young goats or children with two genes for achondroplasia have a severe skeletal disorder that achondroplasics could be viewed as carriers of. Sickle cell anaemia is also considered a recessive condition but carriers that have it by half along with the normal gene have increased immunity to malaria in early childhood which could be described as a related dominant condition.

Subclasses of single gene disorders are as follows:

a. Autosomal Dominant

Only one mutated copy of the gene is needed for a person to be affected by an autosomal dominant disorder. Each affected person usually has one affected parent. There is a 50% chance that a child will inherit the mutated gene. Conditions that are autosomal dominant have low penetrance, which means that, although only one mutated copy is needed, a relatively small proportion of those who inherit that mutation go on to develop the disease later in life *e.g.* Huntingtons disease, Neurofibromatosis, Marfan Syndrome.

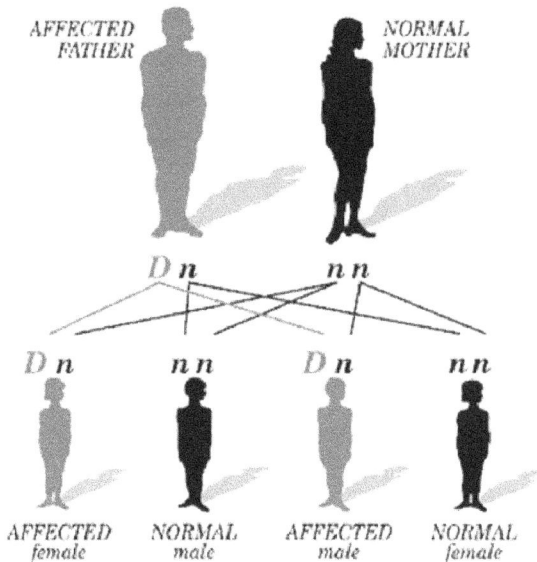

Figure 6.9: Autosomal dominant inheritance pattern: (Parent can be dominant D and normal gene is n, the father is dominant *i.e.* affected. It is possible to construct a pattern with the mother to be dominant too.)

Huntington's disease : Huntington's disease (HD) also known as Huntington disease and previously as Huntington's chorea and chorea maior is a rare inherited neurological disorder affecting up to 8 people per 100,000. It affects 1 out of 20,000 people of Western European descent and 1 out of one million in people of Asian and African descent. It takes its name from Ohio physician George Huntington who described it precisely in 1872. Huntington's disease is caused by a trinucleotide repeat expansion in the Huntingtin (Htt) gene and is one of several polyglutamine or PolyQ diseases. This expansion produces an altered form of Htt protein, mutant Huntingtin (mHtt), which results in neuronal cell death in select areas of the brain and is a terminal illness. Huntington's disease's most obvious symptoms are abnormal body movements called chorea and a lack of coordination but it also affects a number of mental abilities and some aspects of personality. These physical symptoms commonly become noticeable in a person's forties, but can occur at any age. If the age of onset is below 20 years then it is known as Juvenile HD. There is currently no cure but the symptoms are managed with medication and appropriate care. HD is inherited in an autosomal dominant fashion.Huntington's disease is autosomal dominant, needing only one affected allele from either parent to inherit the disease. Although this generally means there is a one in two chance of inheriting the disorder from an affected parent, the inheritance of HD and other trinucleotide repeat disorders is more complex.When the gene has more than 36 copies of the repeated trinucleotide sequence, the DNA replication process becomes unstable and the number of repeats can change in successive generations. If the gene is inherited from the mother, the count is usually similar. Paternal inheritance tends to increase the number of repeats. Because of the progressive increase in length of the repeats, the disease tends to increase in severity and have an earlier onset in successive generations. This is known as anticipation.

The gene involved in Huntington's disease called the HD gene, is located on the short arm of chromosome 4. The end of the HD gene has a sequence of three DNA bases, cytosine-adenine-guanine (CAG) that is repeated multiple times *i.e.* ...CAGCAGCAG...; this is called a trinucleotide repeat. CAG is the codon for the amino acid glutamine, thus a CAG repeat may be termed a polyglutamine (polyQ) expansion. A sequence of fewer than 36 glutamine amino acid residues is the normal form, producing a 348 kDa cytoplasmic protein called huntingtin (Htt). A sequence of 40 or more CAG repeats produces a mutated form of Htt, mHtt. The greater the number of CAG repeats, the earlier the onset of symptoms. In genetically altered knockin mice, the mutant CAG repeat portion of the gene which codes for the N~terminal end of mHtt, is all that is needed to cause disease. Aggregates of mHtt are present in the brains of both HD patients and HD mice, specifically in striatal neurons. These aggregates consist mainly of the amino terminal end of mHtt (CAG repeat) and are found in both the cytoplasm and nucleus of neurons. The presence of these aggregates however does not correlate with cell death. The mHtt acts in the nucleus but does not cause apoptosis through aggregation.

Marfan syndrome: Marfan syndrome is an autosomal dominant genetic disorder of the connective tissue characterized by disproportionately long limbs, long thin fingers, a relatively tall stature and a predisposition to cardiovascular abnormalities, specifically affecting the heart valves and aorta. The disease may also affect numerous other structures and organs including the lungs, eyes, dural sac surrounding the spinal cord and hard palate. It is named after Antoine Marfan, the French pediatrician who first described it in 1899. Marfan syndrome has been linked to a defect in the FBN1 gene on chromosome 15, which encodes a glycoprotein called fibrillin. Fibrillin is essential for the formation of the elastic fibers found in connective tissue, as it provides the scaffolding for tropoelastin. Elastic fibers are found throughout the body but are particularly abundant in the aorta, ligaments and the ciliary zonules of the eye, consequently these areas are among the worst affected. Without the structural supportprovided by fibrillin many connective tissues are weakened which can have severe consequences for supportand stability.

b. Autosomal Recessive

Two copies of the gene must be mutated for a person to be affected by an autosomal recessive disorder. An affected person usually has unaffected parents who each carrya single copy of the mutated gene and are referred to as carriers. Two unaffected people who each carryone copy of the mutated gene have a 25% chance with each pregnancy of having a child affected by disorder *e.g.* cystic fibrosis, sickle cell anemia, Tay Sachs disease, spinal muscular atrophy.

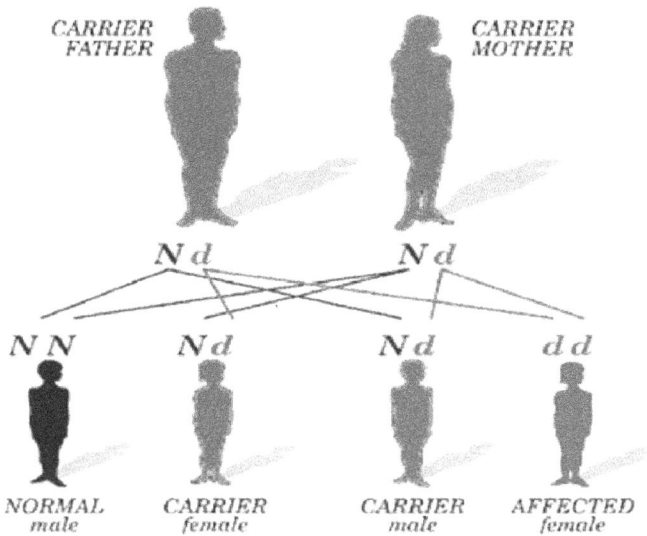

Figure 6.10: Autosomal recessive inheritance pattern : (Recessive gene is d and normal gene is N).

Sickle Cell disease : Sickle cell disease is a group of genetic disorders caused by sickle hemoglobin (Hgb S or Hb S). In many forms of the disease, the red blood cells change shape, usually looking much like that of a banana, upon deoxygenation because of polymerization of the abnormal sickle hemoglobin. The haemoglobin precipitates into long crystals inside the cell making it sickle shaped rather than the normal biconcave disc. This process damages the red blood cell membrane making it fragile leading to anaemia and can cause the cells to become stuck in blood vessels. This deprives the downstream tissues of oxygen and causes ischemia and infarction, which may cause organ damage such as stroke. The disease is chronic and lifelong. Individuals are well but their lives are punctuated by periodic painful attacks. The mutated allele is recessive, meaning it must be inherited from each parent for the individual to have the disease.

Cystic Fibrosis : Cystic fibrosis (CF) also called mucoviscidosis, is a hereditarydisease that affects the entire body, causing progressive disability and early death. Formerly known as cystic fibrosis of pancreas, this entity has increasingly been labeled simply cystic fibrosis. Difficulty breathing and insufficient enzyme production in the pancreas are the most common symptoms. Thick mucus production as well as a low immune system, results in frequent lung infections, which are treated, though not always cured, by oral and intravenous antibiotics and other medications. A multitude of other symptoms, including sinus infections, poor growth, diarrhea and potential infertility mostly in males due to the condition congenital bilateral absence of vas Deferens, result from the effects of CF on other parts of the body. The symptoms of CF appear in infancy and childhood; these include meconium ileus, failure to thrive and recurrent lung infections. Cystic fibrosis is one of the most common life shortening, childhood onset inherited diseases. In the United States, 1 in 3900 children are born with CF. It is most common among Europeans and Ashkenazi Jews; one in twenty two people of European descent carry one gene for CF, making it the most common genetic disease among them. Individuals with cystic fibrosis can be diagnosed prior to birth by genetic testing or in early childhood by a sweat test. Newborn screening tests are increasingly common and effective. There is no cure for CF and most individuals with cystic fibrosis die young many in their 20s and 30s from lung failure although with many new treatments being introduced the life expectancy of a person with CF is increasing. Ultimately, lung transplantation is often necessaryas CF worsens. CF is caused by a mutation in a gene called the cystic fibrosis transmembrane conductance regulator (CFTR). The product of this gene helps create sweat, digestive juices and mucus. Although most people without CF have two working copies of the CFTR gene, only one is needed to prevent cystic fibrosis. CF develops when neither gene works normally. Therefore, CF is considered an autosomal recessive disease. The name cystic fibrosis refers to the characteristic fibrosis (tissue scarring) and cyst formation within the pancreas, first recognized in the 1930s.

c. X -linked Dominant

X-linked dominant disorders are caused by mutations in genes on the X chromosome. Only a few disorders have this inheritance pattern. Males are more frequently affected than females and the chance of passing on an X-linked dominant disorder differs between men and women. The sons of a man with an X~linked dominant disorder will not be affected and his daughters will all inherit the condition. A woman with an X-linked dominant disorder has a 50% chance of having an affected daughter or son with each pregnancy. Some X-linked dominant conditions such as Aicardi Syndrome are fatal to boys.

Aicardi syndrome: Aicardi syndrome is a rare congenital disorder thought to result from an abnormality of the X chromosome and characterized by partial or complete agenesis of the corpus callosum, retinal abnormalities and seizures. It is X linked dominant. Only 500 reported cases in the world.

BOX 6.5

LESS COMMON X=LINKED DISORDERS

1. **Adrenoleukodystrophy:** Leads to progressive brain damage, failure of the adrenal glands and eventually death.

2. **Alport syndrome:** Glomerulonephritis, endstage kidney disease and hearing loss.

3. **Androgen insensitivity syndrome:** Variable degrees of undervirilization and/or infertility in XY persons of either gender

4. **Barth syndrome:** Metabolism distortion, delayed motor skills, stamina deficiency, hypotonia, chronic fatigue, delayed growth, cardiomyopathy and compromised immune system.

5. **Centronuclear myopathy:** Where cell nuclei are abnormally located in skeletal muscle cells. In CNM the nuclei are located at a position in the center of the cell, instead of their normal location at the periphery.

6. **Charcot-Marie-Tooth disease (CMTX2-3):** Disorder of nerves (neuropathy) that is characterized by loss of muscle tissue and touch sensation, predominantly in the feet and legs but also in the hands and arms in the advanced stages of disease.

7. **Coffin Lowry syndrome:** Severe mental retardation sometimes associated with abnormalities of growth, cardiac abnormalities, kyphoscoliosis as well as auditory and visual abnormalities.

8. **Fabry disease:** A lysosomal storage disease causing anhidrosis, fatigue, angiokeratomas, burning extremity pain and ocular involvement.

9. **Glucose-6-phosphate dehydrogenase deficiency:** May exhibit nonimmune hemolytic anemia in response to a number of causes, most commonly infection or exposure to certain medications or chemicals.

10. **Hunter's Syndrome:** Potentially causing hearing loss, thickening of the heart valves leading to a decline in cardiac function, obstructive airway disease, sleep apnea and enlargement of the liver and spleen.

11. **Hypohidrotic ectodermal dysplasia:** Presenting with hypohidrosis, hypotrichosis, hypodontia

12. **Kabuki syndrome:** Multiple congenital anomalies and mental retardation.

13. **Kennedy disease:** Muscle cramps and progressive weakness.

14. **Lesch-Nyhan syndrome:** Neurologic dysfunction, cognitive and behavioral disturbances including self mutilation and uric acid overproduction (hyperuricemia).

15. **Lowe Syndrome:** Hydrophthalmia, cataracts, intellectual disabilities, aminoaciduria, reduced renal ammonia production and vitamin D resistant rickets.

16. **Menkes disease:** Sparse and coarse hair, growth failure and deterioration of the nervous system.

17. **Nonsyndromic deafness and X-linked nonsyndromic deafness:** Hearing loss.

18. **Norrie disease:** Cataracts, leukocoria along with other developmental issues in the eye.

19. **Occipital horn syndrome:** Deformations in the skeleton.

20. **Ornithine transcarbamylase deficiency:** Developmental delay and mental retardation. Progressive liver damage, skin lesions and brittle hair may also be seen.

21. **Rett syndrome:** Reduced head growth and small hands and feet. Stereotypic, repetitive hand movements. Cognitive impairment and problems with socialization.

22. **Simpson-Golabi-Behmel syndrome:** Coarse faces with protruding jaw and tongue, widened nasal bridge and upturned nasal tip.

23. **Spinal muscular atrophy caused by UBE1 gene mutation:** Weakness due to loss of the motor neurons of the spinal cord and brainstem.

24. **Wiskott-Aldrich syndrome:** Eczema, thrombocytopenia, immune deficiency and bloody diarrhea.

25. **X-linked Severe Combined Immunodeficiency (SCID):** Infections, usually causing death in the first years of life.

26. **X-linked sideroblastic anaemia:** Skin paleness, fatigue, dizziness and enlarged spleen and liver.

d. X linked Recessive

X linked recessive disorders are also caused by mutations in genes on the X chromosome. Males are more frequently affected than females and the chance of passing on the disorder differs between men and women. The sons of a man with an X linked recessive disorder will not be affected and his daughters will carry one copy of the mutated gene. With each pregnancy, a woman who carries an X- linked recessive disorder has a 50% chance of having sons who are affected and a 50% chance of having daughters who carry one copy of the mutated gene *e.g.* Hemophilia A, Duchenne muscular dystrophy, Color blindness, Muscular dystrophy androgenetic alopecia and also includes Glucose-6-phosphate dehydrogenase deficiency.

Haemophilia : Haemophilia is X linked recessive genetic disorder. It is more common in men than in women. Blood normally clots during injuries within 5 to 10 minutes, depending on the magnitude of the injury. In haemophilia individuals the normal process of blood clotting is delayed or sometimes blood fails to clot. So blood bleeds continuously leading to the loss of blood, causing even death. It is also called bleeder's disease. It follows the characteristic crisscross inheritance like that of colour blindness, Haemophilia-A is due to the deficiency of antihaemophilic factor (factor VIII), which accounts for 80% of haemophilia. Haemophilia-B is due to the deficiency of plasma thromboplastin component (factor IX), which accounts for 20% of haemophila.

Colour Blindness: Retina of the eye in man contains the cells sensitive to red and green colours. This phenotypic trait is genetically controlled. Its alleles are located on X-chromosome. A man having the recessive gene for the colour blindness can't distinguish either red or green colour. Men are colour blind, if they have a gene for colour blindness on X chromosome. Their vision is normal, if gene for colour blindness is absent on X chromosome. Women have normal vision if gene for colour blindness is absent on both the X chromosomes (homozygous) or if they have only one gene for colour blindness on one of two X chromosomes (heterozygous then she is called a carrier). She will be colour blind, only when she has gene for colour blindness on both the X chromosomes. When a woman with normal vision (homozygous) marries a colour blind man, all the sons and daughters are normal, but the daughters are carriers. If a carrier woman marries a man with normal vision, all the daughters and half of the sons have normal vision and another of half of the sons are colour blind. Colour-blind trait is inherited from male to his grandson through carrier daughter, which is an example of crisscross inheritance.

f. Y-Linked

Y linked disorders are caused by mutations on the Y chromosome. Only males can get them and all of the sons of an affected father are affected. Since the Y chromosome is verysmall, Y linked disorders only cause infertility and may be circumvented with the help of some fertility treatments *e.g.* Male Infertility. In case of male infertility, it is believed to have a genetic predisposition. There are other causes however. It can be treated using fertility treatments.

g. Mitochondrial Inheritance

This type of inheritance also known as maternal inheritance applies to genes in mitochondrial DNA because only egg cells contribute mitochondria to the developing embryo, only females can pass on mitochondrial conditions to their children *e.g.* Leber's hereditary optic neuropathy (LHON).

Leber's Hereditary Optic Neuropathy : Leber's hereditary optic neuropathy (LHON) or Leber optic atrophy is a mitochondrially inherited (mother to all offspring) degeneration of retinal ganglion cells (RGCs) and their axons that leads to an acute or subacute loss of central vision; this affects predominantly young adult males. However, LHON is only transmitted through the mother as it is primarily due to mutations in the mitochondrial (not nuclear) genome and only the egg contributes mitochondria to the embryo. LHON is usually due to one of three pathogenic mitochondrial DNA (mtDNA) point mutations. These mutations affect nucleotide positions 11778, 3460 and 14484, respectively in the ND4, ND1 and ND6 subunit genes of complex I of oxidative phosphorylation chain in mitochondria. Men cannot pass on the disease to their offspring.

Leber hereditaryoptic neuropathy is a condition related to changes in mitochondrial DNA. Although most DNA is packaged in chromosomes within the nucleus, mitochondria have a distinct mitochondrial genome composed of mtDNA.

Mutations in the MT-ND1, MT-ND4, MT-ND4L and MT-ND6 genes cause Leber hereditaryoptic neuropathy. These genes code for the NADH dehydrogenase protein involved in the normal mitochondrial function of oxidative phosphorylation. Oxidative phosphorylation uses a large multienzyme complex to convertoxygen and simple sugars to energy. Mutations in any of the genes disrupt this process to cause a variety of syndromes depending on the type of mutation and other factors. It remains unclear how these genetic changes cause the death of cells in the optic nerve and lead to the specific features of Leber hereditaryoptic neuropathy. A significant percentage of people with a mutation that causes Leber hereditaryoptic neuropathy do not develop any features of the disorder. Specifically, more than 50 percent of males with a mutation and more than 85% of females with a mutation never experience vision loss or related medical problems. Additional factors may determine whether a person develops the signs and symptoms of this disorder. Environmental factors such as smoking and alcohol use may be involved, although studies of these factors have produced conflicting results.

Multifactorial and Polygenic Disorders

Genetic disorders may also be complex, multifactorial or polygenic; this means that they are likely associated with the effects of multiple genes in combination with lifestyle and environmental factors. Multifactoral disorders include heart disease and diabetes. Although complex disorders often cluster in families, they do not have a clear cut pattern of inheritance. This makes it difficult to determine a person's risk of inheriting or passing on these disorders. Complex disorders are also difficult to study and treat because the specific factors that cause most of these disorders have not yet been identified. On a pedigree, polygenic diseases do tend to run in families, but the inheritance does not fit simple patterns as with Mendelian diseases. But this does not mean that the genes cannot eventually be located. There is also a strong environmental component to many of them *e.g.* gout. It is a genetic/acquired disorder of uric acid metabolism that leads to hyperuricemia and consequent acute and chronic arthritis. The recurrent but transient attacks of acute arthritis are triggered by the precipitation of monosodium urate crystals into joints from supersaturated body fluids which accumulate in and around the joints and other tissues causing inflammation. Unknown enzyme defects or known enzyme defects leading to overproduction of uric acid like partial deficiency of hypoxanthine guanine phosphoribosyl transferase (HGPRT) enzyme (as person lacks the genes to produce this enzyme). Also high dietary intake of purines as in pulses, as purines is metabolized to uric acid. Therfore it has both a genetic and environmental predisposition such as diet and multifactorial. Other examples of polygenic disorders are heart disease, hypertension, diabetes, obesity and cancers.

Disorders with Variable Modes of Transmission

Heredity malformations are congenital malformations which may be familial and genetic or may be acquired by exposure to teratogenic agents in the uterus. Heredity malformations are associated with several modes of transmission. Some multifactorial defects are cleftlip, congenital heartdefects, pyloric stenosis etc. Certain congenital malformations are either multifactorial or by a single mutant gene *e.g.* Ehlers Danlos Syndrome. It is characterized by defects in collagen synthesis and structure. These abnormal collagen fibres lack adequate tensile strength and hence the skin is hyperextensible and the joints are hypermobile. Causes include either of the following deficiency of the enzyme lysyl hydroxylase, deficient synthesis of type 3 collagen due to mutations in their coding genes and deficient conversion of procollagen type 1 to collagen due to mutation in the type 1 collagen gene.

Cytogenetic Disorders

These may be from alterations in the number or structure of the chromosomes and may affect autosomes or sex chromosomes *e.g.* fragile X chromosome. It is characterized by mental retardation and an inducible cytogenetic abnormality in the X chromosome. It is one of the most common causes of mental retardation. The cytogenetic alteration is induced by certain culture conditions and is seen as a discontinuity of staining or constriction of in the long arm of the X chromosome.

Eugenics

Eugenics derived from Greek word eugenes meaning wellborn. It is the branch of study concerned with improvement of human race by application of principles of genetics *i.e.* by controlling heredity of genetic traits and improving human genotypes and gene pool. Upto the last century, it was a common notion that better breeds of human beings are produced only in royal and elite families due to ideal conditions of nurture. Therefore, mainly the environmental conditions were given the credit producing better human beings. Sir Francis Galton (1883) first put forth the idea that human race can be improved only by producing human beings possessing better hereditary traits through selective breeding. This was an idea of improving human race by application of genetics. Galton christened this aspect of inheritance as Eugenics. Therefore he is regarded as father of Eugenics. Eugenics seeks the genetic improvement of the human race through selection. This idea became more prominent in the beginning of the 20th century and had another great push during World War II. One of Hitler's main objectives was the purification of the Aryan race. According to the theory of evolution, developed by Charles Darwin in 1859, more fit individuals are capable of leaving a larger number of offspring. However, less fit individuals tend to leave fewer descendants. Therefore, over many generations, genes of less adapted or inferior individuals are gradually eliminated from the population. Darwin called this process natural selection.

Due to the use of medicines and improved medical procedures in the last few centuries, man has evaded natural selection. A classic example is Cesarean section procedure for childbirth. Women that would otherwise die from natural childbirth can produce offspring. Therefore, genes for body shape that prevent natural deliveries are retained in the population. Natural selection for this trait still exists in indigenous populations that do not have access to modern medicine, but this is the exception and not the rule. In some way, less adapted people with low physical resistance, predisposition for genetic diseases and so on, continues to leave offspring with the help of modern medical resources. Proponents of eugenics argue that the human species is accumulating bad genes because man has a slow natural selection. Others argue that people need a license for many activities, such as driving, hunting and fishing, but not to procreate and therefore the government should also control procreation. In China and India, the government regulates population growth. This is a quantitative and not qualitative control. Some people argue that there is sexual discrimination in those two countries and that boys tend to be preferred because they can bring larger revenue for their family.

History of Eugenics

Francis Galton, a cousin of Charles Darwin, coined the term eugenics in 1883, defining it as the science of improving stock, which is by no means confined to ques-tions of judicious mating, but which, especially in the case of man, takes cognisance of all influences that tend in however remote a degree to give to the more suitable races or strains of blood a better chance of prevailing speedily over the less suitable than they otherwise would have had. As Galton's definition suggests, the primary fear of eugenicists was that inferior people were reproducing so quickly that they threatened to infect all of society with their undesirable genes. The eugenics movement quickly became popular, particularly in middle and upper middle class America. Eugenics, as a social program, garnered wide support, with advocates staging multiple exhibitions at the American Museum of Natural History in the early twentieth century. Fitter family awards were handed out at state fairs to encourage the best to breed. Prominent philanthropists such as John D. Rockefeller, Jr. and charities such as the Carnegie Institution funded eugenics re-search. Even feminist pioneer and Planned Parenthood founder Margaret Sanger thoroughly supported eugenics. The eugenics movement of the early twentieth century encom-passed not only positive eugenics (encouraging fit families to reproduce) but also negative eugenics (discouraging the unfit from procreating). Negative eugenics commonly took the form of compulsory sterilization laws in US. Starting with Indiana in 1907, twenty nine states enacted compulsory sterilization laws and a major-ity of states still had such laws as of 1956.

Process of Eugenics

The operative aspect of Eugenics is actually not to change the hereditary traits themselves in individual phenotypes, but to bring about an overall improvement in the gene pool or germplasm of the entire human society by encouraging dissemination of desirable (eugenic) traits and discouraging dissemination of undesirable (dysgenic) traits. The first necessary step to be taken in this direction is to segregate people possessing superior traits from those possessing inferior and unwanted traits. Such segregation is difficult, yet it can be achieved by two methods. Firstly, genealogies of various kindreds can be collected and analyzed to find out which type of traits has persisted in their pedigrees. Secondly, all children can be first provided with identical nurture and segregated into those exhibiting best physical and mental developments from those exhibiting poor physical and mental development. Both these methods can be effectively used only when there is a general social consciousness and faith in eugenics. The second necessary step in eugenics is to discourage people with inferior traits from reproducing, while encouraging people with superior traits to reproduce more and more. Therefore, eugenics is either negative or positive.

Types of Eugenics

Negative Eugenics

Under negative eugenics, people with inferior and undesirable traits are prevented from reproducing, so that the frequency of genes of these traits may gradually diminish in the gene pool of human society. Some methods can be adopted for negative eugenics:

i) **Marriage Control:** Marriage of downtrodden, stupid and diseased people should be legally banned by appropriate Govt. orders.

ii) **Segregation:** Scoundrels, criminals, diseased, immoral and stupid people should be segregated away from others in concentration camps and hospitals etc. to prevent their mixing with and marrying normal, intelligent people. This will reduce the frequency of mixing of good and bad traits in human society.

iii) **Sterilization:** Generation after generation, people possessing dysgenic traits should be motivated, through monetary and other incentives, to accept sterilization. This is an effective method of reducing the frequency of inferior traits and it is sure to lead to a better human society after a few generations. Sterilization of men is done by vasectomy in which the passage of sperms is blocked either by cutting or by putting ligatures (to tie a duct tightly at some point) around the male duct (vasa differentia). Similarly, in women, the passage of ova is blocked in fallopian tubes either by cutting or by ligaturing these tubes. This is called tubectomy or salpingectomy. While vasectomy is a minor operation, tuberctomy is a major and complicated operation, because vasa deferentia are superficially located at the bases of scrotal sacs, while the fallopian tubes are deeply located in the abdomen. However, advanced techno logy available in hospitals has now made even tubectomy a minor affair.

i) **Birth Control:** People possessing more of undesired, dysgenic traits should be encouraged to have small families, if at all allowed to reproduce. This will not only improve the gene pool, but also the rate of increase in human population which is presently a big problem before us. If techniques of detecting genetic traits before birth of a child are developed, fetuses possessing dysgenic traits may be destroyed by abortion.

ii) **Control on Consanguineous Marriage:** Most of the metabolic disease of man is carried by recessive mutant genes. To prevent dissemination of such disease, marriages between close relatives should be banned because like breeding, this increases homozygosity and frequency of recessive traits.

iii) **Immigration Controls:** People with dysgenic traits should not be allowed to migrate from one to another country or population.

Positive Eugenics

Contrary to negative eugenics, positive eugenics aims at improving the human gene pool by increasing frequency of better and desirable traits. Some important methods are:

i) **Better Selection of Mate:** Since it is the offspring produced generation after generation who contribute to the gene pool, an effort should be made to produce more children with better traits. If both parents possess eugenic traits, all their children are likely to have better traits. If only one of the parents possess eugenic traits, some of the children are likely to have inferior traits. Hence the selection of a mate for marriage should be based on eugenic considerations rather than on basis of religion, material gains, caste, social reputation, provincialisms, nationalism etc.

ii) **Better Use of Eugenic Germplasm:** Healthy and intelligent people possessing eugenic traits should be encouraged to reproduces more and more. Today, such people are reproducing less because they are conscious of the benefits of family planning. They spend a major part of their life in education and marry late. Thus contribution of such people to the gene pool has sharply declined. In fact, such people should be encouraged to marry early and to practice polygamy, so that their contribution of better traits to the gene pool might increase.

iii) **Eutelegenesis (Germinal Choice):** Muller (1963) recommended establishment of sperm bank in which the semen of men of excellent hereditary traits might be preserved under deep freeze conditions and might be used for artificial insemination of willing women even after the death of such men. In a modern technique, a woman's ovum is taken out and artificially fertilized in a test tube. The zygote is implanted into woman's uterus for embryonic development. The resulting baby is called test tube baby.

iv) **Genic Surgery (Genic Engineering):** Modern scientists are working to devise methods of artificially changing the genetic material of individuals. Efforts are being made to implants DNA of one individual into the germ cells of the others or to change parts of DNA (Artificial mutations/site directed mutagenesis) with the help of radiations and chemical. Efforts are also being made to suppress reduction division during oogenesis in women possessing eugenic traits and to induce parthenogenesis of ova.

v) **Medical Engineering (Euphenics):** Leiderberg (1963-66) has put forth a novel ideal for improvement in hereditary traits. He recommended modifying the processes of transcription and translation in such a way as to prevent or to change the phenotypic expression of genes of inferior traits.

BOX 6.6

MOLECULAR EVOLUTION

Molecular studies have shed light on the origin of life and its subsequent evolution into a myriad of extinct and extant species. Theories regarding these early events are impossible to prove conclusively with circumstantial evidence. Molecular fossils such as introns within transcriptional units and common biochemcial pathways shared between diverse organisms provide additional support for current models. Living cells possess:

i.   A boundary membrane separating the cell's contents from its external environment;

ii. One or more DNAmolecules that carry genetic information for specifying the structure of proteins involved in replication of its own DNA, in metabolism, in growth and in cell division;

iii. A transcriptional system whereby RNAs are synthesized;

iv. A translational system for decoding ribonucleotide sequences into amino acid sequences;

v.   A metabolic system that provides usable forms of energy to carry out these essential activities.

The first living systems were undoubtedly much simpler than any cells alive today. The transition from nonliving to living was gradual and no single event led to life in all its modern complexity. Even today biologists cannot agree on a definition of life. The following criteria are usually included in attempts to define life. An aggregate of cells is considered alive if it-

a) Can use chemical energy or radiant energy to drive energy-requiring chemical reactions;

b) Can increase its mass by controlled synthesis;

c) Possesses an information coding system and a system for translating the coded information into molecules that maintain the system and allow it to reproduce one or more collections of molecules with similar properties.

The best estimate for the age of the earth is 4.6 billion years. The oldest microfossils superficially resembling bacteria have been dated at about 3.5 billion years ago. Thus, chemical evolution *e.g.* abiotic syntheses of amino acids and their polymerization into peptides during the first 1.0 to 1.5 billion years of earth history probably preceded the appearance of cellular life and its subsequent biological evolution. The major opinion is that earth's atmosphere was nearly neutral, nonoxidizing and contained primarily nitrogen, carbon dioxide, hydrogen sulfide and water. Microfossils resembling modern cyanobacteria (blue-green algae) have been found in limestone rocks called stromalites dated 3.5 billion years ago. Presumably these ancient photosynthetic bacteria produced oxygen as a by product of splitting water, just as cyanobacteria do today. Over more than another billion years, oxygen slowly began to accumulate, eventually causing the primitive atmosphere to become oxidizing.

There are two major scientific theories regarding how life came to be on earth. It either evolved on earth from nonliving chemicals or it evolved elsewhere in the universe and was brought to the earth by comets or meteorites (panspermia theory). The belief that life was created by a supernatural force is impossible to support or refute with factual evidence and hence is outside the realm of science. Amino acids and other precursors of modern biomacromolecules have been found inside meteorites, so chemical evolution of these molecules might have been widespread in the cosmos. In 1953, Stanley Miller, at the suggestion of his mentor

Harold Urey, used a reflux apparatus to simulate early atmospheric conditions in an attempt to reproduce the chemical evolution of biological precursor molecules. He recirculated water vapor and other gases (CH_4, NH_3 and H_2) through a chamber where they were exposed to a continuous high voltage electrical discharge that simulated natural lightning. After a few days, the mixture was analyzed and found to contain at least ten different amino acids, some aldehydes and hydrogen cyanide. Subsequent experiments by Miller and others using different molecular mixtures and energy sources produced a variety of other building blocks of biological polymers. Sidney Fox and his colleagues heated amino acids under water free (anhydric) conditions to temperatures of 160–210°C and found amino acids polymerized into protein like chains which he called proteinoids, which are branched rather than linear. When dissolved in water, these proteinoids exhibit several properties of biological proteins including limited enzymatic activity and susceptibility to digestion by proteases. Protein like peptides can also be synthesized from amino acids on clays. Clays consist of alternating layers of inorganic ions and water molecules.

The highly ordered lattice structure of clays strongly attracts organic molecules and promotes chemical reactions between them. Polypeptides have been detected in laboratory simulations of these processes. When solutions of proteinoids are heated in water and then allowed to cool, small, spherical particles called microspheres are formed. These microspheres are about the same size and shape as spherical bacteria. Some are able to grow by accretion of proteinoids and lipids and subsequently proliferate by binary fission or budding. Lipids can spontaneously organize into double-layered bubbles called liposomes, which are leaky enough to absorb various substances such as proteins from the surrounding medium. Substances trapped within the liposome find themselves in a hydrophobic environment that might provide more favorable conditions for certain kinds of chemical reactions. Thus, lipid bilayers may have promoted both aggregation and catalysis. Vesicles composed of lipid membranes and protein microspheres but devoid of RNA or DNA molecules are hypothesized to have existed in the early stages of life. These entities are called progenotes.

RNA World

A living system must be able to replicate its genetic material and be capable of evolving. Proteins are necessary for DNA replication, but most proteins are synthesized on RNA templates that themselves were synthesized on DNA templates. It has been hypothesized that RNA molecules capable of self-replication arose prebiotically by random condensation of mononucleotides into small polymers. The active sites of most modern proteins and catalytic RNAs constitute relatively small segments of the polymers to which they belong. The smaller primitive RNA replicase polymers, formed abiotically, would probably have only weak catalytic activity and would have been subject to error-prone replication. But such a molecule might have been able to use itself or other RNA molecules as a template for polymerizing RNA nucleotides. The many errors made during replication of the early RNA replicase would create a pool of genetic diversity on which natural selection could act to favor those molecules that were able to replicate faster and/or have greater accuracy. One problem, however, is that no replicase can copy its own active site. It is thus necessary to propose that a minimum of two RNA replicases were synthesized at nearly the same time from the primordial soup of precursors. A primitive type of cell containing an RNA genome, called the eugenote, is hypothesized to have evolved from the progenote population. RNA molecules were probably the primordial genome/enzyme molecules of primitive living systems. Ribose sugars are easier to synthesize under simulated primordial conditions than deoxyribose sugars. The DNA precursors of all extant cells are produced by reduction of RNA nucleoside diphosphates by the highly conserved protein enzyme ribonucleoside diphosphate reductase. This enzyme appears in all modern cells with few structural differences, suggesting that it is an ancient one that has performed the same essential task over a long evolutionary history. Living systems with RNA genomes are presumed to have evolved first. More stable DNA genomes evolved later to store genetic information. Also, ssDNA would have been less likely to form complex three-dimensional configurations due to the lack of the 2 hydroxyl, which may participate in unusual hydrogen bonds. Furthermore, the catalytic activity of some modern ribozymes is known to involve this 2 OH. Lastly, dsDNA molecules have the same unvarying double-helical structure that would not lead us to expect them to have enzymatic properties. However, they can fold back on themselves and ssDNA can fold into tertiary structures. Gradually, proteins took over many of the catalytic functions originally performed by RNA molecules. This would have allowed for greater flexibility in the sequences since there are 20 amino acids and only 4 ribonucleotides. Also, three-dimensional shapes in RNA molecules would require a complementary sequence elsewhere on the strand to form hydrogen bonds. Early life systems that could make a variety of useful proteins would tend to have a selective advantage over those that had a more restrictive repertoire. Selection would promote the early protoribosomes tRNA and tRNA synthetases to diversify. This process is envisioned to have produced a set of peptide-specific ribosomes, each with a different internal guide sequence serving as an mRNA sequence. A primitive genetic code would thus become established as sets of tRNA synthetases and peptide specific protoribosomes evolved.

DNA World

Double stranded DNA molecules are more stable than ssRNA. It would be advantageous for living systems to store heritable information in DNA molecules rather than RNA molecules. The 2' OH of RNA can attack an adjacent phosphodiester bond, rendering RNAs much more labile than DNAs. This autocatalytic process may have been accelerated by the harsh conditions on the primitive earth. As cells became more complex, their genome sizes had to increase. If early eugenotes had segmented RNA genomes, at least one of each segment would have to be present in each daughter cell for its survival. To enhance the probability that progeny cells are provided with a full genome, natural selection would favor production of polycistronic genomes. But the larger the RNA genomic segments are less stable, they would become because of autocatalysis. It would be advantageous for more stable polycistronic DNA molecules to take over genomic functions of RNA, leaving the RNAs to carry out functions that need not require long lived molecules. The earliest anucleate cells containing DNA genomes and all subsequent such cells are known as prokaryotes. At least four major processes were required to complete this transition:

a. Synthesis of DNA monomers by ribonucleoside diphosphate reductase.

b. Reverse transcription of DNA polymers from RNA genomes.

c. Replication of DNA genomes by a DNA polymerase.

d. Transcription of DNA genomes in functional (nongenomic) RNA molecules such as tRNA, mRNA and rRNA.

The split genes of modern eukaryotic cells consist of coding regions (exons) and noncoding regions (introns). The interruption of the gene provided by introns offers an evolutionary advantage. Apparently, exons from different genes can sometimes be recombined by natural mechanisms to code for proteins of different functions but containing related amino acid domains. Each of these domains may have a specific function *e.g.* binding to a receptor, forming x-helix, etc. This process, termed exon shuffling, is inferred to have been used extensively in DNA world of early eukaryotes.

Phylogenetic Analysis

Proteins evolve at different rates because of intrinsic factors (repair mechanisms) and extrinsic factors (environmental mutagens). Highly conserved proteins apparently have only been able to tolerate a few minor changes, whereas some other proteins have been able to absorb many mutations without loss of function. Mutations that occur outside a region involved with normal function of the molecule may be tolerated as a selectively neutral mutation. Over geological time, these neutral mutations tend to accumulate within a geneological lineage. If it is assumed that such neutral mutations accumulate at a fairly constant rate for a highly conserved protein, it is possible to establish the branching pattern of a phylogenetic tree also called a cladogram or an evolutionary tree. The principle of parsimony is commonly used to determine the minimum number of genetic changes required to account for the amino or nucleotide sequence differences between organisms sharing a common ancestor. The evolutionary distances separating organisms in a phylogenetic tree are usually expressed in units of nucleotide mutations or amino acid substitutions along each arm of the tree between branch points.

Evolution of Eukaryotic Cells

At one time, prokaryotes were thought to be more closely related to a postulated progenote, the common ancestor of all cells, before there was a genome, than were eukaryotes and all prokaryotes were thought to be more closely related to one another than to any eukaryote. Most prokaryotic species can be further classified as eubacteria. The other prokaryotic subkingdom, archae, occupies the kinds of environments that were presumed to be widespread when life first evolved. Hence, it was commonly believed that eubacteria evolved from primitive archae and eukaryotes evolved from eubacteria. However, many more differences were found to separate the two subkingdoms. Some archae traits are shared with Eubacteria, they are both prokaryotes, whereas others are shared with eukaryotes *e.g.* genes for rRNA and tRNA contain introns. Based on his analysis of nucleotide sequences in the highly conserved 16S rRNA from many organisms, Carl Woese proposed in 1977 that archae are as different from eubacteria as either group is from the eukaryotes. Now, it is thought that all three lines have descended from the same progenote. Organisms with a nucleus may have evolved as long ago as 3.5 billion years, but how the first nuclear membrane arose remains a mystery. According to the membrane proliferation hypothesis, one or more invaginations of the plasma membrane in the progenote coalesced internally to surround the genome, became severed from the plasma membrane and formed a double-layered nuclear membrane. The origin of mitochondria in younger eukaryotes may be explained by the endosymbiotic theory. Some ancient cells were capable of ingesting food particles by endocytic invaginations of their plasma membranes. It is possible that at least one large, fermenting, feeder cell engulfed one or more smaller respiratory bacteria, but failed to digest them. This endosymbiont was able to survive in an environment where nutrients were abundant and it could hide from other predatory cells. In turn, the host feeder cell gained the energetic advantages of oxidative respiration over fermentation. These complementary advantages evolved into a symbiotic relationship wherein neither entity can survive without the other. Most negatively charged molecules, including mRNA, tRNA, rRNA and some proteins, that cannot cross the membrane of these organelles must still be encoded by the genomes of these organelles. This process is proposed to have given rise to the mitochondria of modern eukaryotic cells at least 1.5 billion years ago. A stronger case can be made for the evolution of chloroplasts by endosymbiosis than that for mitochondria. An aerobic, eukaryotic feeder cell is proposed to have engulfed one or more eubacteria that were capable of oxygenic photosynthesis. In the process of evolving into chloroplasts, the endosymbionts relinquished some of their genes to the nuclear genome, but not as many as did the endosymbionts that evolved into mitochondria. Like the mitochondria, the protochloroplasts had to retain all of the genes specifying tRNA and rRNA for protein synthesis within the chloroplast. Much evidence supports the endosymbiotic theory for the origin of chloroplasts and mitochondria. These organelles are approximately the same size as bacteria. The genomes reside within a single, circular DNA molecule that is devoid of histone proteins, like bacteria. Both organelles reproduce asexually by growth and division of existing organelles in a manner similar to binary fission. Protein synthesis in mitochondria and chloroplasts is inhibited by a variety of antibiotics that inactivate bacterial ribosomes, but have little effect on cytoplasmic eukaryotic ribosomes. Nascent polypeptides in bacteria, mitochondria and chloroplasts have *N*-formylmethionine at their amino ends. Mitochondria and chloroplast genomes encode the tRNA and rRNA molecules for their own protein- synthesizing systems. The ribosomes in both organelles resemble bacterial ribosomes in size and structure. Lastly, the endosymbiotic theory accounts for the fact that both organelles have double membranes. The inner membrane corresponds to the plasma membrane of the ancestral endosymbiont; the outer membrane represents the plasma membrane of the ancestral feeder host cell.

Summary

1. Sex differentiation is a programmed cascade of events in which the indifferent gonad develops as a testis or an ovary with the appropriate urogenital and secondary sex characters.

2. Sex determination is the event that sets this cascade in motion. In placental mammals, there is good evidence that sex is determined by a gene on the Y chromosome (SRY) that initiates testis formation.

3. In humans, differentiation of the testes and ovaries is initiated by 6 weeks and fully achieved by 13 to 14 weeks of fetal development.

4. The phenomenon responsible for mixing maternal and paternal characters in sexually reproducing organisms is said to be recombination.

5. Mutations in a broad sense include all those heritable changes which alter the phenotype of an individual. Mutations may occur spontaneously in nature or they may be artificially induced. A slight slip occurs in the replication of genes and this change in gene duplication is known as gene mutation. Gene mutation also said to be copy-error mutation.

6. The structural changes in chromosome which appear phenotypically are known as chromosomal mutation or aberrations. Chromosomal aberration was first analyzed by H. J. Mullar (1928) in *Drosophila* and by Barbara Mc Clintock (1930) in Zea. It signifies the loss or absence of a section of a chromosome and may involve one or more genes.

7. The presence of a part of a chromosome in excess of the normal complememnt is known as duplication.

8. Translocation involves the transfer of a part of a chromosome or a set of genes to a non homologous chromosome.

9. Inversion involves a relation of a part of a chromosome or a set of genes by 180 degree on its own axis. The net result is neither a gain nor a loss in the genetic material but simply a rearrangement of the gene sequence.

10. The presence of a chromosome number which is different than the multiple of basic chromosome number.

11. Monosomy represents the loss of a single chromosme from the diploid set and they have the chromosome complement 2n-1.

12. Trisomics are those organisms that have an extra chromosome (2n+1) which is homologous to one of the chromosomes of the complement.

13. Variations that involve entire sets of chromosome are known as euploidy.

14. Autopolyploid are those polyploidy which have same basic set of chromosomes multiplied.

15. All forms of energy and certain chemicals which disrupt the chemical structure of chromosomes are mutagens.

16. Mutagenic agents are X-rays, UV rays, Acridin dye, Hydroxylamine, Nitrous acid, Bromouracil and Amino purine etc.

17. Example of Trisomy 21 is Down syndrome; incidence based upon maternal age, though translocation type is familial, features can includes epicanthal folds, simian crease, brachycephaly and cardiac defects.

18. Example of Trisomy 13 is Patau Syndrome also called D-Syndrome. Features include microcephaly, cleft lip and/or palate, polydactyly, cardiac defects, holoprosencephaly.

19. Example of Monosomy X is Turner's syndrome (45, X 0).

20. XXY, a male with 2 X chromosomes is known as Klinefelter's syndromic, features include elongated lower body, gynecomastia, testicular atrophy (incidence: 1/500 males.

21. XYY boys are usually taller than their siblings. Like XXY boys and XXX girls, they are somewhat more likely to have learning difficulties.

22. XXX girls tend to be tall and thin. They have a higher incidence of dyslexia.

23. Health was considered as a state of body and mind where there was a balance of certain hormones. Health is not just the absence of disease. It is a state of complete physical, mental, social and psychological well-being.

24. Disease is any deviation from or interruption of the normal structure and function of any part of the body. It is expressed by a characteristic set of signs and symptoms and in most instances the etiology, pathology and prognosis. A disease caused by a specific pathogenic organism and capable of being transmitted to another individual by direct or indirect contact is known as communicable disease.

25. Some common diseases caused by bacteria are tuberculosis, diphtheria, whooping cough, cholera, diarrhoea, tetanus, typhoid, gonorrhoea and syphilis.

26. Human diseases caused by viruses include mumps, measles, chicken pox, poliomyelitis and trachoma.

27. The disease which don't spread from infected person to a healthy person are known as non-communicable disease *e.g.* diabetes, cardiovascular diseases, heart disease coronary thrombosis, cancer etc.

28. Cancer is a disorder of cell growth in a part of the body. Tumor is a lumpy collection of tissue cells large enough to be seen or felt.

29. Malignancy refers to chaotic cell growth, the invasion and destruction of nearby tissues and distant metastatic spread.

30. Carcinomas are tumors made up principally of epithelial cells that cover or line body organs. Sarcomas are tumors made up principally of connective tissue cells, which are of mesodermal origin. Lymphomas are cancers in which there are excessive production of lymphocytes by the lymph nodes and spleen. Leukaemias result from unchecked proliferation of cell types present in blood and their precursors in the bone marrow.

31. Agents which cause cancers are called carcinogens. Cancer is not a contagious disease nor is it inherited.

32. The diseases which are transferred from generation to generation are called genetic disorder or genetically transmitted diseases.

33. These disorders may be due to incompatible genes, defective genes or abnormalities in the structure or number of chromosomes.

34. The incompatibility may lead to haemolytic disorder in the child and may cause the death of the offspring.

35. The two well studied incompatibilities are those of Rh factor and ABO blood group.

36. Rh factor is an antigenic protein on the surface of R.B.C. inhuman beings.

37. It was first discovered by Karl Landsteiner and A.S. Wiener in 1940 in RBC of rhesus monkeys.

38. Recessively inherited disorders may be autosomal or sex linked. Autosomal recessive disorders include albimism, phenylketonuria, Tay-sachs disease, cystic fibrosis and sickle cell anaemia.

39. Sex linked recessive disorders are caused by defective genes on X-chromosome. They are primarily the disorder of males. Hemophilia, color blindness and muscular dystrophy are sex-linked recessive.

40. The disorders for which genes are dominant over their allele are called dominantly inherited disorder.

41. The area of health care that offers advice on genetic problems is called genetic counseling, the term introduced by Sheldon Reed in 1940.

42. Some sufferes develop Korsakoff's syndrome in which the drinker suffers marked loss of memory which he unwittingly tries to disguise by relating stories of non-existent experiences.

Bibliography

Aguzzi, A. and M. Polymenidou (2004). Mammalian prion biology: One century of evolving concepts. Cell 116: S109.

Allan, V. J., H. M. Thompson and M. A. McNiven (2002). Motoring around the Golgi. Nature Cell Biol. 4:E236.

Bateman, J. F., R. P. Boot-Handford and S. R. Lamande. (2009). Genetic diseases of connective tissue: Cellular and extracellular effects of ECM mutations. Nat. Rev. Genet. 10:173.

Bogorad, L. (2008). Evolution of early eukaryotic cells: Genomes, proteomes and compartments. Photosynth. Res. 95:11.

Boldogh, I. R. and L. A. Pon. (2007). Mitochondria on the move. Trends Cell Biol. 17:502.

Bowman, S. M. and S. J. (2006). Free. The structure and synthesis of the fungal cell wall. Bioessays 28:799.

Brett, C. T. (2000). Cellulose microfibrils in plants: Biosynthesis, deposition and integration into the cell wall. Int. Rev. Cytol. 199:161.

Brinkmann, H. and H. Philippe (2007). The diversity of eukaryotes and the root of the eukaryotic tree. Adv. Exp. Med. Biol. 607:20.

Burke, B. and C. L. Stewart (2006). The laminopathies: The functional architecture of the nucleus and its contribution to disease. Annu. Rev. Genomics Hum. Genet. 7:369.

Cann, A. J. (2001). Principles of Molecular Virology, 3rd ed. San Diego: Academic Press.

Cobb, N. J. and W. K. Surewicz (2009). Prion diseases and their biochemical mechanisms. Biochemistry 48:2574.

Cosgrove, D. J. (2005). Growth of the plant cell wall. Int. Rev. Mol. Cell Biol. 6:850.

Crozet, C., F. Beranger and S. Lehmann (2008). Cellular pathogenesis in prion diseases. Vet. Res. 39:44.

de Duve, C. (1996). The peroxisome in retrospect. Ann. NY Acad. Sci. 804:1.

Dillon, C. and Y. Goda (2005). The actin cytoskeleton: Integrating form and function at the synapse. Annu. Rev. Neurosci. 28:25.

DiMauro, S. (2006). Mitochondrial myopathies. Curr. Opin. Rheumatol. 18:636.

Ding, B., A. Itaya and X. Zhong (2005). Viroid trafficking: A small RNA makes a big move. Curr. Opin. Plant Biol. 8:606.

Dinman, J. D. (2009). The eukaryotic ribosome: Current status and challenges. J. Biol. Chem. 284:11761.

Erickson, H. P. (2007). Evolution of the cytoskeleton. Bioessays 29:668.

Fan, J., Z. Hu, L. Zeng, W. Lu, X. Tang, J. Zhang and T. Li (2008). Golgi apparatus and neurodegenerative diseases. Int. J. Dev. Neurosci. 26:523.

Flores, R. et al. Viroids and viroid-host interactions. Annu. Rev. Phytopathol. 43 (2005): 117.

Glick, B. S. (2000). Organization of the Golgi apparatus. Curr. Opin. Cell Biol. 12:450.

Gould, S. J. and D. Valle (2000). Peroxisome biogenesis disorders: Genetics and cell biology. Trends Genet. 16:340.

Grabowski, G. A. and R. J. Hopkins (2003). Enzyme therapy for lysosomal storage diseases: Principles, practice and prospects. Annu. Rev. Genomics Hum. Genet. 4:403.

Hall, A. (2009). The cytoskeleton and cancer. Cancer Metastasis Rev. 28:5.

Howard, J. (2001). Mechanics of Motor Proteins and the Cytoskeleton. Sunderland, MA: Sinauer Associates.

Jackson, C. L. (2009). Mechanisms of transport through the Golgi complex. J. Cell Sci. 122:443.

Jamet, E., C. Albenne, G. Boudart, M. Irshad, H. Canut and R. Pont-Lezica (2008). Recent advances in plant cell wall proteomics. Proteomics 8:893.

Kassen, R. and P. B. Rainey (2004). The ecology and genetics of microbial diversity. Annu. Rev. Microbiol. 58:207.

Kiselyov, K. (2007). Autophagy, mitochondria and cell death in lysosomal storage diseases. Autophagy 3: 259.

Kreis, T. and R. Vale, eds. (1999). Guidebook to the Extracellular Matrix, Anchor and Adhesion Proteins, 2nd ed. Oxford: Oxford University Press.

Leigh, R. A. and D. Sanders, eds. (1997). The Plant Vacuole. San Diego: Academic Press.

Marastoni, S., G. Ligresti, E. Lorenzon, A. Colombatti and M. Mongiat (2008). Extracellular matrix: A matter of life and death. Connect. Tissue Res. 29:203.

Máximo, V., J. Lima, P. Soares and M. Sobrinho-Simoes (2009). Mitochondria and cancer. Virchows Arch. 454: 481.

Michie, K. A. and J. Lowe (2006). Dynamic filaments of the bacterial cytoskeleton. Annu. Rev. Biochem. 75:467.

Moore, R. A., L. M. Taubner and S. A. (2009) Priola. Prion protein misfolding and disease. Curr. Opin. Struct. Biol. 19 14.

Morava, E. (2006). Mitochondrial disease criteria: Diagnostic applications in children. Neurology 67:1823.

Ni, M. and A. S. Lee (2007). ER chaperones in mammalian development and human diseases. FEBS Lett. 581: 3641.

Okamoto, K. and J. M. Shaw (2005). Mitochondrial morphology and dynamics in yeast and multicellular eukaryotes. Annu. Rev. Genet.39: 503.

Pace, N. R. (2006). Time for a change. Nature 441:289.

Pogliano, J. (2008). The bacterial cytoskeleton. Curr. Opin. Cell Biol. 20:19.

Prusiner, S. B. and M. R. Scott. (1997). Genetics of prions. Annu. Rev. Genet. 31:139.

Prusiner, S. B., ed. (2004).Prion Biology and Diseases, 4th ed. Cold Spring Harbor, New York: Cold Spring Harbor Laboratory Press,

Reeve, A. K., K. J. Krishnan and D. Turnbull (2008). Mitochondrial DNA mutations in disease, aging and neurodegeneration. Ann. NY Acad. Sci. 1147:1147.

Reisner, D. and H. H. Gross. (1985). Viroids. Annu. Rev. Biochem. 54:531.

Reumann, S. (2000). The structural properties of plant peroxisomes and their metabolic significance. Annu. Rev. Genet. 34:623.

Rippe, K. (2007). Dynamic organization of the cell nucleus. Curr. Opin. Genet. Dev. 17:373.

Sabatini, D. D. and G. E. Palade (1999). Charting the secretory pathway. Trends Cell Biol. 9: 413.

Sapp, J. (2005). The prokaryote-eukaryote dichotomy: Meanings and mythology. Microbiol. Mol. Biol. Rev. 69:292.

Schröder M. (2008). Engineering eukaryotic protein factories. Biotechnol. Lett. 30:187.

Shorter, J. and G. Warren (2002). Golgi architecture and inheritance. Annu. Rev. Cell Dev. Biol. 18:379.

Strelkov, S. V., H. Herrmann and U. Aebi (2003). Molecular architecture of intermediate filaments. BioEssays 25:243.

Strnad, P., C. Stumptner, K. Zatloukal and H. Denk (2008). Intermediate filament cytoskeleton of the liver in health and disease. Histochem. Cell Biol. 129:735.

Stürmer M., H. W. Doerr and L. Gürtler. (2009). Human immunodeficiency virus: 25 years of diagnostic and therapeutic strategies and their impact on hepatitis B and C virus. Med. Microbiol. Immunol.198:147.

Tanaka, S., M. R. Sawaya and T. O. Yeates (2010). Structure and mechanisms of a protein-based organelle in *Escherichia coli*. Science 327:81.

Tchélidzé P., A. Chatron-Colliet, M. Thiry, N. Lalun, H. Bobichon and D. Ploton (2009). Tomography of the cell nucleus using confocal microscopy and medium voltage electron microscopy. Crit. Rev. Oncol. Hematol. 69:127.

Trotsenko, Y. A. and V. N. Khmelenina (2002). Biology of extremophilic and extremotolerant methanotrophs. Arch. Microbiol. 177:123.

Voeltz, G. K., M. M. Rolls and T. A. (2002). Rapoport. Structural organization of the endoplasmic reticulum. EMBO Rep. 3:944.

Waters, M. T. and J. A. Langdale (2009). The making of a chloroplast. EMBO J. 28:2861.

Webster, M., K. L. Witkin and O. Cohen-Fix (2009). Sizing up the nucleus: Nuclear shape, size and nuclear envelope assembly. J. Cell Sci. 122:1477.

Wlodkowic, D., J. Skommer, D. McGuinness, C. Hillier and Z. Darzynkiewicz. (2009). ER-Golgi network—a future target for anti-cancer therapy. Leuk. Res. 33:1440.

Woese, C. R. and G. E. Fox (1977). Phylogenetic structure of the prokaryotic domain: The primary kingdoms. Proc. Nat. Acad. Sci. USA74:5088.

Woese, C. R., O. Kandler and M. L. Wheelis (1990). Towards a natural system of organisms: Proposal for the domains Archaea, Bacteria and Eucarya. Proc. Nat. Acad. Sci. USA87:4576.

Yeates, T. O., Crowley, C. S. and S. Tanaka (2010). Bacterial microcompartment organelles: Protein shell structure and evolution. Annu. Rev. Biophys. 39:185.

Yoshida, H. (2007). ER stress and diseases. FEBS Lett. 274:630.

Glossary

Adenine (A): One of the bases present in DNA and RNA; adenine is a purine.

Adenosine diphosphate (ADP): Adenosine with two phosphates attached to the 5′ carbon of ribose.

Adenosine monophosphate (AMP): Adenosine with one phosphate attached to the 5′ carbon of ribose.

Adenosine triphosphate (ATP): Adenosine with three phosphates attached to the 5′ carbon of ribose. ATP is a coenzyme and one of the cell's energy currencies.

Adenosine: Adenine linked to the sugar ribose. Adenosine is a nucleoside.

Adenyl cyclase: Enzyme that converts ATP to the intracellular messenger cyclic AMP

ADP/ATP exchanger: Carrier in the inner mitochondrial membrane. ADP is moved in one direction and ATP in the other.

Anabolism: Those metabolic reactions that build up molecules: biosynthesis.

Anaphase I: Anaphase of the first meiotic division (meiosis I).

Anaphase II: Anaphase of the second meiotic division (meiosis II).

Anaphase: The stage of mitosis or meiosis during which centromeres split and chromatids separate and chromatids move to opposite poles.

Anion: Negatively charged ion, *e.g.* chloride, Cl^- or phosphate, HPO_4^{2-}.

Anode: Positively charged electrode, *e.g.* in a gel electrophoresis apparatus used for SDS-PAGE.

Antenna chlorophyll: Chlorophyll molecules that capture light and pass the energy to reaction center chlorophylls.

Antibiotics: Chemical that is produced by one type of organism and kills others by inhibiting protein synthesis. The most useful antibiotics to humans are those that are selective for prokaryotes.

ATP synthase: Carrier of the inner mitochondrial membrane that is built around a rotary motor. Ten H$^+$ enter the mitochondrial matrix for every three ATP made.

ATP synthetase: Another name for ATP synthase; a carrier of the inner mitochondrial membrane that is built around a rotary motor. Ten H$^+$ enter the mitochondrial matrix for every three ATP made.

Autoradiography: Process that detects a radioactive molecule. In Southern blot experiment, the membrane that has been hybridized to a radioactive gene probe is placed in direct contact with a sheet of X-ray film. Radioactive decay activates the silver grains on the emulsion of the X-ray film. When the film is developed, areas that have been in contact with radioactivity will show as black.

Axon: Long process of a nerve cell, specialized for the rapid conduction of action potentials.

BAC (Bacterial Artificial Chromosome): Cloning vector used to propagate DNAs of about 300,000 bp in bacterial cells.

Bacteriophage: A virus that infects bacterial cells.

BAD: A bcl-2 family protein that causes the release of cytochrome c from mitochondria, triggering apoptosis. BAD is phosphorylated and thereby inactivated by protein kinase B.

Basal body: Structure from which cilia and flagella arise; has the same structure as the centriole.

Base pair: The Watson Crick model of DNA showed that guanine in one DNA strand would fit nicely with cytosine in another strand while adenine would fit nicely with thymine. The two hydrogen-bonded bases are called a base pair. RNA can also participate in base pairing; instead of thymine it is uracil that now pairs with adenine. The rare base inosine, found in some tRNAs, can base pair with any of uracil, cytosine or adenine.

Basement membrane: Thin layer of extracellular fibers that supports epithelial cells.

B-DNA: Right handed DNA double helix.

B-DNA: Right handed DNA double helix.

Binding site: Region of a protein that specifically binds a ligand.

Bioluminescence: Production of light by a living organism.

Bisphosphate: Bearing two independent phosphate groups (as opposed to a diphosphate, which bears a chain of two phosphates in a line). Fructose-1, 6-bisphosphate is an example.

Blastocyst: Early embryo.

Bloom's syndrome: Disease resulting from a deficiency in helicase. Affected individuals cannot repair their DNA and are susceptible to developing skin cancer and other cancers.

Blue-green algae: Old name for the photosynthetic prokaryotes now known as cyanobacteria.

Bright field microscopy: Most basic form of light microscopy. The specimen appears against a bright background and appears darker than the background because of the light it has absorbed or scattered.

Bulky Lesion: Distortion of the DNA helix caused by a thymine dimer.

C (cytosine): One of the bases present in DNA and RNA; cytosine is a pyrimidine.

Ca^{2+} ATPase: Carrier that uses the energy released by ATP hydrolysis to move calcium ions up their concentration gradient out of the cytosol. Different isoforms of calcium ATPase are located at the plasma membrane and in the membrane of the endoplasmic reticulum.

Cadherin: Cell adhesion molecule that helps form adherens junctions.

Calcineurin: Calcium-calmodulin activated phosphatase *i.e.* an enzyme that removes phosphate groups from proteins, opposing the effects of kinases. Calcineurin is inhibited by the immunosuppressant drug cyclosporin.

Calcium action potential: Action potential driven by the opening of voltage-gated calcium channels and the resulting calcium influx.

Calcium ATPase: Carrier that uses the energy released by ATP hydrolysis to move calcium ions up their concentration gradient out of the cytosol. Different isoforms of calcium ATPase are located at the plasma membrane and in the membrane of the endoplasmic reticulum.

Calcium pump: Carrier that moves calcium ions up their electrochemical gradient out of the cytosol into the extracellular medium or into the endoplasmic reticulum. There are two important calcium pumps: the sodium/calcium exchanger is found on the plasma membrane, while different isoforms of the calcium ATPase are found on the plasma membrane and on the membrane of the endoplasmic reticulum.

Calcium-binding protein: Any protein that binds calcium. Calmodulin, troponin and calreticulin are examples found in the cytosol, attached to actin filaments in striated muscle and in the endoplasmic reticulum respectively.

Calcium-calmodulin–activated protein kinase: Important regulatory enzyme, activated when calcium-loaded calmodulin binds, which phosphorylates target proteins on serine and threonine residues.

Calcium-induced calcium release: Process in which a rise of calcium concentration in the cytoplasm triggers the release of more calcium from the endoplasmic reticulum. The best understood mechanism of calcium-induced calcium release is via ryanodine receptors.

Calmodulin: Calcium binding protein found in many cells. When calmodulin binds calcium, it can then activate other proteins such as the enzymes calcineurin and glycogen phosphorylase kinase.

CAP (catabolite activator protein): Protein found in prokaryotes that bind to cAMP. The CAP–cAMP complex then binds within the promoter region of some bacterial operons and helps RNA polymerase to bind to the promoter.

Carbohydrates: Monosaccharides and all compounds made from monosaccharide monomers.

Catabolism: Metabolic reactions that break down molecules to derive chemical energy.

Cation: Positively charged ion *e.g.* Na^+, K^+ and Ca^{2+}.

Cdc25: Protein phosphatase involved in the regulation of CDK_1.

Cdk1 (cyclin-dependent kinase 1): Protein kinase involved in the regulation of the G_2/M transition of the cell cycle and associates with cyclin B to form MPF.

Cdk2 (cyclin-dependent kinase 2): Protein kinase involved in the regulation of G_1 phase of the cell cycle and associates with cyclin E.

Cdk4 (cyclin-dependent kinase 4): Protein kinase involved in the regulation of G_1 phase of the cell cycle and associates with cyclin D.

cDNA (complementary DNA): DNA copy of an mRNA molecule.

cDNA Library: Collection of bacterial cells each of which contains a different foreign cDNA molecule.

Cell adhesion molecule: Integral membrane protein responsible for sticking cells together. The extracellular domain binds a cell adhesion molecule on another cell while the intracellular domain binds to the cytoskeleton, either directly or via a linker protein.

Cell center: Point immediately adjacent to the nucleus of eukaryotes where the centrosome and Golgi apparatus are located.

Cell cycle (cell division cycle): Ordered sequence of events that must occur for successful cell division; consists of G_1, S, G_2 and M phases.

Cell division cycle: Another name for the cell cycle: the ordered sequence of events that must occur for successful cell division; consists of G1, S, G2 and M phases.

Cell junctions: Points of cell–cell interaction in tissues; includes tight junctions; anchoring junctions and gap junctions.

Cell membrane: Membrane that surrounds the cell; also known as the plasmalemma or plasma membrane.

Cell surface membrane: Another name for the plasma membrane.

Cell wall: Rigid case that encloses plant and fungal cells and many prokaryotes. The cell wall lies outside the plasma membrane. Plant cell walls are composed of cellulose plus other polysaccharide molecules such as hemicellulose and pectin.

Cell: Fundamental unit of life. A membrane-bound collection of protein, nucleic acid and other components that is capable of self replication using simpler building blocks.

Cellulose synthase: Multiprotein complex of the plant plasma membrane that makes cellulose.

Cellulose: Major structural polysaccharide of the plant cell wall; with the formulan, a polysaccharide consisting of a linear chain of seeral humnared to over tenthousand B linked d-guicose units.

Centriole: Structure found at the centrosome of animal cells; composed of microtubules.

Centromere: Region of the chromosome at which the kinetochore where the microtubules of the mitotic or meiotic spindle attach is formed.

Centrosome: Structure from which cytoplasmic microtubules arise.

CF (cystic fibrosis): Inherited disease characterized by failure of the pancreas and by thick sticky mucus in the lungs leading to fatal lung infection unless treated. Cystic fibrosis is caused by failure to make or properly target, plasma membrane chloride channels.

Channel: Integral membrane protein that forms a continuous water-filled hole through the membrane.

Chaperone: Protein that helps other proteins to remain unfolded for correct protein targeting or to fold into their correct 3D structure.

Chiasmata (chiasma): Structures formed during crossing over between the chromatids of homologous chromosomes during meiosis; the physical manifestation of genetic recombination.

Chimera: Structure formed from two different parts. Chimeric proteins are generated by joining together all or part of the protein coding sections of two distinct genes. Chimeric organisms are formed by mixing two or more distinct clones of cells.

Chimeric protein: Proteins generated by joining together all or part of the protein coding sections of two distinct genes, GFP and a protein of interest.

Chiral: Structure whose mirror image cannot be superimposed on it. Organic molecules will be chiral if a carbon atom has four different groups attached to it and is therefore asymmetric.

Chlorophyll: Major photosynthetic pigment of plants and algae.

Chloroplast: Photosynthetic organelle of plant cells.

Chromatid: Complete DNA double helix plus accessory proteins subsequent to DNA replication in eukaryotes. At mitosis, the chromosome is seen to be composed of two chromatids; these separate to form the chromosomes of the two progeny cells.

Chromatin: Complex of DNA and certain DNA-binding proteins such as histones.

Chromatophore: Pigment cell in the skin of fish and amphibia.

Chromosome: Single, enormously long molecule of DNA, together with its accessory proteins. Chromosomes are the units of organization of the nuclear chromatin and carry many genes. In eukaryotes chromosomes are linear; in prokaryotes they are circular.

Cilium (cilia): Locomotory appendage of some epithelial cells and protozoa.

Cisternae: Flattened membrane-bound sacs, *e.g.* those that make up Golgi apparatus.

CKI (cyclin-dependent kinase inhibitor): Type of cell cycle regulatory protein. Binds to and inactivates CDKs.

Clathrin adaptor protein: Protein that binds to specific transmembrane receptors and which in turn recruits clathrin to form a coated vesicle. The vesicle therefore contains the molecule for which the receptor is specific.

Clathrin: Protein that functions to cause vesicle budding in response to binding of specific ligand.

Cleavage furrow: The structure that constricts the middle of the cell during cytokinesis in animal cells.

Clone: A number of genetically identical individuals.

Cloning: It is the creation of a number of genetically identical organisms. In molecular genetics, the term is used to mean the multiplication of particular sequences of DNA by an asexual process such as bacterial cell division.

Codon: Sequence of three bases in an mRNA molecule that specifies a particular amino acid.

Coenzyme: Molecule that acts as a second substrate for a group of enzymes. ATP/ADP,

Cofactor: Nonprotein molecule or an ion necessary for the activity of a protein. Cofactors are associated tightly with the protein but can be removed. Examples are pyridoxal phosphate in aminotransferases and zinc in zinc finger proteins.

Cohesin: Protein that holds two chromatids together. Degradation of cohesin allows the two chromatids to separate at the start of anaphase in mitosis and in meiosis II.

Colchicine: Plant alkaloid from the autumn crocus, *Colchicum autumnale;* binds to tubulin.

Collagen: Major structural protein of the extracellular matrix.

Columnar: Taller than it is broad. Used as a description of some types of epithelial cells.

Complementary DNA (cDNA): DNA copy of an mRNA molecule.

Connective tissue: Tissue that contains relatively few cells within a large volume of extracellular matrix.

Covalent bond: Strong bond between two atoms in which electrons are shared.

Cristae: Name given to the folds of the inner membrane of mitochondria.

Crossing over: Physical exchange of material that takes place between homologous chromosomes during recombination and is manifest in the formation of chiasmata.

Cyanobacteria: photosynthetic prokaryotes that were formerly known as blue green algae.

Cyclin: One of a family of proteins whose level oscillates (cycles) through the cell division cycle. Cyclins associate with and activate cyclin dependent kinases and hence allow progression through cell cycle control points.

Cystic fibrosis (CF): Inherited disease characterized by failure of the pancreas and by thick sticky mucus in the lungs leading to fatal lung infection unless treated. Cystic fibrosis is caused by failure to make or properly target, plasma membrane chloride channels.

Cystine: Double amino acid formed by two cysteine molecules joined by a disulfide bond.

Cytochemistry: Use of chemical compounds to stain specific cell structures and organelles.

Cytochrome C: Soluble protein of the mitochondrial intermembrane space, often found loosely associated with the inner mitochondrial membrane. Cytochrome C transports electrons between components of the electron transport chain. If it is allowed to escape from mitochondria cytochrome *c* activates caspase 9 and hence triggers apoptosis.

Cytochrome: Proteins with a heme prosthetic group that is able to transfer electrons. Cytochromes form a critical part of the electron transport chain of mitochondria and also form part of the cytochrome P450 detoxification system in the liver.

Cytokinesis: Process by which a cell divides in two; part of the M phase of the cell division cycle.

Cytology: Study of cell structure by light microscopy.

Cytoplasm: Semiviscous ground substance of the cell. All the volume outside the nucleus and inside the plasma membrane is cytoplasm.

Cytoplasmic dynein: Motor protein that moves organelles along microtubules in a retrograde direction.

Cytoplasmic streaming: Movement of cytoplasm that is commonly seen in plant cells and in amoebae; generated by actin and myosin.

Cytosine: One of the bases present in DNA and RNA; cytosine is a pyrimidine.

Cytoskeleton: Cytoplasmic filament system consisting of microtubules, microfilaments and intermediate filaments.

Cytosol: Viscous, aqueous medium in which the organelles and the cytoskeleton are bathed.

Death domain: Domain found on proteins concerned with regulating apoptosis, such as Fas and the p75 neurotrophin receptor. When activated, death domain proteins turn on caspase 8 and hence initiate apoptosis.

Dendrite: Branching cell process. The term is commonly used to name those processes of nerve cells that are too short to be called axons.

Deoxyribonucleic acid (DNA): Polymer of deoxyribonucleotides. DNA specifies the inherited instructions of a cell.

Deoxyribonucleotide: Building block of DNA made up of a nitrogenous base and the sugar deoxyribose to which a phosphate group is attached.

Deoxyribose: Ribose that instead of —OH has only —H on carbon 2. Deoxyribose is the sugar used in the nucleotides that make up DNA.

Depolarization: Any positive shift in the transmembrane voltage, whatever its size or cause.

Desmin: Protein that makes up the intermediate filaments in muscle cells.

Desmosome: Type of anchoring junction that joins the intermediate filaments of neighboring cells. Desmosomes are common in tissues such as skin.

Diabetes: The word diabetes simply refers to conditions in which a patient produces lots of urine. The only form of diabetes we discuss in this book is diabetes mellitus in which the patient produces large volumes of urine containing sugar. Diabetes mellitus is caused by either a failure in the endocrine gland that produces insulin or a failure of the tissues to respond adequately to insulin.

Diakinesis: This is the final stage of meiotic prophase I in which the chromatids break at the chiasmata and exchange their parts. During this phase the chromosomes are fully condensed and the meiotic spindle is assembled to prepare the homologous chromosomes for sepration.

Dideoxyribonucleotide: Man made molecule similar to a deoxyribonucleotide but lacking a 3-hydroxyl group on its sugar residue. Used in DNA sequencing.

Differentiation: Process whereby a cell becomes specialized for a particular function.

Diphosphate: Bearing a chain of two phosphates in a line as opposed to a bisphosphate, which bears two independent phosphate groups *e.g.* Adenosine diphosphate.

Diploid: Containing two sets of chromosomes, in humans, this means two sets of 23, one from the father, one from the mother. Most of the cells of the body (somatic cells) are diploid.

Dogma: The central dogma of molecular biology is that DNA makes RNA makes protein: the concept that the sequence of bases on DNA defines the sequence of bases on RNA and the sequence of bases on RNA defines the sequence of amino acids on protein.

Domain: Separatrly folded segment of the polypeptide chain of a protein.

Dominant: Gene that exerts its effect even when only one copy is present. Most dominant genes are dominant because they produce functional protein while the recessive gene does not. However, some mutant genes are dominant because even having 50% of one's protein as the mutant form is enough to cause an effect; the gene causing familial Creutzfeldt-Jacob disease is an example.

Donor: In a hydrogen bond, the donor is the atom (oxygen, nitrogen or sulfur) to which the hydrogen is covalently bonded and that gives up some of its share of electrons to a second electron grabbing atom.

Double helix: Structure formed when two filaments wind about each other, most commonly applied to DNA, but also applicable to, *e.g.* F-actin.

Duplication: Doubling-up of a particular sequence of the genetic material.

Dynamic instability: Term that describes the behavior of microtubules in which they switch from phases of growth to phases of shortening.

Ectoplasm: Viscous, gel like outer layer of cytoplasm.

Effective stroke: Part of the beat cycle of a cilium that pushes on the extracellular medium.

Electron gun: Source of electrons in electron microscopes.

Electron microscope: Microscope in which the image is formed by passage of electrons through or scattering of electrons by, the object.

Electron transport chain: Series of electron acceptor/donator molecules found in the inner mitochondrial membrane which transport electrons from the reduced carriers NADH and $FADH_2$ to oxygen. The entire complex forms a carrier that uses the energy of NADH and $FADH_2$ oxidation to transport hydrogen ions up their electrochemical gradient out of the mitochondrion.

Embryonic stem cell: Cells derived from an early embryo. Embryonic stem cells have the capability to divide indefinitely and to become any cell type in the body.

Endocytosis: Inward budding of plasma membrane to form vesicles. Endocytosis is the process by which cells retrieve plasma membrane and take up material from their surroundings.

Endoplasm: Fluid, inner layer of cytoplasm that streams during cytoplasmic streaming.

Endoplasmic reticulum (ER): Network (reticulum) of membrane-delimited tubes and sacs that extends from the outer membrane of the nuclear envelope almost to the plasma membrane. There are two types of ER, rough endoplasmic reticulum (RER) with a surface coating of ribosomes and smooth endoplasmic reticulum (SER).

Endosome: Organelle to which newly formed endocytotic vesicles are translocated and with which they fuse.

Endosymbiotic theory: Proposal that some of the organelles of eukaryotic cells originated as free-living prokaryotes.

Endothelial cells: Cells that line blood vessels and other body cavities that do not open to the outside.

Endothelium: Layer of cells that lines blood vessels and other body cavities that do not open to the outside.

Energy currency: Source of energy that the cell can use to drive processes that would otherwise not occur because their G is positive. Energy currencies can be coenzymes such as ATP and NADH, which give up energy on conversion to, respectively, ADP and NAD^+ or electrochemical ion gradients such as the hydrogen ion gradient across the mitochondrial membrane and the sodium gradient across the plasma membrane.

Enzyme: Catalyst made mainly of protein. Like all catalysts, enzymes work by reducing the activation energy of the reaction.

Epidermis: Protective outer cell layer of an organism.

Epithelial cells: Cells that make up an epithelium.

Epithelium: Sheet of cells covering the surface of the human body and those internal cavities such as the lungs and gut that open to the outside. In contrast endothelium lines internal spaces such as blood vessels.

ES (embryonic stem) cell: Cell derived from a very early embryo. ES cells have not yet determined their developmental fate and can depending on the conditions generate the entire range of tissue types.

Euchromatin: The portion of the nuclear chromatin that is not tightly packed. Euchromatin contains genes that code for proteins that are being actively transcribed.

Eukaryotic: Organisms whose cells contain distinct nuclei and other organelles; includes all known organisms except prokaryotes (bacteria and cyanobacteria).

Exocytosis: Fusion of a vesicle with the plasma membrane. Exocytosis causes the soluble contents of the vesicle to be released to the extracellular medium, while integral membrane proteins of the vesicle become integral membrane proteins of the plama membrane.

Extracellular matrix: Meshwork of filaments and fibers that surrounds and supports mammalian cells. The major protein of the extracellular matrix is collagen.

Extracellular medium: Aqueous medium outside cells. For a unicellular organism the extracellular medium is the outside world. For a multicellular organism such as a human being the extracellular medium is the fluid between the cells.

Extragenic DNA: DNA that can neither be identified as coding for protein or RNA nor as being promoters or enhancers regulating transcription.

Ferredoxin: Protein component of the electron transport system of chloroplasts.

Fibroblast growth factor: Paracrine transmitter that opposes apoptosis and promotes cell division in target cells. Although named for its effect on fibroblasts, FGF triggers proliferation of many tissues and plays critical roles in determining cell fate during development.

Fibroblast: Cell found in connective tissue. Fibroblasts synthesize collagen and other components of the extracellular matrix.

Fission: Breakage into two parts. The word is used for prokaryote replication. In addition it describes the division of a single membrane-bound organelle into two and the process whereby a vesicle breaks away from a membrane.

Flagellin: Protein that is the bacterial flagellum.

Flagellum: Swimming appendage. In eukaryotes flagella are extensions of the cell that use a dynein/microtubule motor system. In prokaryotes flagella are extracellular proteins rotated by a motor at their base.

Fluid mosaic model: Generally accepted hypothesis of how cell membranes are formed from a lipid bilayer plus protein.

G_0: Describes the quiescent state of cells that have left the cell division cycle.

G_1 **(gap 1):** Period of the cell division cycle that separates mitosis from the following S phase.

G_2 **(gap 2):** Period of the cell division cycle between the completion of S phase and the start of cell division or M phase.

G-actin: Globular, subunit form of actin.

Gamete: Sperm or egg. Gametes are haploid; that is, they contain just one set of chromosomes.

Gap junction channel (connexon): Channel in the plasma membrane with a central hole about 1.5 nm in diameter. Gap junction channels only open when they contact a second channel on another cell, in this case they open and form a water filled tube that runs all the way through the plasma membrane of the first cell, across the small gap between the cells and through plasma membrane of second cell, so allowing passage of solute from cytosol of one cell to the cytosol of other.

Gap junction: Type of cell junction that allows solute to pass from the cytosol of one cell to the cytosol of its neighbor without passing through the extracellular medium. Gap junctions consist of many paired gap junction channels or connexons.

Gastrocnemius muscle: Muscle at the back of the shin. When it contracts the toes move down.

Gelsolin: Type of actin-binding protein that binds to and fragments actin filaments.

Gene chip: Tiny glass wafer to which cloned DNAs are attached, also known as microarrays or DNA chips.

Gene family: Group of genes that share sequence similarity and usually code for proteins with a similar function.

Gene probe: The cDNA or genomic DNA fragment used to detect a specific DNA sequence to which it is complementary in sequence. The probe is tagged in some way to make it easy to detect. The tag could be a radioactive isotope or a fluorescent dye.

Gene: Fundamental unit of heredity. In many cases a gene contains the information needed to code for a single polypeptide.

Genome: Complete set of genes in an organism.

Genomic DNA library: Collection of bacterial clones each of which contains a different fragment of foreign genomic DNA.

Germ cells: Cells that give rise to the eggs and sperm.

Glial cells: Electrically inexcitable cells found in the nervous system.

Glucocorticoid receptor: Intracellular receptor to which glucocorticoid hormone binds.

Glucocorticoid: Steroid hormone produced by the adrenal cortex that forms part of the system controlling blood sugar levels.

Gluconeogenesis: Synthesis of glucose from noncarbohydrate precursors such as amino acids and lactate.

Glucose: Hexose monosaccharide. Glucose is the commonest sugar in the blood and is the dominant cellular fuel in animals, being used in glycolysis to generate ATP and pyruvate, the latter fueling Krebs cycle.

Glycolysis: Breakdown of glucose to pyruvate.

Glyoxisome: Type of peroxisome found in plant cells that is concerned with the conversion of fatty acids to carbohydrate.

Golgi apparatus: System of flattened cisternae concerned with glycosylation and other modifications of proteins.

Grana: Distinctive structures within the chloroplast formed by the stacking of the thylakoid membranes.

Green fluorescent protein: Fluorescent protein made by the jellyfish *Victoria victoria*. Unlike other colored or fluorescent proteins, it contains no prosthetic groups and therefore will fluoresce when expressed by any cell in which the gene is successfully inserted and expressed.

Growth factor: Paracrine transmitter that modifies the developmental pathway of the target cell, often by causing cell division.

Guanine: One of the bases found in DNA and RNA; guanine is a purine.

Guthrie test: Test for phenylketonuria. Newborn babies' blood is tested for the presence of phenylalanine at unusually high concentration.

Hairpin loop: Loop in which a linear object folds back on itself. It is used to describe the loop formed in a RNA molecule due to complementary base pairing.

Haploid: Containing a single copy of each chromosome, in humans, this means 23 chromosomes. Sperm and eggs are haploid while somatic cells contain one set of 23 from each parent and are referred to as being diploid.

Hemoglobin: Oxygen-carrying, iron containing protein of the blood.

Heterochromatin: That portion of the nuclear chromatin that is tightly packed. Much of the heterochromatin is repetitive DNA with no coding function.

Heterozygote: Individual whose two copies of a gene differ *e.g.* one may be mutant.

Histone: Positively charged protein that binds to negatively charged DNA and helps to fold DNA into chromatin.

Homologous recombination: Process in which a length of DNA with ends that is homologous to a section of chromosome swops in, replacing the existing length of DNA in the chromosome. Homologous recombination occurs naturally at chiasmata during crossing over during meiosis. It can also occur in some cells when they transfected with the appropriate exogenous DNA.

Homozygote: Individual whose two copies of a gene are identical. Most of us are homozygous for most of our genes.

Hormone: Long lived transmitter that is released into the blood and travels around the body before being broken down.

Housekeeping gene: Gene that is transcribed intomRNAin nearly all the cells of a eukaryotic organism; in bacterial cells a housekeeping gene is one that is always being transcribed.

Hypoxanthine: Purine that is used to make the nucleotide inosine. Inosine can pair with any of uracil, cytosine or adenine.

Imino acid: Organic molecule containing both carboxyl (—COOH) and imino (—NH—) groups. Proline is an imino acid although it is usually called an amino acid.

Insulin receptor: Receptor tyrosine kinase specific for insulin, which acts mainly through activation of PI-3-kinase and hence protein kinase B.

Insulin: Hormone produced by endocrine cells in the pancreas. It activates its own receptor tyrosine kinase, which in turn acts mainly through activation of PI-3-kinase and hence protein kinase B.

Integrin: Dimeric proteins with an extracellular domain that binds to extracellular matrix proteins and an intracellular domain that attaches to actin microfilaments.

Intermediate filament: One of the filaments that make up the cytoskeleton; composed of various subunit proteins.

Interphase: Period of synthesis and growth that separates one cell division from the next; consists of the G1, S and G2 phases of the cell division cycle.

Ion: Charged chemical species. A single atom that has more or less electrons than are required to exactly neutralize the charge on the nucleus is an ion *e.g.* Na^+, Cl^-. A molecule with one or more charged regions is also an ion *e.g.* phosphate, HPO_4^{2-} leucine, "OOC— H (CH_2.CH (CH_3)$_2$)—NH_3^+.

Karyokinesis: The indirect division of cells in which, prior to division of the cell protoplasm, complicated changes take place in the nucleus, attended with movement of the nuclear fibrils. The nucleus becomes enlarged and convoluted, and finally the threads are separated into two groups, which ultimately become disconnected and constitute the daughter nuclei.

Kinetochore: These are disc shaped structures present on the sides of centromere.

Leptotene: This is the stage of meiosis in which the chromosomes are slender, like threads.

Linkage: Physical association of genes on the same chromosome. Linked genes tend to be inherited together.

Linker DNA: Stretch of DNA that separates two nucleosomes.

Lipid bilayer: Two layers of lipid molecules that form a membrane.

Lumen: Inside of a closed structure or tube.

Lysosome: Membrane bound organelle containing digestive enzymes.

Macrophage: Phagocytic housekeeping cell that engulfs and digests bacteria and dead cells.

Major groove (of DNA): Larger of the two grooves along the surface of the DNA double helix.

Mannose: Hexose monosaccharide.

Matrix: Very vague term meaning a more or less closed location, often but not exclusively one that is a solid basis on which things can grow or attach. The term is used of the extracellular matrix in animals, formed of collagen and other fibers and of the aqueous volume inside various organelles.

Meiosis I and II: First and second meiotic divisions.

Meiosis: Form of cell division that produces gametes, each with half the genetic material of the cells that produce them.

Metaphase plate: The plane of the equator (a plane that is equally distant from the two spindle poles) of the spindle into which chromosomes are positioned during metaphase.

Minisatellite DNA: Repetitious DNA of unknown function comprising up to 20,000 repeats of a unit of about 25 base pairs.

Minor groove (of DNA): Smaller of the two grooves along the surface of the DNA double helix.

Mitochondrial inner membrane: Inner membrane of mitochondria that is elaborated into cristae. The electron transport chain and ATP synthase is integral membrane proteins of the mitochondrial inner membrane.

Mitochondrial matrix: Aqueous space inside the mitochondrial inner membrane, where the enzymes of Krebs cycle are located.

Mitochondrial outer membrane: Outer membrane of mitochondria, permeable to solutes of Mr <10,000 because of the presence of the channel porin.

Mitochondrion: Cell organelle concerned with aerobic respiration.

Mitogen: Anything that promotes cell division. FGF and PDGF (fibroblast growth factor and platelet derived growth factor) are potent mitogens for endothelial and smooth muscle cells.

Mitosis: Type of cell division found in somatic cells, in which each daughter cell receives the full complement of genetic material present in the original cell.

Mitotic spindle: microtubule-based structure upon which chromosomes are arranged and translocated during mitosis.

Mole: Amount of substance comprising 6.023×10^{23} (Avogadro's number) molecules. One mole has a mass equal to the value of the relative molecular mass expressed in grams.

Monomer: Single unit, usually used to refer to a single building block of a larger molecule. Thus DNA is formed of nucleotide monomers.

M-phase: The period of the cell division cycle during which the cell divides; M phase consists of mitosis and cytokinesis.

Muscle: Tissue specialized for generating contractile force.

Myelin: Fatty substance that is wrapped around nerve cell axons by glial cells.

Myosin: Type of motor protein that moves along or pulls on, actin filaments. The thick filaments in skeletal muscle are formed of myosin II molecules.

Necrosis: Cell death that is due to damage so severe that the cell cannot maintain the level of its energy currencies and therefore falls apart, distinct from apoptosis.

Nine plus two (9+2) axoneme: Structure of cilium or flagellum; describes the arrangement of nine peripheral microtubules surrounding two central microtubules.

Node (of a myelinated axon): Gap between adjacent lengths of myelin sheath, where the nerve cell plasma membrane directly contacts the extracellular medium. It is also called node of Ranvier after its discoverer Louis Ranvier.

Nonsister chromatids: Nonsister chromatids are not identical to each other as they represent different but homologous chromosomes and they will carry the same type of genetic information, but not exactly the same information.

Nuclear envelope: Double membrane system enclosing the nucleus; it contains nuclear pores and is continuous with the endoplasmic reticulum.

Nuclear lamina: Meshwork of proteins lining the inner face of the nuclear envelope.

Nuclear pore complex: Multiprotein complex that lies within and around the nuclear pore and that regulates import into and export from the nucleus in a process called gated transport.

Nuclear pores: Holes running through the nuclear envelope that regulate traffic of proteins and nucleic acids between the nucleus and the cytoplasm.

Nuclease: Enzyme that degrades nucleic acids.

Nucleic acid: Polymer of nucleotides joined together by phosphodiester bonds; DNA and RNA are nucleic acids.

Nucleoid: Region of a bacterial cell that contains the chromosome.

Nucleolar organizer regions: Region of one or more chromosomes at which the nucleolus is formed.

Nucleolus: Regions of the nucleus concerned with the production of ribosomes.

Nucleoside: Purine, pyrimidine or nicotinamide attached to either ribose or deoxyribose.

Nucleosome: Beadlike structure formed by a stretch of DNA wrapped around a histone octamer.

Organism: Cell or clone of cells that functions as a discrete and integrated whole to maintain and replicate itself.

p38: A stress activated protein kinase related to mitogen associated protein kinase (MAP kinase) but with a very different role. The p38 is activated by cell stress and stimulates both cell repair and apoptosis.

p53: Transcription factor that stimulates cell repair but also apoptosis. Cancer cells are frequently found to have mutated, nonfunctional p53 genes.

p75 neurotrophin receptor: Death domain receptor for neurotrophins. Upon binding neurotrophins p75 activates caspase 8 and hence initiates apoptosis unless a countermanding signal to survive is present.

Pachytene: In meiosis, the stage following synapsis (zygotene) in which the homologous chromosome threads (synaptonemal complex) shorten, thicken, and continue to intertwine, and each of the conjoined (bivalent) chromosomes separate into two sister chromatids, which are held together by a centromere, to form a tetrad. During this phase the chromatids break up and corresponding regions of the nonsister chromatids of the paired chromosomes are exchanged in a process known as crossing over.

Peripheral membrane protein: Class of protein that is easily detached from a cell membrane, unlike integral membrane proteins, which can only be isolated by destroying the membrane, *e.g.* with detergent.

Peroxisome: Class of cell organelles of diverse function. Peroxisomes frequently contain the enzyme catalase, which breaks down hydrogen peroxide into oxygen and water.

pH: Measure of the acidity of a solution, equal to minus the logarithm to base 10 of the hydrogen ion concentration in moles per liter. A neutral solution has a pH of 7 *i.e.* the H^+ concentration is 10^{-7} mol per liter or 100 nmol per litre.

Phase contrast microscopy: Type of light microscopy in which differences in the refractive index of a specimen are converted into differences in contrast.

Plasma membrane: Membrane that surrounds the cell, also called the plasmalemma or the cell membrane.

Plasmalemma: Membrane that surrounds the cell, also called the plasma membrane or the cell membrane.

Plasmid: Circular DNA molecule that is replicated independently of the host chromosome in bacterial cells.

Plasmodesmata (plasmodesma): Type of cell junction unique to plant cells, which provides a much bigger hole for passage of substances between the cytoplasm of the two cells than gap junctions do.

Plastoquinone: Quinone electron carrier found in chloroplasts.

Platelet: Small fragment of cell that contains no nucleus but that has a plasma membrane and some endoplasmic reticulum. Platelets are critical in the process of blood clotting and they also release platelet derived growth factor.

Platelet-derived growth factor (PDGF): Paracrine transmitter that opposes apoptosis and promotes cell division in target cells such as endothelial cells and smooth muscle.

Polycistronic mRNA: The mRNA that yields more than one polypeptide when translated.

Progeny: Children, offspring.

Programmed cell death (apoptosis): It is a process in which a cell actively promotes its own destruction, as distinct from necrosis. Apoptosis is important in vertebrate development, where tissues and organs are shaped by the death of certain cell lineages.

Prokaryotic: Type of cellular organization found in bacteria in which the cells lack a distinct nucleus and other organelles.

Prometaphase: Period of mitosis or meiosis that sees the breakdown of the nuclear envelope and the attachment of the chromosomes to the mitotic spindle.

Pronuclei: Nuclei of the egg and sperm prior to fusion.

Prophase I: First prophase of meiosis.

Prophase II: Second prophase of meiosis.

Prophase: Period of mitosis or meiosis in which the chromosomes condense.

Recombination: Cut and paste of DNA. Recombination occurs at chiasmata during meiosis and also in embryonic stem cells, allowing insertional mutagenesis.

Repetitious DNA: DNA sequence that is repeated many times within the genome.

Replication (of DNA): The process whereby two DNA molecules are made from one.

Replication fork: Y shaped structure formed when the two strands of the double helix separate during replication.

RER (rough endoplasmic reticulum): Portion of the endoplasmic reticulum associated with ribosomes and concerned with the synthesis of secreted proteins. Proteins destined to remain within the majority of single membrane bound organelles such as Golgi, lysosomes are also made on the rough ER, as are integral proteins of these organelles and of the plasma membrane.

Retinoblastoma: Cancer of the eye, usually caused by a mutation in the *RB* gene.

Retrovirus: Virus whose genetic information is stored in RNA.

S phase: Period of the cell division cycle during which DNA replication occurs.

S value (sedimentation coefficient): A value that describes how fast macromolecules and organelles sediment in a centrifuge.

S value (sedimentation coefficient): Value that describes how fast macromolecules and organelles sediment in a centrifuge.

Sarcomere: contractile unit of striated muscle.

Sarcoplasmic reticulum: Type of smooth endoplasmic reticulum found in striated muscle; concerned with the regulation of the concentration of calcium ions.

Satellite DNA: DNA sequence that is tandemly repeated many times.

Scanning electron microscope (SEM): Type of electron microscope in which the image is formed from electrons that are reflected back from the surface of a specimen as the electron beam scans rapidly back and forth over it. The scanning electron microscope is particularly useful for providing topographical information about the surfaces of cells or tissues.

Schwann cell: Glial cell of the peripheral (outside the brain and spinal cord) nervous system. **Secondary antibody:** In immunofluorescence, a labeled antibody that is used to reveal the location of an unlabeled primary antibody. Secondary antibodies are produced by one species of animal in response to the injection of another animal's antibodies, thus a goat antirabbit secondary will bind to any primary antibody that has been generated by a rabbit. Labeled secondary antibodies can be used to study many different questions because the specificity in the final image or western blot is provided by the primary antibody, not by the secondary.

Secondary cell wall: Layers of a plant cell wall formed external to the primary cell wall.

Secondary structure: Regular, repeated folding of the backbone of a polypeptide. The side chains of the amino acids have an influence but are not directly involved. There are two common types of secondary structue: á helix and the â sheet.

Sister chromatids: During S phase of the cell cycle the DNA is replicated and an identical copy of the chromatid is made. These identical copy of chromatids are called sister chromatids.

Skeletal muscle cells: Large multinucleate muscle cells that are attached to bone. Most cuts of meat are mainly skeletal muscle.

Small nuclear RNAs (snRNAs): Small RNA molecules found in the nucleus that plays a role in RNA splicing.

Smooth endoplasmic reticulum (SER): Portion of the endoplasmic reticulum without attached ribosomes, among its functions are the synthesis of lipids and the storage and stimulated release of calcium ions.

Smooth muscle: Nonstriated muscle, found in many places in the body including blood vessels and the intestine.

SNARES: Proteins that mediate fusion of vesicles with other membranes.

snRNAs (small nuclear RNAs): Small RNA molecules found in the nucleus that play a role in RNA splicing.

Somatic cells: Cells that make up all the normal tissues of the human body; distinct from the germ cells that form the gametes (eggs and sperm).

SOS: Guanine nucleotide exchange factor for a GTPase called Ras. SOS is recruited to the plasma membrane by binding to growth factor receptor binding protein number 2, which in turn binds activated receptor tyrosine kinases.

Spermatid: Cell formed by meiosis that differentiates to form a spermatozoon.

Spermatozoon: Motile male gamete.

Spindle fibres: It is a group of microtubules that extend from the centromere of chromosomes to the poles of the spindle or from pole to pole in a dividing cell.

Splicesome: Complex of proteins and small RNA molecules involved in RNA splicing.

Squamous: Flat. A term used of epithelial cells.

Stratified epithelium: It is type of epithelium consisting of several layers, such as the skin.

Striated muscle: Striped muscle; includes skeletal and cardiac muscle.

Stroma: Volume within the chloroplast inner membrane but outside the thylakoids.

Supercoiling: Organization of a linear structure into coils at more than one spatial scale.

Svedberg unit (S value): Value that describes how fast macromolecules and organelles sediment in a centrifuge.

Synapse: Structure formed from the axon terminal of a nerve cell and the adjacent region of the postsynaptic cell. Transmitter released by the axon terminal diffuses across the synapse gap and acts upon the postsynaptic cell.

Synapsis: The pairing of homologous chromosomes along their length; synapsis usually occurs during prophase I of meiosis, but it can also occur in somatic cells of some organisms.

Synaptonemal complex: A ribbon like protein structure formed between synapsed homologues at the end of the first meiotic prophase, binding the chromatids along their length and facilitating chromatid exchange.

T (thymine): One of the four bases found in DNA; thymine is a pyrimidine.

Tandem repeats: Many copies of the same DNA sequence that lie adjacent to each other on the chromosome.

TATA box: Sequence found about 20 bases upstream of the beginning of many eukaryotic genes that forms part of the promoter sequence and is involved in positioning RNA polymerase for correct initiation of transcription.

Taxol: Compound obtained from the bark of the Pacific yew, *Taxus brevifolia;* binds to tubulin. Taxol is a powerful anticancer drug.

Telomeres: Specialized regions at the ends of eukaryotic chromosomes. Telomeres are rich in minisatellite DNA.

Telophase I: Telophase of the first meiotic division (meiosis I).

Telophase II: Telophase of the second meiotic division (meiosis II).

Thick filament: One of the two filaments that form the cytoskeleton of striated muscle; composed of the motor protein myosin II.

Thin filament: One of the two filaments that form the cytoskeleton of striated muscle; composed of actins.

Thylakoid: Folded inner membrane of the chloroplast; site of the light reaction of photosynthesis. Thylakoids are arranged in stacks called grana.

Tight junctions: Type of cell junction in which a tight seal is formed between adjacent cells occluding the extracellular space.

Tissue: Group of cells having a common function.

Transfer RNA (tRNA): RNA molecule that carries an amino acid to an mRNA template.

Transmembrane proteins: class of proteins that span the plasma membrane.

Transmembrane translocation: Form of protein transport in which unfolded polypeptide chains are threaded across one or more membranes as a simple polypeptide chain and then refolded at their final destination.

Transmission electron microscope: Type of microscope in which the image is formed by electrons that are transmitted through the specimen.

Transmitter: Chemical that is released by one cell and that changes the behavior of another cell.

Transpiration: Loss of water from plant leaves.

Transport vesicle: Membrane vesicle that transports proteins from one membrane compartment to another.

Troponin: Calcium-binding protein found in muscle cells.

Tryptophan (*trp*) operon: Cluster of five bacterial genes involved in the synthesis of the amino acid tryptophan.

Tubulin: Protein that forms microtubules; exists as α, β and γ subunits.

Tumour: Proliferative cell mass associated with many cancers.

U (uracil): One of the four bases found in RNA; uracil is a pyrimidine.

Ultramicrotome: Machine for cutting thin sections (<100 nm) for electron microscopy.

Ultrastructure: Fine structure of the cell and its organelles revealed by electron microscopy.

Upstream: General term meaning the direction from which things have come. When applied to the DNA within and adjacent to a gene, it means lying on the side of the transcription start site that is not transcribed into RNA. When applied to signaling pathways, it means opposite to the direction in which the signal travels; thus the insulin receptor is upstream of protein kinase B.

Vacuole: Large membrane bound compartment. Plant cells often contain a large vacuole filled with sugars and pigments.

Van der Waals force: Weak close range attraction between atoms.

Vascular tissue: Blood vessels. The term is also used to describe the water transporting and support tissue of plants that is composed of xylem and phloem.

Vasoconstrictor: Substance that constricts blood vessels.

Vasodilator: Substance that dilates (widens) blood vessels.

Vesicle: Small closed bags made of membrane.

Vesicular trafficking: Precisely controlled movement of vesicles between different organelles and/or the plasma membrane.

Villin: Type of actin-binding protein those crosslinks actin filaments.

Villus (plural villi): Finger like extension of an epithelial surface that increases the surface area.

Virus: Packaged fragment of DNA or RNA that uses the synthetic machinery of a host cell to replicate its component parts.

VNTRs (variable number tandem repeats): DNA sequences that occur many times within the human genome. Each person carries a different number of these repeats.

Wobble (in tRNA binding): Flexibility in the base pairing between the 5′ position of the anticodon and the 3′ position of the codon.

Xeroderma pigmentosum: Inherited human disease caused by defective DNA repair enzymes; affected individuals are sensitive to ultraviolet light and contract skin cancer when exposed to sunlight.

Xylem: Part of the plant vascular system; transports water from the roots to the leaves.

Z-DNA: Left handed helical form of DNA.

Zellweger's syndrome: Inherited human disease resulting from aberrant targeting of proteins to the peroxisome.

Zinc fingers: Structural motif in some families of DNA binding proteins in which a zinc ion coordinated by cysteines and/or histidines stabilizes protruding regions that touch the edges of the base pairs exposed in the major groove of DNA.

Zygotene: This is the synaptic stage of the first meiotic prophase in which the two leptotene chromosomes undergo pairing by the formation of synaptonemal complexes to form a bivalent structure.